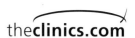

# CLINICS IN SPORTS MEDICINE

The Interface Between
Sport Psychiatry and
Sports Medicine

GUEST EDITORS
Ian R. Tofler, MB, BS
Eric D. Morse, MD

CONSULTING EDITOR
Mark D. Miller, MD

October 2005 • Volume 24 • Number 4

SAUNDERS

An Imprint of Elsevier, Inc.
PHILADELPHIA    LONDON    TORONTO    MONTREAL    SYDNEY    TOKYO

**W.B. SAUNDERS COMPANY**
*A Division of Elsevier Inc.*

1600 John F. Kennedy Blvd. · Suite 1800 · Philadelphia, Pennsylvania 19103

http://www.theclinics.com

CLINICS IN SPORTS MEDICINE                     Volume 24, Number 4
October 2005                                             ISSN 0278-5919
Editor: Debora Dellapena                          ISBN 1-4160-2771-8

*Reprints:* For copies of 100 or more, of articles in this publication, please contact the Commercial
Reprints Department, Elsevier Inc., 360 Park Avenue South, New York, New York 10010-1710. Tel.
(212) 633-3813; Fax: (212) 462-1935 e-mail: reprints@elsevier.com.

The ideas and opinions expressed in *Clinics in Sports Medicine* do not necessarily reflect those of the
Publisher. The Publisher does not assume any responsibility for any injury and/or damage to persons or property arising out of or related to any use of the material contained in this periodical. The
reader is advised to check the appropriate medical literature and the product information currently
provided by the manufacturer of each drug to be administered to verify the dosage, the method
and duration of administration, or contraindications. It is the responsibility of the treating physician
or other health care professional, relying on independent experience and knowledge of the patient,
to determine drug dosages and the best treatment for the patient. Mention of any product in this
issue should not be construed as endorsement by the contributors, editors, or the Publisher of the
product or manufacturers' claims.

*Clinics in Sports Medicine* (ISSN 0278-5919) is published quarterly by W.B. Saunders Company.
Corporate and Editorial Offices: 1600 John F. Kennedy Blvd., Suite 1800, Philadelphia, PA 19103-
2899. Accounting and Circulation Offices: 6277 Sea Harbor Drive, Orlando, FL 32887-4800.
Periodicals postage paid at Orlando, FL 32862, and additional mailing offices. Subscription prices
are $190.00 per year (US individuals), $295.00 per year (US institutions), $95.00 per year (US stu-
dents), $215.00 per year (Canadian individuals), $350.00 per year (Canadian institutions), $125.00
(Canadian students), $245.00 per year (foreign individuals), $350.00 per year (foreign institutions),
and $125.00 per year (foreign students). Foreign air speed delivery is included in all *Clinics* sub-
scription prices. All prices are subject to change without notice. POSTMASTER: Send address
changes to *Clinics in Sports Medicine*, W.B. Saunders Company, Periodicals Fulfillment, Orlando,
FL 32887-4800. **Customer Service: 1-800-654-2452 (US). From outside of the US, call 1-407-345-
4000.** E-mail: hhspcs@harcourt.com.

*Clinics in Sports Medicine* is covered in *Index Medicus, Current Contents/Clinical Medicine, Excerpta Medica,*
*and ISI/Biomed.*

Printed in the United States of America.

# CLINICS IN SPORTS MEDICINE

ELSEVIER
SAUNDERS

# The Interface Between Sport Psychiatry and Sports Medicine

## CONSULTING EDITOR

MARK D. MILLER, MD, Professor, Department of Orthopaedics; Director, Division of Sports Medicine, University of Virginia Health System, Charlottesville, Virginia

## GUEST EDITORS

IAN R. TOFLER, MB, BS, Associate Professor, Department of Psychiatry, Charles R. Drew University of Medicine and Science/University of California, Los Angeles, Los Angeles, California

ERIC D. MORSE, MD, Team Psychiatrist, University of Maryland Baltimore County, Catonsville; Staff Psychiatrist, Mental Health Services, University of Maryland College Park, College Park; Division of Alcohol and Drug Abuse, Department of Psychiatry, University of Maryland School of Medicine, Baltimore, Maryland

## CONTRIBUTORS

DAVID BARON, DO, Professor and Chair, Department of Psychiatry, Temple University School of Medicine, Philadelphia, Pennsylvania

ANTONIA L. BAUM, MD, Vice President, International Society for Sport Psychiatry; Clinical Faculty, George Washington University Medical Center, Washington, DC

DAVID F. BOGACKI, PhD, Assistant Professor and Head, Division of Psychology, Cooper University Hospital, Robert Wood Johnson Medical School, Camden, New Jersey

ROBERT W. BURTON, MD, Assistant Professor, Department of Psychiatry and Behavioral Sciences, The Feinberg School of Medicine, Northwestern University, Chicago, Illinois

GRANT J. BUTTERBAUGH, PhD, Associate Professor of Clinical Psychiatry; Director of Neuropsychology, Louisiana State University, Health Sciences Center School of Medicine, New Orleans, Louisiana

JOSHUA W. CALHOUN, MD, Associate Medical Director, United Behavioral Health; Assistant Clinical Professor, Department of Psychiatry, St. Louis University Medical School, St. Louis, Missouri

TERRENCE P. CLARK, MD, Assistant Professor of Psychiatry, Department of Psychiatry and Behavioral Sciences, James H. Quillen College of Medicine, East Tennessee State University, Mountain Home, Tennessee

DAVID O. CONANT-NORVILLE, MD, Assistant Clinical Professor of Psychiatry, Division of Child and Adolescent Psychiatry, Oregon Health and Sciences University, Beaverton, Oregon

ALAN CURRIE, MD, MPhil, MRCPsych, Consultant Psychiatrist, The Hadrian Clinic; Clinical Lecturer, University of Newcastle, Newcastle; Medical Officer (Psychiatry), United Kingdom Athletics, Birmingham, England

IRA D. GLICK, MD, Professor, Department of Psychiatry and Behavioral Sciences, Stanford University School of Medicine, Stanford, California

JON HELLSTEDT, PhD, Professor, Department of Psychology, University of Massachusetts, Lowell, Massachusetts

KENNISE M. HERRING, PhD, Assistant Professor of Clinical Psychology, Roosevelt University, Chicago, Illinois

JESSICA L. HORSFALL, PhD, Project Coordinator, Department of Psychiatry and Behavioral Sciences, Stanford University School of Medicine, Stanford, California

TERESA L. IADEVITO, BS, High Risk Coordinator, United Behavioral Health, St. Louis, Missouri

RONALD L. KAMM, MD, Clinical Assistant Professor of Psychiatry, Drexel University School of Medicine, Philadelphia, Pennsylvania; Director, Sport Psychiatry Associates, Oakhurst, New Jersey; Vice President, Fighters Initiative for Support and Training, New York, New York; President, International Society for Sport Psychiatry, Chicago, Illinois

PENELOPE KRENER KNAPP, MD, Professor Emerita, Psychiatry and Pediatrics, Department of Psychiatry, University of California, Davis, Davis, California

MICHAEL T. LARDON, MD, Associate Clinical Professor of Psychiatry, School of Medicine, University of California at San Diego, San Diego, California

DAVID R. McDUFF, MD, Clinical Associate Professor, Division of Alcohol and Drug Abuse, Department of Psychiatry, University of Maryland School of Medicine, Baltimore, Maryland

ERIC D. MORSE, MD, Team Psychiatrist, University of Maryland Baltimore County, Catonsville; Staff Psychiatrist, Mental Health Services, University of Maryland College Park, College Park; Division of Alcohol and Drug Abuse, Department of Psychiatry, University of Maryland School of Medicine, Baltimore, Maryland

THOMAS S. NEWMARK, MD, Professor and Chair, Department of Psychiatry, Cooper University Hospital, Robert Wood Johnson Medical School, Camden, New Jersey

IAN R. TOFLER, MB, BS, Associate Professor, Department of Psychiatry, Charles R. Drew University of Medicine and Science/University of California, Los Angeles, Los Angeles, California

ROBERT K. WHITE, MA, Division of Alcohol and Drug Abuse, Department of Psychiatry, University of Maryland School of Medicine, Baltimore, Maryland

# CLINICS IN SPORTS MEDICINE

## The Interface Between Sport Psychiatry and Sports Medicine

**CONTENTS**   VOLUME 24 · NUMBER 4 · OCTOBER 2005

### Foreword   xiii
Mark D. Miller

### Preface   xv
Ian R. Tofler and Eric D. Morse

### Interviewing Principles for the Psychiatrically Aware Sports Medicine Physician   745
Ronald L. Kamm

This article describes how sports medicine physicians can best approach the diagnosis of mental illness in athletes. Examples of psychiatric problems common to athletes, their incidences in the population, and diagnostic tips to ferret them out are given. Vignettes of well-known athletes who have had these problems are included. Each highlights how a lack of diagnostic awareness and the stigma of having a "mental illness" prevented the athlete from getting treatment sooner.

### Diagnosis and Psychiatric Treatment of Athletes   771
Ira D. Glick and Jessica L. Horsfall

Although enormous amounts of time and money have been invested in enhancing performance for college and professional athletes, their psychiatric needs have been minimally addressed. Given the virtual absence of controlled scientific literature, in this article the authors detail the diagnostic issues and delineate treatment principles, including: (1) making an accurate diagnosis; (2) setting realistic goals; (3) delivering psycho-education; (4) inducing the patient to undergo treatment, including involving the family and significant others; and (5) delivering appropriate treatment (the most difficult task). The objective is to improve performance and quality of life by treating the problem or psychiatric illness. A special concern is minimizing countertransference feelings and avoiding undertreatment, because by definition the athlete needs to perform.

### Developmental Overview of Child and Youth Sports for the Twenty-first Century   783
Ian R. Tofler and Grant J. Butterbaugh

This article presents an overview of sporting participation for children and adolescents from psychological, physical, social, developmental, and historical perspectives. The following areas are reviewed: (1) normal developmental readiness and sporting participation; (2) benefits and risks of athletic participation for the child and adolescent; (3) self-concept and sporting participation; (4) adverse psychophysiological and somatoform effects of sports; (5) interactional and systemic contributions to adverse physical and psychological effects; (6) a historical/social perspective of sport in the United States; (7) the current and future role of psychiatrists in conjunction with sports medicine physicians; (8) the sports psychiatry interview of the child, family, and coach; and (9) summary and future challenges.

### Achievement by Proxy Distortion in Sports: A Distorted Mentoring of High-Achieving Youth. Historical Perspectives and Clinical Intervention with Children, Adolescents, and their Families 805

Ian R. Tofler, Penelope Krener Knapp, and Michael Larden

This article describes potentially pathogenic behavior in youth sports. It delineates the four stages of achievement by proxy distortion (ABPD) behavior and attempts to raise awareness of that behavior and to facilitate communication among sports medicine and psychiatry professionals of the potential for exploitation and abuse of children and adolescents by parents, mentors, coaches, and the systems that nurture and develop these children. Information is presented to distinguish motivations behind normal parenting from those that lead to risky sacrifice, objectification of the child, and potential abuse. Distinct abuse stages of ABPD are described. The authors identify "red flags" that indicate distorted views and potentially harmful behavior toward children.

### Attention Deficit/Hyperactivity Disorder and Psychopharmacologic Treatments in the Athlete 829

David O. Conant-Norville and Ian R. Tofler

It is conjectured that attention deficit/hyperactivity disorder (ADHD) symptoms adversely impacting academics, family functioning, social relationships, and vocational performance might also negatively affect athletic and sport performance and enjoyment; this warrants further scientific inquiry. Children, adolescents, and adults participate in organized and impromptu sport activities, both team and individual. With the concern about an epidemic of obesity in the United States, barriers to participation in sport and exercise such as ADHD need to be better understood. This article approaches ADHD in sports by providing a brief introduction to ADHD, first reviewing general clinical findings, then discussing recreational youth sports and psychopharmacological treatment risks and benefits for the elite athlete.

## Aggression and Sport
**845**

Robert W. Burton

Viewing aggression in its healthy form, in contrast to its extreme and inappropriate versions, and sport as a health-promoting exercise in psychological development and maturation may allow participants and spectators alike to retain an interest in aggression and sport and derive further enjoyment from them. In addition, it will benefit all involved with sport to have a broader understanding of human aggression. Physicians, mental health professionals, and other health care providers can be influential in this process, and should be willing to get involved and speak out when issues and problems arise.

## Suicide in Athletes: A Review and Commentary
**853**

Antonia L. Baum

Not only are athletes at risk for psychiatric illness, but they are at risk of suicide. In an effort to learn more about suicide in athletes and those connected to the sports arena, a review of the medical literature from 1960 to 2000 was conducted through Medline, and a review of the periodical literature from 1980 to 2000 was conducted through Infotrac. These reviews revealed 71 cases of athletes who have either contemplated, attempted, or completed suicide. In this article, these cases are analyzed by sport, gender, and age. Through inference, an attempt to establish the etiologic basis for these behaviors is undertaken. Intervention and prevention strategies are discussed, based on the available data.

## Eating Disorders in Athletes: Managing the Risks
**871**

Alan Currie and Eric D. Morse

Athletes risk injuries and make personal sacrifices in their education, careers, and personal relationships in pursuit of excellence. Well-prepared athletes and their support teams take steps to minimize these risks. Since the 1980s, it has been apparent that development of an eating disorder is a risk associated with considerable morbidity and significant mortality, and with shorter careers characterized by inconsistency and recurrent injury. How likely is it that an athlete will develop an eating disorder? Who is at risk? Can eating disorders be prevented? How can eating disorders be identified? What are the consequences of developing an eating disorder? What can be done to help an athlete who has an eating disorder? This article attempts to answer these questions.

## Substance Use in Athletics: A Sports Psychiatry Perspective
**885**

David R. McDuff and David Baron

Athletes use substances to produce pleasure, relieve pain and stress, improve socialization, recover from injury, and enhance performance.

Therefore, they use some substances in substantially higher rates than nonathletes. Despite these higher rates of use, rates of addiction may in fact be lower in athletes. This article reviews the prevalence and patterns of use, health and performance effects, and preventive and treatment interventions for alcohol, tobacco, stimulants, and steroids. Each substance is considered from the differing perspectives of abuse/addiction and performance enhancement models. Similarities and differences between college and professional athletes are discussed. Finally, suggestions for future research are made.

## Invisible Players: A Family Systems Model     899
Jon Hellstedt

This article attempts to demonstrate that the family is a key player in the athlete's development and performance, sometimes invisible, but often all too visible. The practice of clinical sport psychology is enriched by a family-based orientation to the assessment and treatment of athletes. Creating a workable family system is a challenge for parents. They have many difficult decisions to make, and are often without support and direction in making those choices. Sport psychiatrists and psychologists can be helpful to parents as well as athletes by using family-based assessments and treatment interventions that provide education, challenge, and support as they negotiate the tasks and transitions in the family life cycle.

## Systemic Issues Involved in Working with Professional Sports Teams     929
Joshua W. Calhoun, Kennise M. Herring, and Teresa L. Iadevito

Sport psychiatrists face a number of systemic and intra-psychic issues when treating professional athletes. Although only a modicum of literature exists to aid sport psychiatrists, there are several steps they may take to become an integral part of an athletic organization and to be successful in the treatment of the athletes themselves. The ability to delineate their role within the sports club is crucial to mental health professionals' organizational success. Equally important, it is incumbent upon sport psychiatrists to recognize and transcend intra-psychic issues that occur between athlete and physician.

## Professional and Collegiate Team Assistance Programs: Services and Utilization Patterns     943
David R. McDuff, Eric D. Morse, and Robert K. White

Elite professional and collegiate athletes underuse stress control, mental health, and substance abuse treatment services. Behavioral health services use can be increased by establishing on-site, sports-specific services. Like Employee Assistance Programs of industry and government, Team Assistance Programs (TAPs) address critical issues such as substance abuse prevention, tobacco cessation, stress recognition, mental illness management, injury rehabilitation, performance enhancement, and cultural support. Strong links with the team's medical and conditioning staff can ensure a steady stream of TAP referrals and build trust with players and team staff. This article describes nine years of operation for two professional TAPs and three years for one college TAP. Use patterns and linkage strategies with team physicians, trainers, strength staff, chiropractors, and nutritionists are discussed.

## The Sport Psychiatrist and Golf      959
Terrence P. Clark, Ian R. Tofler, and Michael T. Lardon

The sport psychiatrist is well-positioned to consult to competitive golfers. The interrupted pace of play in golf provides ample time for the golfer's thoughts to go awry. The sport psychiatrist can work with competitive golfers in refining their strategies for dealing with these myriad distractions and stressors. The authors review pre-performance routine and methods for optimizing focus, and discuss the science behind being "in the zone." The authors also discuss how acute performance failure, or "choking," is best understood as being three separate disorders. The sport psychiatrist's unique role in competitive, professional golf is discussed by employing the concept of a sports mental health continuum and its relation to psychiatric disorders.

## The Use of Relaxation, Hypnosis, and Imagery in Sport Psychiatry      973
Thomas S. Newmark and David F. Bogacki

Hypnosis is a procedure during which a mental health professional suggests that a patient experience changes in sensations, perceptions, thoughts, or behavior. The purpose of this article is to briefly describe the use of various methods of relaxation, hypnosis, and imagery techniques available to enhance athletic performance. The characteristics that these techniques have in common include relaxation, suggestibility, concentration, imaginative ability, reality testing, brain function, autonomic control, and placebo effect. Case studies are provided for illustration.

## Erratum      979

## Cumulative Index 2005      981

# CLINICS IN SPORTS MEDICINE

## FORTHCOMING ISSUES

January 2006

**Stress Fractures**
Christopher Kaeding, MD
*Guest Editor*

April 2006

**Hip Injuries**
Marc Phillipon, MD, and
Srino Bharam, MD
*Guest Editors*

July 2006

**Imaging of Upper Extremities**
Tim Sanders, MD
*Guest Editor*

## RECENT ISSUES

July 2005

**Training Room Management of Medical Conditions**
John M. MacKnight, MD
*Guest Editor*

April 2005

**Sports Chronobiology**
Teodor T. Postolache, MD
*Guest Editor*

January 2005

**Osteoarthritis**
Eric C. McCarty, MD
*Guest Editor*

Clin Sports Med 24 (2005) xiii

# CLINICS IN SPORTS MEDICINE

## FOREWORD

# The Interface Between Sport Psychiatry and Sports Medicine

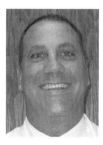

Mark D. Miller, MD

*Consulting Editor*

S ports psychiatry—are you crazy? No, but sometimes our athlete patients need a little professional help. Drs. Ian Tofler and Eric Morse have put together an outstanding issue for *Clinics in Sports Medicine* that I think will provide some new insights for most of us who take care of athletes. They have successfully recruited experts in their area to share everything from interviewing to treatment of common (and not-so-common) problems in our athletes. I found it particularly interesting to learn about eating disorders and substance abuse from a different perspective. I appreciate the outstanding effort made by Drs. Tofler and Morse—please enjoy some free counseling without the couch time!

Mark D. Miller, MD
Department of Orthopedic Surgery
University of Virginia Health System
P.O. Box 800753
Charlottesville, VA 22903-0753, USA
E-mail address: mdm3p@hscmail.mcc.virginia.edu

0278-5919/05/$ – see front matter
doi:10.1016/j.csm.2005.06.008

Clin Sports Med 24 (2005) xv–xvi

# CLINICS IN SPORTS MEDICINE

ELSEVIER
SAUNDERS

## PREFACE

# The Interface Between Sport Psychiatry and Sports Medicine

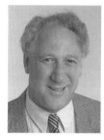
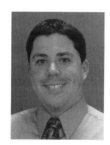

Ian R. Tofler, MB, BS, Eric D. Morse, MD

*Guest Editors*

P sychiatrists have worked with athletes for many years. Their involvement in professional sports teams has been primarily focused on working with the perennial issues of substance abuse and substance abuse prevention. It was not until 1992, however, that the International Society for Sport Psychiatry was created, with Dan Begel as its inaugural president. Since then, active involvement with the American Academy of Child and Adolescent Psychiatry and the American Psychiatric Association has also been fostered, as has psychiatric participation within the sport psychology and sports medicine fields.

There have been many developments in this emerging field. Among them, raising awareness of the potential problems in women's gymnastics during the 1996 Olympics in the *New England Journal of Medicine* by Tofler, Stryer, and others, and International Society for Sport Psychiatry (ISSP) immediate past president Ron Kamm's work with transitional issues in ex-boxers in the New York/New Jersey area.

The foundations of sport psychiatry literature have been gradually laid down. First, with the publication in 1998 of the *Clinics of Child and Adolescent Psychiatry* issue on sport psychiatry guest-edited by Ian Tofler, with the encouragement of editor Melvin Lewis. The first textbook, *Sport Psychiatry: Theory and Practice* (Norton press), edited by Daniel Begel and Bob Burton, the first two ISSP presidents, came out in 2000, and has had a galvanizing effect on developing further interest in the area. As empirical research continues to lag, the editors hope this new issue will help encourage further contributions.

0278-5919/05/$ – see front matter
doi:10.1016/j.csm.2005.06.009

The editors have brought together a strong collection of authors for this issue, which we hope and trust will facilitate the interface, communication, understanding, and sense of collegiality between sports medicine physicians and sport psychiatrists in the practical day-to-day work with youth, college, and professional athletes and in the academic arena.

In this issue, the athlete is considered from the points of view of the initial interview, the developing athlete, and the normal, nurturing, and potential pathogenic contributions of the family and other systems involved in achievement-by-proxy situations with the child and adolescent athlete. Psychopathology that can develop in conjunction with sporting participation, including attention deficit disorder, substance abuse, depression, suicidality, and eating disorders, are all introduced or re-examined from a psychiatric perspective for the sports medicine professional.

Golf, one of the most influential sports in the past decades, is reinterpreted from a psychiatric standpoint, and hypnosis as a form of performance enhancement is reconsidered.

Guest editors Ian Tofler and Eric Morse wish to thank all contributors for their hard work, and also to thank *Clinics in Sports Medicine* editor Mark D. Miller and edition editor Deb Dellapena for their support and participation in bringing this edition to the light of day.

Ian R. Tofler, MB, BS
Charles R. Drew University of Medicine and Science/
University of California, Los Angeles
8835 Key Street
Los Angeles, CA 90035, USA
E-mail address: robertoff@aol.com

Eric D. Morse, MD
Mental Health Services
University Health Center
140 Campus Drive
University of Maryland College Park
College Park, MD 20742, USA

Sports Medicine
University of Maryland Baltimore County
1000 Hilltop Circle
Catonsville, MD 21250, USA
E-mail address: ericmorse@comcast.net

Clin Sports Med 24 (2005) 745–769

# CLINICS IN SPORTS MEDICINE

ELSEVIER
SAUNDERS

# Interviewing Principles for the Psychiatrically Aware Sports Medicine Physician

Ronald L. Kamm, MD[a,b,c,d,*]

[a]Sport Psychiatry Associates, 257 Monmouth Road, A-5, Oakhurst, NJ 07755, USA
[b]Fighters Initiative for Support and Training (FIST), 265 W. 14th Street, Second Floor, New York, NY 10011, USA
[c]International Society for Sport Psychiatry, Chicago, IL, USA
[d]Department of Psychiatry, Drexel University School of Medicine, Philadelphia, PA, USA

The charge of the sports medicine physician (SMP) is to prepare athletes for the realization of their full potential by reducing their incidence of mental and physical injury. To accomplish the mental side of this task effectively, the physician must create an atmosphere in the consulting room that conveys psychological safety to the athlete. This "holding environment" [1] encourages injured athletes to voice their fears and concerns.

To best create this atmosphere, whether performing a preparticipation physical examination, (PPE), or following the athlete over the course of an injury, the physician should convey the following to the patient:

1. Patience—it is essential not to appear rushed, even within a very circumscribed time frame.
2. Interest—paraphrase what the athlete says; try not to take calls in the midst of the consultation.
3. Connectedness—make good eye contact.
4. Confidentiality—where this is possible, assure athletes that you answer only to them. When employed by a team, the SMP should, at the outset, disclose mixed allegiances and define the bounds of confidentiality.
5. Understanding— many child and adolescent athletes are guarded in the presence of a physician, but an athlete who feels understood will readily open up. The SMP who, through experience, can give voice to an athlete's inner fears, encourages the athlete to speak to deeper issues [2]. Example: an athlete whose recovery from an injury was proceeding more slowly than anticipated said, "You know, it really bugs me. It seems like I've been at this level in my recovery forever." The SMP said, "and you really don't know how quickly you're going to get better, and you're a little worried about that, aren't

* Sport Psychiatry Associates, 257 Monmouth Road, A-5, Oakhurst, NJ 07755. E-mail address: rlkamm@monmouth.com

0278-5919/05/$ – see front matter
doi:10.1016/j.csm.2005.06.002

you?" The athlete replied with a sigh, "Yeah, doc, and I'll tell you some other things I'm worried about ... "

6. Support—be accepting and nonjudgmental of where the patient is. Functional pain, for example, is still pain, and the emotional pain behind it may be massive.

If, in the end, the SMP conveys these qualities to the athlete, there is a good chance that a therapeutic relationship based on trust and rapport will evolve.

The PPE may be the only time all year that an athlete sees a physician. It has therefore been argued that the PPE is the optimal time to counsel athletes regarding such issues as smoking, alcohol and drug use, failure to use seat belts, and violence, because all of the aforementioned (except for smoking) have a higher incidence in athletes compared with the nonathletic population [3,4]. The SMP can therefore function as an important gatekeeper in the prevention, diagnosis, and, if necessary, the referral of emotional disorders and injuries in athletes [5].

## THE EXAMINATION

It is essential that the SMP understands the stigma facing many athletes when it comes to admitting that they have an emotional problem or disorder. Indeed, the very word "psychiatrist" in sporting circles can provoke a stigma reaction. Consequently, many athletes suffer needlessly, stoically ignoring their symptoms.

Terry Bradshaw, the Hall of Fame quarterback for the Pittsburgh Steelers, used to sweat profusely and break into tears after a game, but never realized he was suffering from depression. Nor did those around him, who focused on his stellar performance on the field. Only after growing more melancholy after retirement, seeking therapy, and then being placed on paroxetine has Bradshaw stopped experiencing his inexplicable lows [6]. The following are some of the entities that the psychiatrically savvy SMP should have in the back of his or her mind when examining an athlete. The incidence of these entities in athletes seems to mirror their incidence in society, unless otherwise noted.

## DEPRESSION

Insomnia, weight loss, and fatigue, in particular, should alert the SMP to the possibility of depression, which has a lifetime prevalence of 15% in the general population and 25% in women.

The case of ex-New York Mets pitcher Pete Harnisch illustrates the low index of suspicion that exists in the athletic community regarding the existence of emotional disorder.

Coming off shoulder surgery, Harnisch was expected to be the ace of the 1997 Mets pitching staff. He stopped chewing tobacco in spring training, and soon found himself unable to sleep, losing weight, and fatigued. Unsure of himself, Harnisch approached manager Bobby Valentine and told him he didn't feel he could pitch on opening day. According to Harnisch, he was ridiculed by his manager in front of the team, poisoning the relationship between the two. When Harnisch approached other team personnel he was prescribed diphenhydramine for insomnia, and then thought to have Lyme disease, before the proper diagnosis of depression was finally made. Harnisch was prescribed paroxetine and made an excellent recovery, feeling that his pitching was just as good on paroxetine as off [7]. In retrospect, more careful interviewing by team trainers and physicians would have revealed Harnisch's feelings of sadness and guilt, lack of joy, and the fact that there was a history of depression in his family, thereby making him more susceptible to a depressive episode. Interestingly, abrupt tobacco cessation can also be a precipitating factor in depression.

A depressive disorder can best be ferreted out by the SMP through observation if the patient seems down, slumped, and sad. Through history, the SMP can determine if there is sleep, appetite, and concentration disturbance; irritability; lack of energy or fatigue; loss of interest and lack of pleasure from things; or guilt. There may be crying and suicidal ideation. A cluster of at least five of these symptoms has to be present more often than not for a 2-week period to make the diagnosis. All SMPs should have a reference copy of the 4th edition of the American Psychiatric Association's *Diagnostic and Statistical Manual of Mental Disorders* (DM-IV-TR) [8] manual in their offices.

## BIPOLAR DISORDER

Though bipolar disorder is prevalent in only 1% of the population [9], several high-profile athletes have been diagnosed with this disorder, including Illie Nastase, John Daly, and Muffin Spencer-Devlin. In the hypomanic (less severe) phase, athletes may seem only gregarious, outrageous or "overaggressive." In the frankly manic or depressed phase, severe behavioral dysfunction occurs, as when Miami Dolphins defensive tackle Dimitrius Underwood took a knife to his neck in 1999.

Pro Bowl center Barret Robbins of the Oakland Raiders missed the 2003 Super Bowl when he went to Tijuana on a drinking binge the evening before the big game. Though Raider officials were aware that Robbins had been diagnosed as having bipolar disorder since 1996, Robbins' teammates were never told. According to the San Francisco Chronicle, Robbins had stopped taking his medication during preseason summer camp (typical of many patients who suffer from bipolar disorder) [10]. Though his mood and behavior became erratic during his Pro Bowl season, and though he started drinking (substance abuse can precipitate a bipolar episode), no one on the Raiders' staff effectively intervened [10]. His recent arrest for attempted murder of a police officer in Miami, again after discontinuing medication and apparently in conjunction with polysubstance abuse (including steroids), suggests a continuation of this labile behavior at an even more dangerous level [11].

This case underscores the importance of the SMP being attuned to the nuances of mental illness. In retrospect, the Raiders, with Robbins' permission, should have had a "buddy system" in place for their center, through which a trainer or teammate could have been assigned to be on the lookout for gross changes in behavior and report back to the team physician, especially when stress on players peaked as the team began its Super Bowl run. The presence on the team staff of an astute, proactive, sport psychiatrist would also have been helpful.

Bipolar disorder can be diagnosed by noting escalated or irritable mood that causes discomfort in colleagues and friends, overspending, little need for food and sleep, pressured speech, inflated self-esteem or grandiosity, and boundless energy. Judgment becomes impaired and athletes frequently turn to drugs or alcohol, especially if there is a prior history of alcohol abuse, as seems to have been the case with Robbins. In childhood and adolescence, aggressiveness and irritability, and attention deficit/hyperactivity (ADHD) symptoms may be the first indications of an underlying bipolar disorder. The diagnosis becomes more probable when there is a history of bipolar disorder among blood relatives, or when family history reveals the existences of an "eccentric" relative who was a gambler, a criminal, or a prostitute.

## ANXIETY DISORDER

Generalized anxiety disorder (GAD) is characterized by excessive worry and anxiety, but not by gross panic attacks. It is a common condition, with a 1-year prevalence range of 3% to 8% [12]. Many athletes have normal "state" anxiety–they get anxious during the state of preparedness that precedes a big meet. But some athletes also have "trait" anxiety–from an early age, often beginning in adolescence, they have been worriers, stressed out before examinations and frequently projecting ahead catastrophically regarding an upcoming youth sport contest: "What if I drop the pass?; What if I strike out?" Such individuals should raise the SMP's index of suspicion regarding GAD.

Perhaps the best way to distinguish between GAD and normal anxiety is to ask the athlete whether she feels that her anxiety is "excessive" or "difficult to control." One must be aware that athletes sometime present more with the psychosomatic manifestations of anxiety–headache, palpitations, upset stomach, and diarrhea–than with the anxiety itself. Fatigue, difficulty concentrating ("My mind went blank during the meet") and insomnia may be present, but the prominent feature is the "what iffing"–either regarding upcoming athletic performance, or about the meaning of somatic symptoms: "Gee, Doc, I've been getting these headaches; what if I have a brain tumor?"

## PANIC DISORDER

There is a lifetime prevalence rate of 5% for panic disorder and panic attacks [13]. Panic attacks are characterized by spontaneous, unexpected bouts of sheer terror, during which patients will state, "I felt totally out of control, like I was going to die, like I was going to go crazy." They also often feel trapped, and feel they must leave a situation immediately, or they feel that they are having a heart attack and need to call 911. There is often no cue for the first attack.

On history, one may find that there have been previous attacks. In panic attacks, the patient will usually remember their first episode very well and be able to relate it in detail.

Common physical symptoms include tachycardia, palpitations, shortness of breath, and sweating. Feelings of choking or smothering can lead to feelings of weakness and fatigue. During an attack, memory can be impaired and dissociation can occur (the individual feels removed from himself). Panic attacks can also be associated with substance intoxication. The unrestricted use of amphetamines ("greenies") in baseball suggests that there could be an increased rate of anxiety and panic in baseball players.

Almost as debilitating as the panic attack is the anticipatory anxiety that can exist between attacks. The patient lives in fear that if he goes back to the place where the initial attack occurred, another will happen. Panic attacks can be differentiated from anxiety attacks because they are unexpected, uncued, and the patient feels "out of control" and in an intense state of fear. Possible medical reasons for the physical symptoms, such as mitral valve prolapse, thyrotoxicosis, paradoxical atrial tachycardia, pheochromocytoma, and so forth, must of course be ruled out.

If a team physician suspects that an athlete is having a panic attack during a game, bring him to the sidelines and narrow his visual and auditory input. Cup your hands on both sides of the athlete's face, like blinders, have him look you in the eye and reassure him that everything is all right. Having the athlete rebreathe his own exhaled air with increased carbon dioxide in a paper bag can help alleviate many of the immediate symptoms. A short break in the locker room may be even more beneficial.

A boxer inexplicably quit in the middle of an important fight. Interestingly, he had a history of strange behavior in the ring and had been disqualified more than once for repeatedly fouling his opponent, even while ahead on the judges' cards. Those around him openly wondered if he had an anxiety disorder, and one could speculate that the boxer did indeed suffer a form of panic attack in all of these instances. As Clark and Lardon mention in their golf article [14], when in a state of panic, an athlete's cognitive abilities are greatly diminished, judgment is impaired, and the athlete frequently reverts to instinct.

One could speculate that, in this instance, the boxer was no longer cognizant of the rules of boxing (ie, hit above the belt), and reverted to instinct, slugging away without regard to which areas were fair or foul.

A women's-eight rower stopped rowing as her team approached the last leg of its race in a major international competition. The athlete had behaved similarly 2 years before, but sport psychiatry services were never offered to her. Though exceptionally well-trained (but not overtrained), the athlete reported complete exhaustion at that pivotal point in the race. The sport psychology/psychiatry community in the rower's home country felt, in retrospect, that her behavior was the result of an emotional disorder, not a "quitter's mentality," as many in the rowing community were saying. There were reports of the athlete throwing up before the race, and one could again speculate that her sudden experience of exhaustion was a manifestation of a panic attack.

## SOCIAL ANXIETY DISORDER

The best known example of social anxiety disorder is Ricky Williams, star running back for the Miami Dolphins, who, early in his career, gave postgame interviews to reporters while still wearing his helmet with his visor down. In retrospect, Williams always knew he was "wired differently" from his classmates, even in high school. He would recoil from social situations, even from speaking in class, and believes that because he was a football star, his extreme introversion was shrugged off as aloof behavior typical of a coddled athlete [6]. Williams' case illustrates how society's tendency to place a gifted athlete on a pedestal can impede the diagnosis of psychiatric conditions in these athletes. As Williams says, "If I didn't want to honor an obligation, I always knew someone would cover for me. A lot of people made it easy for me to hide."

Williams broke his ankle during his second National Football League (NFL) season, while still with the New Orleans Saints, and although trainers and rehabilitation specialists oversaw his every move, he states that no one paid attention to his psyche.

With the stress of an injury now adding to his anxiety, Williams went to the Internet, and finally diagnosed himself with social anxiety. He then sought out a therapist and had the diagnosis confirmed. When he went to Coach Jim Haslet to explain that he was seeking treatment for psychological issues, however, Williams says that Haslet yelled at him to "stop being a baby and just play football" [6]. This vignette illustrates how an injury can make an underlying psychiatric condition more manifest, and how seeking help for treatment for an emotional disorder tends to still be seen as a weakness by many in the sports establishment. With the help of a selective serotonin re-uptake inhibitor (SSRI) and psychotherapy, Williams became one of the most productive running backs in Miami Dolphin history. New Orleans fans are correct to wonder whether Williams might have stayed with the Saints and changed that franchise's luck if he had been diagnosed and successfully treated when he was with the team.

Taking a good history is important in the diagnosis of social anxiety disorder, and will usually reveal that the patient has been self-conscious about entering social situations for many years, especially if it means being among strangers. Often the individual will use alcohol or marijuana to self-medicate before entering such situations, and the SMP must remain ever mindful of the common coexistence of anxiety disorders, substance abuse, and alcoholism.

Williams' apparently selfish late withdrawal from the 2004–5 season at Miami, which provoked great anger from teammates, seems, in retrospect, to have been classical social anxiety behavior. Social anxiety patients have a marked fear of public humiliation or embarrassment and will do anything to avoid being "on the spot" in their personal lives [58]. In a *60 Minutes* interview with Mike Wallace in December of 2004, Williams stated that public disclosure of marijuana smoking was "my biggest fear of my whole entire life; I was scared to death of that" [59]. Of course, another part of William's motivation for withdrawing from his team may have been due to his desire to continue smoking marijuana thereby continuing to self-medicate his social anxiety.

Social anxiety disorder can also be manifested by performance anxiety, when, for example, a softball pitcher throws well in practice but "freezes up" before a game. Another form of performance anxiety is the sudden, inexplicable inability to perform what should be a routine athletic task (Chuck Knoblauch, Steve Sax, Mackie Sasser, Steve Blass).

## POST-TRAUMATIC STRESS DISORDER

Post-traumatic stress disorder (PTSD) is a common psychiatric disorder that, unfortunately, often goes unrecognized by general physicians and psychiatrists alike.

The lifetime prevalence of PTSD is estimated to be about 8% of the general population, but an additional 5% to 15% (up to 23% of the population) may experience subclinical forms of the disorder [15]. Vietnam veterans, of course, have a higher incidence (30% of RVN veterans have experienced PTSD; an additional 25% experienced subclinical forms of the disorder), and athletes, particularly in sports with high risks of serious injury or even death (auto racing, horse racing, football, boxing) seem to be at higher risk.

Hall of Fame Jockey Julie Krone detailed her experience with PTSD at a psychiatric symposium chaired by the author [16]. Partly because she had a reputation for being so tough—as a woman in a man's sport must be—her symptoms went unnoticed and she almost committed suicide.

Julie suffered a spill at Saratoga in the summer of 1993, just a few months after becoming the first and only woman rider to win a Triple Crown race—the Belmont. At Saratoga, Julie fell under the heels of the several horses and her injuries were almost fatal. She suffered heart contusions, and a fractured ankle that needed to be rebuilt with two plates and 14 screws. Julie recovered well from that injury, however, taking it as a challenge.

The spill that precipitated her PTSD was actually much less serious (not uncommon in PTSD), and occurred 2 years later at Gulf Stream Park when her horse broke down in the middle of a race and pitched her off. Rolling on the turf, she covered her head with her hands, which were broken. "It fried me," she said, "I couldn't talk. The straw didn't break the camel's back; it gutted the sucker, left the camel for dead. I was numb, couldn't think. I was afraid of horses, hated riding" [17].

Julie's quotes illustrate some crucial important points about PTSD. Note that the stressor in this case was not of the magnitude of the Saratoga spill. The previous spill had, however, sensitized her, and events in her life were such that this spill took on devastating psychological meaning, and was "the last straw." As Julie told me (personal communication, April, 2000), "The heart and the hands are a jockey's biggest organs. The first spill got my heart, but this one got my hands—my trademark; the way I uniquely communicated with my mounts."

The diagnostic features of PTSD include experiencing a traumatic event that is perceived as a major threat to one's life or self, or viewing a scene (human body parts) outside the realm of normal human experience. This is followed by the painful re-experiencing of the traumatic event. When Julie went to the starting gate, she had actual flashbacks of the spill. She then became anxious, and communicated this to the horse, resulting in a performance decline. Julie also had recurrent nightmares of the spill, and even re-experienced the event when someone swung a golf club near her, the swish of the wind made by the club making her feel again that horses were passing over her. Characteristics of PTSD include:

- Avoidance—as Julie was quoted as saying above, for the first time in her life she became afraid of horses and riding.
- Emotional numbing—Julie felt numb and detached and did not care about riding.
- Increased arousal—Julie manifested symptoms of insomnia, difficulty concentrating, and irritability. The latter caused her difficultly when, after a race, she uncharacteristically attacked a jockey who had cut her off. This resulted in a 7-day suspension. Julie consulted with various physicians over this time period, but no one picked up on her PTSD. She even went to an optometrist for blurred vision at the starting gate (actually anxiety), but was told there was nothing wrong. By luck, Julie ran into a psychiatrist friend at the race track, just as she was contemplating committing suicide that evening. He suggested that she talk to him, and psychotherapy eventually led to medication (an SSRI), which returned Julie to full function.

This case highlights many important features of PTSD, which should be suspected when an athlete has a minor injury that takes longer than expected to resolve. It should be suspected when the presentation is one of vague medical/psychophysiological complaints (headaches, stomachaches, backaches, soreness of muscles, blurred vision). History should focus on events known to have traumatic or tragic consequences in a sport—having been beaned in baseball, or having been tackled particularly hard while crossing over the middle to make a reception in football, for example. Gymnasts should specifically be asked about recurrent nightmares and avoidance of the apparatus if they present with an injury after falling from the high bar or hurt their neck while vaulting.

## OBSESSIVE-COMPULSIVE DISORDER

In obsessive-compulsive disorder (OCD), patients cannot get certain thoughts that bother them or make them anxious out of their minds, regardless of how hard they try. They may have compulsions such as compulsive checking, hand washing, counting, or hoarding. These symptoms have to be inquired about, because the patient will rarely volunteer them. Because OCD is an anxiety disorder, any situation that increases stress will worsen it.

As a senior, Julian Swartz was the Associated Press high school basketball player of the year in Wisconsin and had been diagnosed and treated for OCD since the ninth grade.

As a freshman at the University of Wisconsin, however, Julian's team made the Final Four, and his anxiety mushroomed. Julian doubted he was good enough (doubt is a common symptom of this disorder) and, being a perfectionist, he also felt he wasn't working hard enough. A bout of depression followed, as did a suicide attempt.

Finally, Julian transferred to a Division III school, where he felt less pressure to perform, and his symptoms became controllable again. In retrospect, a small school would probably have been a better initial choice for Julian, given his disorder [18].

OCD is to be distinguished from the superstitious rituals that are common in athletics. The distinction can be rather easily made, because OCD grossly interferes with important areas of the patients' life. Obligatory running [19] or obligatory exercise may also be seen as part of the OCD spectrum. It is compulsive in that the patient "has to" do it. If affected athletes do not run a certain distance, or swim a certain number of laps, they feels very anxious. Such individuals organize their lives around their exercise, and it can severely impact interpersonal relations. Though patients realize on a certain level that they don't "have to" run, they still feel that they must, and usually rationalize by saying to themselves that running will help them maintain their weight or tone their cardiovascular system. These individuals will train even when advised by the SMP to rest because of injury.

## EATING DISORDERS

### Anorexia

Athletes are at greater risk for developing eating disorders than the general population [20]. Often coaches or parents will have praised another athlete within earshot of the patient regarding how much weight the other athlete has lost, how much better she now looks, and how much faster she is. The vulnerable teen or preteen then embarks on a crash program to also lose weight. Interestingly, male athletes are much more at risk for developing eating disorders compared with the general population of males than female athletes are when compared with nonathletic females. In making the diagnosis of eating disorder in an athlete, one must not be bound strictly by weight. In anorexia athletica [21], which can be considered a part of eating disorder not otherwise specified (NOS) in DSM-IV-TR nomenclature, athletes are able to keep themselves above 85% of their accepted minimum body weight because of their intense training and increased muscle mass, while still exhibiting many of the other signs and symptoms of anorexia nervosa. Athletes at greater risk are those engaged in sports that value or demand a certain esthetic look, such as gymnastics, figure skating, sports dance, and diving; as well as those involved in sports with various weight classifications, such as lightweight football, boxing, wrestling, and lightweight crew.

On the other end of the spectrum, some positions in sports put a premium on weight gain—linemen in football, shot putters, heavyweight wrestlers. These athletes may indulge in binge eating to keep their weight up.

Anorexia nervosa should be suspected when a patient appears overly thin to the physician. Questions regarding body image should then follow: "When you look in the mirror, how do you see yourself?" The anorectic will say that he is fat when to the neutral observer he is clearly thin. This syndrome is frequently associated with compulsive exercise, intense fear of gaining weight, and meticulous dietary restriction. In postmenarchical females, as body fat drops, the patient will have missed at least three consecutive periods. Not all anorectics purge to control weight; some use laxatives, diuretics and enemas. Others only restrict intake (restricting type). When the athlete becomes anorectic, weakness eventually affects performance. Patients who have anorexia are very secretive and often wear bulky clothes to conceal their thinness. A high index of suspicion is therefore often necessary to make the diagnosis, and collateral visits with family members are usually necessary.

Because anorectics have perfectionist tendencies and engage in denial, they have a hard time admitting that they have a serious problem. Yet early detection and intervention are associated with a better outcome [22,23], essential in an illness with a significant mortality rate (5%–18%) [24]. Successful referral, then, is of the utmost importance.

Because patients will resist the idea that they have an eating disorder that requires psychotherapy, Murphy [21] advises the referring SMP to focus on the distress the athlete is currently feeling—distress from decreased athletic performance, and from pressure from their family to eat and see a doctor— rather than focusing on weight. Suggesting that the athlete go for a consultation to assess whether there is a problem is often better received than a direct referral for therapy.

## Bulimia Nervosa

Women with bulimia nervosa are often normal or slightly overweight. This disorder is more common than anorexia nervosa, and affects between 1 to 3% of young women.

Bulimia is defined as eating more food than most persons would in similar circumstances and in a similar period of time, and is accompanied by a strong sense of loss of control. Bulimics are frequently concerned about body shape and weight, and often attempt to counteract the "fattening" effects of food by self-induced vomiting, appetite suppressants, or diuretics. As with anorectics, there is the self perception of being too fat, and an intrusive dread of fatness. During a binge, patients eat food that is sweet, high in calories, and generally soft and smooth in texture, such as donuts. The family may report suspicious behavior, such as the patient eating frequently alone, taking numerous trips to the bathroom when at restaurants, and returning from the bathroom with bloodshot eyes. Bulimics frequently have wide fluctuations in weight, and are often depressed, particularly after a binge. As with anorexics, not all binge eaters purge, and pure bingers are felt to have less body image disturbance and less anxiety concerning eating than binge/purgers. Bulimics, like anorectics, are very secretive about their illness, so confirmatory history usually needs to be obtained from family. Particularly when there is purging, laboratory studies may show electrolyte imbalances, hypomagnesaemia, and hypermaylasemia. Bulimia, unlike anorexia, may not directly affect the athlete's performance, but the associated guilt, depression, and conflicts within the family regarding the bulimia will stress the athlete. Some psychoanalysts believe that bulimia is a symptom of the struggle that a young woman is having between merging with the maternal figure and separating from it. The eating may represent a wish to fuse with the caretaker mother, and regurgitating may unconsciously express the wish for separation [24].

## ALCOHOLISM AND SUBSTANCE ABUSE HISTORY

Recent evidence indicates that high school athletes, though they get better grades than their nonathletic classmates, are more likely to use drugs and alcohol [25]. Among athletes, particularly at the high school level, male athletes have been found to drink to intoxication significantly more often than female athletes. Since it has been found that 0.2% of Americans have indulged in heavy alcohol use in the past month, if the SMP is the team physician for a football team, it is likely that at least 3–4 players will be affected [26]. In a study by Nattiv and Puffer [4], undergraduate college student athletes were found to be more likely than their nonathletic peers to consume large quantities of alcohol per sitting, and were also found to have three times as many citations for driving under the influence of alcohol. A family history of alcohol or drug abuse was also greater in the athlete group (athletes, 22%; nonathletes, 9.5%). Diagnostically, in alcohol abuse there is recurrent use that results in failure to fulfill major role obligations (school, home, team), recurrent use in hazardous situations, recurrent alcohol-related legal problems, or continued use despite social or interpersonal problems caused and exacerbated by the alcohol.

The diagnosis of alcohol dependence includes tolerance–the athlete needs increased amounts to achieve the same effect. The athlete experiences withdrawal and a great deal of time is spent trying to obtain alcohol, in using it, or in recovering from its effects. Alcohol dependence impacts the athlete's performance and allegiance to the team, and persistent efforts to cut down or control the alcohol use prove unsuccessful. The patient continues to use alcohol, despite the knowledge that it is causing him psychological and physical problems (denial). There may also be periods of amnesia for heavy drinking bouts (blackouts). The CAGE questionnaire [27] is a brief and straightforward instrument that has been widely used as a screening device. CAGE is an acronym derived from the following four questions:

1. Have you ever felt you ought to **C**ut down on your drinking?
2. Have people **A**nnoyed you by criticizing your drinking?
3. Have you ever felt bad or **G**uilty about your drinking?
4. Have you ever had a drink first thing in the morning (**E**ye opener) to steady your nerves or to get rid of a hangover?

John Ewing, the scale developer, found that answering yes to at least two of these questions was a strong indicator for alcohol abuse by men. In the screening for substance abuse, use of the patients' drug of choice can be substituted for the word "drinking." Because marijuana and alcohol use usually begin in high school, and cocaine thereafter, it is important that the SMP specifically ask about the use of these agents.

Jonas and colleagues [28] describe the crucial role of the team physician in the diagnosis of drug or alcohol abuse:

Identification of the use or abuse of therapeutic (and illicit) agents in athletes often requires little more than a careful clinical history during the athlete's preparticipation evaluation. ...[Young] athletes are often unaware of the abuse potential of many of these agents and need to be counseled regarding their appropriate use, not only as it relates to athletic competition, but also regarding the appropriate use of medication to treat medical illnesses and their symptoms. Athletes frequently use over-the-counter products without considering them to be medications. It is especially important for athletes who are competing in events where drug screening is performed and detection of banned substances is possible that they are carefully counseled regarding what medicines they may or may not be permitted to take. (For a complete listing of the NCAA and United States Olympic Committee [USOC] banned and restricted drug list, refer to the Athletic Drug Reference '99 [29] or go to www.antidoping.org.) When it is not readily apparent from the history, it becomes much more difficult to detect inappropriate use of therapeutic agents other than through random drug screening programs. The use of these medications should be tightly controlled by the team physician. Athletes who need these potent medications should be counseled regarding their appropriate use. Most of these compounds are on a banned substance list of many athletic governing bodies. Athletes' access to most prescription medications is through either their team or primary care physician. Education programs encouraging athletes to communicate with members of the health care team regarding their use of any drug are important. Primary care physicians should be aware of the appropriate use of therapeutic drugs [in] athletes and participate as active members of the health care team to ensure safe, ethical, and legal participation of athletes who require medical treatment.

## ANABOLIC STEROID ABUSE

An estimated one million people in the United States have used illegal steroids at least once [30]. Alarmingly, half the users start before the age of 16, and a recent survey [31] showed that 6% of all high school students have used steroids. The highest use is seen among 18- to 25-year-olds, with 26- to 34-year-olds having the next highest rate. Estimates for the rate of use in body builders have ranged from 50% to 80%, and athletes who abuse steroids have, in the past, tended to come from those sports emphasizing strength and endurance (track and field, weight lifting); however, as the performance enhancement benefits of steroids have become known over the past 40 years, athletes in all sports have been magnetically drawn to them.

While an athlete is cycling on steroids, he will often note affective lability—euphoria, irritability, and grandiose feelings, even to the point of feeling invincible. The athlete may also experience anger, arousal, irritability, hostility, and anxiety. "Roid rage" has become a popular term for the violence and behavior that steroid users sometime engage in. Somatization and depression may be present, particularly during times where steroids are not used. Changes in personality are not uncommon, and steroid abusers who have no record of antisocial behavior or violence have been known to commit murder and other violent crimes. Steroids are both psychologically and physically addictive, and when an abuser stops using he may become depressed, anxious, and overly concerned about his body's physical shape.

It is assumed that the SMP is well aware of the physical stigmata of steroid use in young men and women, so these will not be listed here.

Even more than their ego-syntonic use of alcohol and drugs, athletes may have difficulty perceiving steroid use as problematic, asking "How can anything be wrong with something that actually makes me faster, stronger, and able to jump higher?" Jose Canseco's justification of steroid use in baseball [32] is a recent example of this. Indeed, even the athlete's coach and parents may view the use of anabolic agents positively and as perfectly acceptable, seeing their use as a "laudable" conformity to the sports ethic of "win at all costs." Such performance-enhancement and "gaining a competitive edge" practices have been referred to by sport sociologist Jay Coakley [33] as "positive deviance," and they are on the rise. Ominously, a survey that recently appeared in *Pediatrics* [34] revealed that 2.9% of middle-schoolers (fifth to eighth grade) were using steroids. That number increased to 9% when serious gymnasts and weight-lifters in the same age group were polled.

Steroid users are reluctant to give up a drug that they feel makes their bodies look and feel so good, and increases their performance. The SMP should therefore reframe the choice of whether or not to use performance-enhancing agents by placing it into the larger context of how sports participation can help an athlete develop "decision-making skills." After all, one of the hallmarks of great athletes is their ability to make difficult decisions under duress, good decisions for themselves and their team, or good decisions during a match. Asking the athlete to reflect on whether the use of steroids is really a good decision, and whether it meshes with the moral lessons that one ideally learns from sports participation (fairness, integrity, compassion, sportsmanship), is to give an adolescent or young adult a say in the unfolding of his own moral development. Canseco's recently published book on steroid use in professional baseball [32] promises to keep this issue on the front burner.

## MUSCLE DYSMORPHIA

Muscle dysmorphia, also known as "reverse anorexia," is a disorder of distorted body image. Though the patients are extremely well built and solid, they feel that they are small. They check their appearance dozens of times a day in the mirror, and become anxious if they miss even 1 day of working out in the gym. Their preoccupation with weight lifting costs them social and occupational opportunities. For example, though their bodies are extremely well developed, athletes who have muscle dysmorphia feel that they will look "too small" when seen in a bathing suit, and often will not go to the beach. Muscle dysmorphia is a subtype of body dysmorphic disorder. Bodybuilders seem to be more at risk than other athletes, and there is a higher incidence in female bodybuilders than in their male counterparts [35].

## SUPPLEMENTS AND OVER-THE-COUNTER MEDICINES

All athletes should be asked whether they are taking creatine or other over-the-counter supplements. Some supplements, especially those containing stimulants, can precipitate a manic episode in those prone to bipolar disorder. Sometimes athletes will refrain from abusing substances if the SMP stresses strongly enough that the governing body of their sport will disqualify them for continued use.

## PATHOLOGICAL GAMBLING AND FANTASY LEAGUE INVOLVEMENT

More and more athletes are involved in multiple fantasy leagues. Athletes are not only competing with each other on the field, but also on their computers. In professional sports, ethical conflicts of interest may arise. If you are a defensive tackle or linebacker in football, should you stop an opposing running back cold if he is the mainstay of your fantasy league?

Pathological gambling is present in up to 3% of the general population, and has been responsible for the destruction of several professional athletes' careers, most notably those of baseball's Pete Rose and Art Schlichter, the great quarterback from Ohio State and the Indianapolis Colts. According to DSM-IV-TR [8], the prevalence of pathological gambling may be as high as 8% in adolescents and college students; in 1999 the National Research Council [36] estimated that 20% of adolescents were either pathological or problem gamblers, and that was before the onset of the current poker craze. This disorder is more common in men than women, and on history, approximately one fourth of pathological gamblers have a parent who has a gambling problem [37].

Pathological gamblers make no serious attempts to budget or save money. Like substance abusers, when their borrowing resources are strained, they are likely to engage in antisocial behavior (eg, forging checks) to obtain money to sustain their habit. In sports, they may be subject to fixing athletic contests. At times they will bet on their own team, as Pete Rose did. The criteria for the diagnosis of pathological gambling are similar to those for the diagnosis of alcohol dependence: preoccupation with gambling, the need to gamble with increasing amounts of money to achieve the desired degree of excitement, repeated unsuccessful efforts to cut back, gambling despite the loss of personal and vocational relationships, and the like. Social gambling is distinguished from pathological gambling in that the former occurs with friends, on special occasions, and with predetermined, acceptable, and tolerable losses [37].

## ATTENTION DEFICIT/HYPERACTIVITY DISORDER

The ADHD athlete will probably not come to you complaining of ADHD, but careful history or history obtained from parents will reveal that the athlete has difficulty finishing projects, often loses things, is forgetful, has difficulty organizing tasks and activities, and is easily distracted. A good question to ask the athlete to tease out the diagnosis is: When you were in grammar school and a fire engine went by, or it started to snow, did you get so lost in the distraction that you forgot about the teacher? These symptoms will have been present before age 7 or second grade. In the hyperactive type, the athlete will have a history of having been "always on the go," like the energizer bunny. Early report cards will be full of teacher descriptions of the patient fidgeting, leaving his seat in the classroom, or interrupting the teacher (or coach) in the middle of a question. There may well have been a history of difficulty playing quietly or of engaging in quiet leisure activities. Lack of impulse control may also be part of this syndrome (impulsive type), as in a soccer goalie who, unable to wait for a play to fully develop, would run out and tackle the opposing forward, at one point breaking an opponent's leg. It might seem counterintuitive that a goalie could have ADHD, but goalies have to be aware of everything that is going on around them, and if they can also keep their focus on the field of play, the ADHD can work to their advantage.

One ice hockey goalie, however, had his performance impaired by ADHD when people in the stands would yell his name. When the goalie would turn and look at them, he would allow the puck to slide into the goal. Michael Stabeno [38] feels that ADHD athletes do best in "continuous chaos" sports (soccer, ice hockey), in which there is a high degree of unpredictability and the athlete is continuously reacting to and needs to be aware of the entire surface of the contest. ADHD athletes do less well in slow-paced sports, such as American football or baseball, in which more time is spent waiting for the next play than is spent actually playing the sport. Referral to a sport psychiatrist and prescription of medication (one must be careful regarding banned substances), in addition to psychotherapy and family therapy are extremely effective in treating ADHD. Stabeno's book and an article by Kamm [39], which maybe found on www.mindbodyandsports. com, offer helpful guides to parents and coaches of ADHD athletes.

## NEUROPSYCHIATRY

### Postconcussion Syndrome

Pat LaFontaine, the all-star hockey player, suffered a severe concussion while playing for Buffalo in 1996. Following the concussion, LaFontaine experienced severe migraine headaches, depression, sleepless nights, confusion, and wild mood swings. He was shocked one day to find that hockey no longer mattered to him. Though LaFontaine's symptoms continued to worsen, a number of physicians, apparently misdiagnosing overtraining, told him that all he needed was "rest." One physician, minimizing the player's complaints, even told him, "You know, I'm sure if you go out and score a couple of goals, you'll feel better and everything will be fine" [10]. LaFontaine remembers looking at the physician and saying, "Doc, I don't care about scoring goals anymore. I'm scared." Afterward, realizing that he had just told a doctor that he didn't care about scoring goals, LaFontaine knew that something was drastically wrong. He went to the Mayo Clinic, where postconcussion syndrome (PCS) was diagnosed.

LaFontaine's symptoms make him a textbook case for PCS. In addition to the symptoms described above, one may also see fatigue, vertigo or dizziness, irritability, aggression with little or no provocation, and a change in personality. Postconcussional disorder causes significant impairment in social or occupational functioning, and there is a noticeable decline from previous levels of functioning. When deciding to treat, it is essential that the SMP be mindful of the fact that head trauma patients may be particularly susceptible to the side effects associated with psychotropic medication. Therefore, if the SMP elects to treat the anxiety or depression component of PCS with an SSRI or with a benzodiazepine, treatment with these agents should be initiated in lower doses than usual, and they should be titrated upward very slowly [40].

### Dementia Pugilistic

Dementia pugilistic or punch-drunk syndrome is typically found in boxers. Symptoms ultimately affect one boxer in five [41].

This syndrome is also known as chronic traumatic brain injury (CTBI), and is the most serious public health concern in modern boxing [42]. CTBI is thought to represent the long-term and cumulative neurological consequences of repetitive head trauma. It has most typically been used to describe active or retired boxers after a long exposure to the sport (number of rounds sparred seems to be one of the greatest risk factors, even more than number of fights), but CTBI may be found in individuals who have participated in other sports in which head trauma, or the use of the head, is common, such as football, soccer, or ice hockey. Clinically, the diagnosis is made through history of repeated head trauma and the presence of cognitive impairment, Parkinsonism, ataxia, pyramidal tract dysfunction, and behavioral changes. It has long been a mystery why some boxers who have many brutal fights do not develop CTBI, whereas some who have relatively short careers do. Recent research points to the fact that possession of the apolipoprotein E ε4 (APOE) gene type predisposes boxers to the development of CTBI, which is very similar to Alzheimer's disease.

## OVERTRAINING

Overtraining [43] refers to a negative response to training stress, often due to chronically high training levels without periods of lower training loads. The overtraining syndrome consists of a variety of psychophysiological signs and symptoms.

Often athletes push themselves to train so intensively because they do not feel as talented as others on their team, but feel they can compensate by intensive, excessive training. The syndrome is dubbed overtraining because despite the lengthy and diligent workouts, the athlete's performance actually drops off (particularly noticeable in running, cycling, or swimming).

Physiological symptoms described in literature [43–46] include:

- Elevated resting heart rate and blood pressure
- Muscle soreness
- Weight loss and loss of body fat
- Changes in serum hormonal levels
- Sleep disturbance
- Increased incidence of sickness and injury

Asking athletes to keep a training log can be a useful method to determine how much they are training and whether it is excessive. Consulting with the coach and parents can also be very helpful in making the diagnosis. Overtraining can certainly lead to fatigue and depression, so athletes need to be informed that by overtraining they are not increasing their performance potential, but are increasing their potential for injury and illness.

Noakes [47] makes the point that endogenous depression can be differentiated from depression secondary to overtraining by asking the athletes how they feel about training and exercising. The moderately to severely depressed athlete will have lost interest in training, whereas the victim of overtraining will still desperately want to exercise, only to become profoundly fatigued when doing so. The diagnosis of overtraining is confirmed when a reduction in training intensity yields a beneficial response.

On the other hand, exercise can be an effective therapeutic agent in preventing and treating mild to moderate depression [48]. In fact, the incidence of depression may be lower among active athletes than in the general population because of the athletes' intense training. Both Derrick Adkins, the 1996 Gold Medalist in the 400 meter hurdles, and Gerry Cooney, the former top heavyweight contender, both feel that the intense training associated with their sports successfully warded off bouts of depression that they experienced, or started to experience, while competing [49].

Adkins' case is interesting in that fluvoxamine, the only antidepressant that helped him, also slowed his times in the 400. Adkins' psychiatrist had the creative job of titrating his fluvoxamine dosage to adequately treat his depression without negatively impacting his running. The collaboration was successful, and Adkins won gold before his hometown crowd in Atlanta, proudly circling Olympic Stadium with the American flag draped around his shoulders. Unfortunately, in the euphoria that followed the victory, like many athletes, Adkins decided to stop his medication. He soon descended into deep depression again, a fact noticed by his mother, who watched him on television racing in Europe without his usual flair. In an effort to improve his times on the track, rather than use fluvoxamine, Adkins had tried the serotonin precursor 5-hydroxy-Tryptophan (5HT), an alternative, nonprescription remedy. Though 5HT's side effects were more amenable to good racing times, the benefits to the depression were not as robust.

## CAREER TERMINATION ISSUES

It is often said that a professional athlete dies twice. Certainly retirement is a major problem for a person whose identity is based primarily on athletic prowess. When an athlete ends his or her career, by definition it is premature, and this makes an adverse reaction more likely. Over one third of people in the general population who retire become depressed, and after 2 years 50% are back in the work place in some capacity [50]. Athletes fare even less well. They engage in denial, and one must counsel athletes along a death-and-dying model to help them grieve the loss of their career. This is most serious in the professional athlete, but a depression can follow the end of a college or high school career as well.

Kamm's study [51] of 152 retired boxers found that 14% (considered gross under-reporting on a screening interview) had turned to alcohol or drugs to soothe the depression and anxiety attendant to giving up a sport that had been like a religion for a good part of their lives. Interestingly, those boxers who had been world champions or top contenders were less likely to have abused alcohol and drugs after retirement than their lesser-achieving counterparts. The study described the Fighters' Initiative for Support and Training (FIST), founded by former top heavyweight contender Gerry Cooney. FIST provides medical, psychological, and vocational assistance to this underserved population of "independent contractors" as they try to make the difficult transition from boxing to the real world.

## LEARNING DISABILITIES

In the course of examining an athlete's thought processes, the interviewer may discover that the athlete has been pushed along in the educational process, not because of academic merit, but because of his or her highly valued athletic prowess. Alan Page [52], the Hall of Fame defensive lineman for the Minnesota Vikings and current associate justice of the Minnesota Supreme Court, related the following: late in Page's career, the Vikings got a new defensive line coach. Though the players were part of one of the greatest units in NFL history, the coach insisted that each defensive line meeting consist of one player reading plays from the Vikings defensive playbook to the others. As the playbook was passed around the room, it became apparent to Page that four of the seven linemen in his unit could not read.

Like Page, the SMP may uncover illiteracy during a routine examination. Detecting this condition and helping the athlete overcome it can only enhance the player's self-esteem and lessen anxiety about being "found out."

## DREAMS

Occasionally a patient may sheepishly relate a dream to the SMP. One does not have to be a psychiatrist to explore what the athlete feels the meaning of such a dream is. Dreams are important to explore because athletes, as a group, tend to be superstitious, and more than a few believe that dreams can foretell their future. For example, before he fought Lou Del Valle in their July 1998 bout, light heavyweight champion Roy Jones dreamt that the soft-punching Del Valle would knock him down. Though Jones won the fight, Del Valle did, in fact, knock him down, the first time in his career that Jones had ever been knocked off his feet [53].

## SPORTS PARENTS INTERVIEW

When dealing with a child or adolescent athlete, it is important to involve the parents in an assessment of the athlete and the athlete's problem. A meeting with the parents should be held, and parameters of confidentially should be laid out. If the athlete is an adolescent, the teen's permission should be sought before having the parental interview. Child athletes greatly appreciate having their permission sought out as well, and the request shows interest and understanding on the part of the SMP.

In the interview, the parents should be asked for their version of the presenting problem, and an athletic and developmental history of the patient should be taken. The interview can be particularly helpful in uncovering disorders about which the athlete might be secretive—eating disorders, or alcohol, drug, or steroid abuse.

One should make an assessment of the degree of parental involvement. Though many parents say they "just want their athlete to have fun," the athlete may give a much different account of the achievement orientation of her parents.

It is crucial to the identity and status of some parents that their athlete be a high achiever. Tofler and colleagues [54] have termed this phenomenon "achievement by proxy distortion," and parents who manifest it often push their children into early single-sport specialization and year-round training, signing them up for several travel teams and several private coaches as well as extra practice sessions. Little wonder then that overuse injuries in children are increasing in number and severity. Dr. James Andrews, the noted sports ortho-pedist, has observed, "You get a kid on the operating table and you say to yourself, it's impossible for a 13-year-old to have this kind of wear and tear. We've got an epidemic going on" [55].

If achievement by proxy distortion is suspected, the following signs of it should be inquired about:

1. Did the athlete have many overuse injuries in latency and preadolescence?
2. Have the parents ever been told that they might be pushing their child too hard?
3. How do the parents view each other's spectator and coaching decorum?
4. Has either parent every been
   (a) asked by child, spouse, coach, or league official not to attend a practice or game?
   (b) disciplined or suspended by the league for behavior at their child's ath-letic event?
   (c) accused of abusive behavior toward their own or someone else's child (verbal, emotional, physical, sexual)?
5. Has a coach ever been given inordinate power or "say" in the child's life?
6. Has there been an inordinate economic or geographic sacrifice made for the athlete (mortgaging house for special training, equipment, or private coaching; moving, or allowing the athlete to move, to another city so that the athlete can train with a special coach)?

In the sport parent interview it is also important to inquire if there is a history of emotional disorder in the family, and what treatment has been successful. One should ask if the parents themselves are currently involved in competitive athletics (tennis, golf, bowling, other), and to what degree? Such involvement may ameliorate a parent's overinvolvement in the child's' ex-ploits. Are there family problems that are adding to the stress in the house-hold, such as difficulties with other children, previous marriages, in-laws, or finances? How do siblings react to the elite athlete's stardom? And finally, what is each parent's theory as to what might be at the root of the athlete's current problem?

## TRANSFERENCE

Speaking of parents, an athlete's attitude toward a physician is apt to be a repetition of the attitude the athlete has had toward authority figures. It is the set of expectations, beliefs, and emotional responses that a patient brings to the doctor–patient relationship. Transference, therefore, does not necessarily reflect the reality of who a doctor is or how a doctor acts, but rather what persistent experiences the patient has had with all important authority figures throughout life.

The athlete's attitude may therefore range from one of realistic basic trust, with the expectation that the doctor has the patient's best interest at heart, to one of overidealization; or, conversely, to one of basic mistrust, with an expectation that the doctor will be contentious and potentially abusive [56].

SMPs will do well to remember that they are probably not as talented or "good" as an overidealizing athlete makes them out to be, nor as "bad" and intrusive as an athlete who has been abused by authority figures all of his life seems to make them feel.

## COUNTERTRANSFERENCE

Physicians, too, have unconscious or unspoken expectations of patients. They might think of patients as "good" when their expressed severity of symptoms correlates with an overtly diagnosable biological disorder. Patients are appreciated when they are compliant and do not challenge the treatment, when they are emotionally controlled, and when they are appropriately grateful [56]. If these expectations are not met, physicians may blame patients and experience them as unlikable, untreatable, or bad. The physician's sense of job satisfaction may even be impaired by a string of such patients.

In working with particularly elite or famous athletes, the SMP must guard against the dangers of "countertransference awe" and of needing the consultation and treatment to lead to improved performance or complete remission of symptoms, so that the physician can take credit for a great athlete's career. The more elite and famous the athlete, the more the physician must guard against the temptations of overidentification, basking in achievement by proxy distortion reflected glory, and using the athlete in the service of the physician's own narcissistic needs.

## PSYCHIATRIC DIAGNOSIS AND REFERRAL

The SMP may make a formal psychiatric diagnosis, if he is comfortable with doing so, or he can speak to the athlete and family in general terms ("Emily seems down; perhaps she's depressed," or "Rick's feeling like he's under too much pressure; he may be having anxiety"). Treatment for emotional problems may be undertaken if the SMP is comfortable in that arena, or referral to a sport psychiatrist can be made. At times, if the SMP feels that the athlete might feel a stigma from being diagnosed with a mental illness or seeing a psychiatrist, she can refer the patient to "a colleague who specializes in behavioral sports medicine" or to a "mental skills training specialist."

## THIRD-PARTY PAYMENT

If the SMP decides to undertake psychotherapy, the therapy could be submitted to insurance using the diagnoses of an Axis I disorder, such as anorexia nervosa. Often a DSM-IV Axis I diagnosis of "adjustment disorder" is applicable [57], especially if the athlete's performance problem is causing a "significant impairment in their social (including sports), academic, occupational, or family functioning." If the athlete has a medical condition (asthma, diabetes, headache) that worsens when she is experiencing great competitive stress or a performance problem, a diagnosis of "psychological factors affecting medical condition" would certainly seem warranted.

## SUMMARY

The SMP must function as an important gatekeeper in the diagnosis and prevention of emotional disorders and injuries. The preparticipation physical, the only time all year that many athletes see a physician, provides the opportunity. Examples of psychiatric problems common to athletes, their incidence in the population, and diagnostic tips to ferret them out have been given. Vignettes about well known athletes who have had these problems are included. Each highlights how the lack of diagnostic awareness of mental health issues in the athletic community and the stigma of "mental illness" prevented the athlete from getting treatment sooner. When dealing with a child or adolescent athlete, a sport parent interview is suggested, as it can be particularly helpful in uncovering disorders about which the athlete might be secretive—eating disorders, alcohol, drugs, or steroid abuse.

In addition, traditional psychiatric concepts such as transference and countertransference have been discussed with relevance to the SMP.

After reading this article, the SMP should be more attuned to the psychiatric entities existing in the athlete population that he or she routinely examines, and be in a better position to diagnose the athletes.

### Acknowledgments

Deepest appreciation to Judy Brown for research assistance and transcription, and to Ian Tofler, MB, BS, for editing assistance.

### References

[1] Winnicot DW. Maturational processes and the facilitating environment. London: Inst of Psa and Karnac Books; 1990.

[2] Heil J, Bowman JJ, Bean B. Patient management and the sports medicine team. In: Heil J, editor. Psychology of sport injury. Champaign (IL): Human Kinetics; 1993. p. 237–49.

[3] Eccles J, Barber B. The student council volunteering basketball or marching band: what kind of extracurricular involvement matters? Journal of Adolescent Research 1999;14(1): 10–43.

[4] Nattiv A, Puffer JC. Lifestyles and health risks of collegiate athletes. N Engl J Med 1991;33(6):585–90.

[5] Armsey TD, Hosey RG. Medical aspects of sports: epidemiology of injuries, preparticipation physical examination, and drugs in sports. Clin Sports Med 2004;23(2): 255–79.

[6] Wertheim LJ. Prisoners of depression. Sports Illustrated Magazine September 8, 2003; 71–9.

[7] Harnish P. Psychopharmacological approaches to the athletic and exercise population. Interview shown at Sport Psychiatry Symposium #54, American Psychiatric Association Annual Convention. Chicago, Illinois, May 16, 2000.

[8] American Psychiatric Association. Diagnostic and statistical manual of mental disorders. 4th edition. Washington (DC): American Psychiatric Association; 1994.

[9] Kaplan HI, Sadock BJ, Sadock VA. Mood disorders. In: Sadock BJ, Sadock VA, editors. Kaplan & Sadock's synopsis of psychiatry. 9th edition. Philadelphia: Lippincott, Williams & Wilkins; 2003. p. 534–78.

[10] Saunders P. Fearsome opponent—athletes who have spent years fine-tuning their bodies, find it difficult to accept mental illness and its stigma. Saturday Denver Post March 10, 2003.

[11] Nobles C. Pro football; former Raider faces charges after struggle. New York Times January 20, 2005;Sports Thursday:Section D. p. 2.

[12] Kaplan HI, Sadock BJ, Sadock VA. Generalized anxiety disorder. In: Sadock BJ, Sadock VA, editors. Kaplan & Sadock's synopsis of psychiatry. 9th edition. Philadelphia: Lippincott, Williams & Wilkins; 2003. p. 632–5.

[13] Kaplan HI, Sadock BJ, Sadock VA. Panic disorder and agoraphobia. In: Sadock BJ, Sadock VA, editors. Kaplan & Sadock's synopsis of psychiatry. 9th edition. Philadelphia: Lippincott, Williams & Wilkins; 2003. p. 599–608.

[14] Clark TP, Lardon MT. The sport psychiatry and golf. Clin Sports Med 2005;24:959–71.

[15] Kaplan HI, Sadock BJ, Sadock VA. Posttraumatic stress disorder and acute stress disorder. In: Sadock BJ, Sadock VA, editors. Kaplan & Sadock's synopsis of psychiatry. 9th edition. Philadelphia: Lippincott, Williams & Wilkins; 2003. p. 591–636.

[16] Krone J. Psychopharmacological approaches to the athletic and exercise population. Presentation at Sport Psychiatry Symposium #54, American Psychiatric Association Annual Convention. Chicago, Illinois, May 16, 2000.

[17] Lipsyte R. Julie Krone's race against depression. New York Times May 21, 2000:13.

[18] Rhoden WC. Road after the final four was his hardest journey. New York Times March 22, 2003;Sports of the Times:2.

[19] Yates A, Leehey K, Shisslak CM. Running—an analogue of anorexia? N Engl J Med 1983;308(5):251–5.

[20] Sungot-Borgen J. Risk and trigger factors for the development of eating disorders in female elite athletes. Med Sci Sports Exerc 1994;26:414–9.

[21] Swoap RA, Murphy SM. Eating disorders and weight management in athletes. In: Murphy SM, editor. Sport psychology interventions. Champaign (IL): Human Kinetics; 1995. p. 307–26.

[22] Kaplan HI, Sadock BJ, Sadock VA. Anorexia nervosa. In: Sadock BJ, Sadock VA, editors. Kaplan & Sadock's synopsis of psychiatry. 9th edition. Philadelphia: Lippincott, Williams & Wilkins; 2003. p. 739–45.

[23] Morse E, Currie A. Eating disorders in athletes: managing the risks. Clin Sports Med 2005;24:871–83.

[24] Kaplan HI, Sadock BJ, Sadock VA. Bulimia nervosa and eating disorders not otherwise specified. In: Sadock BJ, Sadock VA, editors. Kaplan & Sadock's synopsis of psychiatry. 9th edition. Philadelphia: Lippincott, Williams & Wilkins; 2003. p. 746–50.

[25] Carr CM, Murphy SM. Alcohol and drugs in sport. In: Murphy SM, editor. Sport psychology interventions. Champaign (IL): Human Kinetics; 1995. p. 283–304.

[26] Anonymous. National household survey on drug abuse. Rockville (MD): National Clearinghouse for Alcohol and Drug Information; 1994.

[27] Marder SP. Scales for assessing alcoholism and substance abuse. In: Kaplan HI, Sadock BJ, editors. Comprehensive textbook of psychiatry, vol. I. 6th edition. Baltimore (MD): Williams & Wilkins; 1995. p. 619–35.

[28] Jonas AP, Sickles RT, Lombardo JA. Substance abuse. Clin Sports Med 2004;11(2): 379–401.

[29] Rosenberg JM. Banned drug list. In: Fuentes RJ, editor. Athletic drug reference. Durham (NC): Clean Data Inc.; 1999. p. 314–408.

[30] Kaplan HI, Sadock BJ, Sadock VA. Anabolic steroid abuse. In: Sadock BJ, Sadock VA, editors. Kaplan & Sadock's synopsis of psychiatry. 9th edition. Philadelphia: Lippincott, Williams & Wilkins; 2003. p. 466–8.

[31] Steroid scandal. Good Morning America, ABC News. New York: WABC; February 25, 2005.

[32] Canseco J. Juiced: wild times, rampant 'roids, smash hits, and how baseball got big. New York: Regan Books; 2005.

[33] Coakley J. Sport in society: issues and controversies. 6th edition. New York: McGraw-Hill; 1998.

[34] Faigenbaum AD, Zaichkowsky ID, Gardner DE, et al. Anabolic steroid use by male and female middle school students. Pediatrics 1998;101(5):E6.

[35] Pope H, Gruber A, Choi P, et al. Muscle dysmorphia: an underrecognized form of body dysmorphic disorder. Psychosomatics 1997;38:548–57.

[36] National Research Council. Pathological gambling: a critical review. Washington (DC): National Academy Press; 1999.

[37] Kaplan HI, Sadock BJ, Sadock VA. Impulse-control disorders not elsewhere classified. In: Sadock BJ, Sadock VA, editors. Kaplan & Sadock's synopsis of psychiatry. 9th edition. Philadelphia: Lippincott, Williams & Wilkins; 2003. p. 782–94.

[38] Stabeno M. The ADHD affected athlete. Victoria (Canada): Trafford; 2004.

[39] Kamm RL. Tips for coaching a child with attention deficit/hyperactivity disorder. Technique 1999;19(10):22–8.

[40] Sadock BJ, Sadock VA. Delirium, dementia, and amnesic and other cognitive disorders and mental disorders due to a general medical condition. In: Saddock BJ, Saddock VA, editors. Kaplan & Saddock's synopsis of psychiatry. 9th edition. Philadelphia: Lippincott, Williams & Wilkins; 2003. p. 319–70.

[41] Kolata G. Research hints at a gene link to brain afflictions of boxers. New York Times July 9, 1997;section A:18.

[42] Jordan B, Relkin N, Ravdin L, et al. Apolipoprotein E ε4 association with chronic traumatic brain injury in boxing. JAMA 1997;278(2):136–40.

[43] McCann S. Overtraining and burnout. In: Murphy SM, editor. Sport psychology interventions. Champaign (IL): Human Kinetics; 1995. p. 347–65.

[44] Callister R, Callister RK, Fleck SJ, et al. Physiological and performance responses to overtraining in elite judo athletes. Medicine and Science in Sports and Exercise 1989; 22:816–24.

[45] Costill DL, Flynn MG, Kirwin JP, et al. Effects of repeated days of intensified training on muscle glycogen and swimming performance. Med Sci Sports Exerc 1998;20: 249–54.

[46] Hackney AC, Pearman SN, Nowacki JM. Physiological profiles of overtrained and stale athletes: a review. Applied Sport Psychology 1990;2:21–33.

[47] Noakes TD. Denial of mental illness in athletes. Br J Sports Med 2000;34:315.

[48] Morgan. Affective benefits of vigorous physical activity. Med Sci Sports Exerc 1985; 17:94–100.

[49] Adkins D. Psychopharmacological approaches to the athletic and exercise population. Presented at the Sport Psychiatry Symposium #54, American Psychiatric Association Annual Convention. Chicago, Illinois, May 16, 2000.

[50] Atchley WR. The sociology of retirement. Cambridge (MA): Schenkman; 1975.

[51] Kamm R. A Unique program for boxers at career end. Presented at Symposium 35, contemporary issues in sport psychiatry, American Psychiatric Association Annual Convention. New York, May 4, 2004.

[52] Page A. Keynote address at The Summit: The International Conference on Ethical Issues in Sport. Ethics Center, University of South Florida, Tampa, FL, May 28, 1998.

[53] Eskenazi G. First knockdown breaks the monotony for Jones. New York Times July 20, 1998;Sports Monday.

[54] Toffler I, Knapp P, Drell M. The achievement by proxy spectrum in youth sports: historical perspective and clinical approach to pressured and high-achieving children and adolescents. Child Adolesc Psychiatr Clin N Am 1998;7(4):803–20.

[55] Pennington B. Doctors see a big rise in injuries as young athletes train nonstop. New York Times February 22, 2005;D:1, 7.

[56] Kaplan HI, Sadock BJ, Sadock VA. The doctor-patient relationship and interviewing techniques. In: Sadock BJ, Sadock VA, editors. Kaplan & Sadock's synopsis of psychiatry. 9<sup>th</sup> edition. Philadelphia: Lippincott, Williams & Wilkins; 2003. p. 1–15.

[57] Sachs M. Professional ethics in sport psychology. In: Singer R, Murphy M, Tennant L, editors. Handbook of research on sport psychology. New York: Macmillan; 1993. p. 929.

[58] Kaplan HI, Sadock BJ, Sadock VA. Specific phobia and social phobia. In: Sadock BJ, Sadock VA, editors. Kaplan & Sadock's synopsis of psychiatry. 9<sup>th</sup> edition. Philadelphia: Lippincott, Williams & Wilkins; 2003. p. 609–16.

[59] Crouse K. Sports Monday, D5. NY Times, Monday, July 25, 2005.

Clin Sports Med 24 (2005) 771–781

# CLINICS IN SPORTS MEDICINE

ELSEVIER
SAUNDERS

# Diagnosis and Psychiatric Treatment of Athletes

Ira D. Glick, MD*, Jessica L. Horsfall, PhD

*Department of Psychiatry and Behavioral Sciences, Stanford University School of Medicine, 401 Quarry Road, Suite 2122, Stanford, CA 94305-5723, USA*

Although much time and money have been invested in treating the physical injuries of college and professional athletes, their associated psychiatric problems have been minimally addressed [1,2]. Even at the most basic level–at the entry level of family or team sports medicine physician–psychiatric treatment, including psychotropic medication and psychotherapy, has been overlooked. If recognized, patients may be undertreated. Perhaps this is related in part to the fact that although there is some anecdotal evidence in this population, there is no controlled evidence to suggest that psychiatric intervention is efficacious in improving performance or treating symptoms. Of course there is evidence that psychiatric treatment works in the general population [3]. Athletes (like anyone else) are at risk for both psychological problems or psychiatric illness (including substance abuse), but unlike others, for the most part there is a perception by those physicians working in the field that athletes generally do not seek out or connect with sports psychiatric providers to receive appropriate intervention. This is due in part to the social stigma regarding psychiatric illness [4]. Furthermore, treatment (especially of men) denotes weakness to athletes and coaches, who in some cases do not have mature coping strategies, whereas others naively believe they have the ability to conquer mental illness without medical help [5]. The authors present an initial case, by way of example, of the potential consequences of undertreatment or lack of care.

## CASE 1

Mr. X was a professional basketball player in his mid-30s. He had had a 13-year career in the National Basketball Association (NBA). He had a history of lowered mood, (ie, "depression") since his teens, for which he had never sought treatment. He did, however, use alcohol, but never to excess, throughout his career as a way of coping with the lowered mood. On being released by his team, he felt that his life had no future. He drank steadily for several months, and

* Corresponding author. *E-mail address:* iraglick@stanford.edu (I.D. Glick).

0278-5919/05/$ – see front matter
doi:10.1016/j.csm.2005.03.007

refused therapy or help from former players. He died of a self-inflicted gunshot wound within the year.

## GOALS

Psychiatric interventions for athletes have been made for many years, but psychiatric contributions to the sports medicine literature have been sparse [6]. In 1992, Begel [1] wrote a seminal overview article, and a few articles have appeared in some clinical journals during the past few years [5,6], but sports psychiatry is clearly still evolving as a professional specialty [7]. In part this is because it lacks a knowledge base or fellowship program, and in part it is because the incidence and prevalence of psychiatric illness in the athletic population are low. Therefore, very few clinicians have the experience, nor has anyone had a large enough sample, to do systematic surveys of incidence or prevalence, or controlled studies with adequate sample sizes. An excellent overview article on "sport psychiatry" was published in 1998 [6], but focused on substance abuse, eating disorders, and brain injury. Likewise, Begel and Burton [8] have now published the first text on sport psychiatry, and Tofler [9] has compiled a volume on sport psychiatric issues in children and adolescents. The authors' aim with this article is to introduce sports psychiatry to sports medicine professionals.

Accordingly, our objectives are (1) to provide an overview of psychiatric problems and illness (in the broadest sense) associated with this population, and (2) to discuss diagnosis and psychiatric treatment to aid sports medicine physicians, sports psychiatrists, sports psychologists, or general psychiatrists as they work with adult athletes [10]. For issues in children or adolescents, we suggest the overviews by Stryer et al [11] and Eppright and associates [12]. The field of sports psychology is not the focus of this article, except as some of the controlled literature bears on psychiatric issues. We will not cover the vast literature on exercise science or performance sports psychology, because these topics are concerned with very different issues. In that context, in 1996, Myers and colleagues [13] published an extensive review of cognitive behavioral strategies and performance enhancement.

## METHODOLOGY

This article offers a review of the literature in the field of college and professional sports psychiatry. Searches conducted in Medline and Psychlit for the period from 1980 to 1999 included (but were not limited to) the terms "athlete, professional, treatment, elite, depression, anxiety, substance, eating disorder, sport, gender, psychiatry, psychology, medication, therapy, counseling, exercise, intervention, brain, basketball, football, Olympic," and "boxing." The search revealed a paucity of empirical data relating to characteristics or psychiatric treatment of college and professional athletes. In addition, to supplement the literature, the authors have summarized experience from an adult, sports psychiatry practice located in two academic centers–Cornell University Medical College and the Stanford University School of Medicine. The areas covered include problems of living, such as problems in relationships and work; Diagnostic and Statistical Manual of Mental Disorders, 4th Edition (DSM-IV) Axis I disorders, such as substance abuse, mood disorder, and anxiety disorders; and Axis II personality disorders. Salient issues specific to team sports (football, basketball, baseball, soccer, and the like) and individual sports (boxing, weight lifting, tennis, track, and so on.) are also addressed.

The major limitations of the article are the lack of scientific literature and paucity of epidemiological and empirical data. The situation with athletes is similar to that in the field of suicidology; that is, controlled studies of treatment of athletes [1], like studies of those who have suicidal ideation, are relatively rare. Very few mental health professionals have had enough experience to make strong treatment recommendations (although there are some who have worked with athletes for over 25 years), nor have many controlled studies been done.

## DIAGNOSTIC ISSUES
For the psychiatric clinician, accurate diagnosis is an essential first step to lay the groundwork for successful treatment. This includes the process of the clinical evaluation/work-up, methods of evaluation, and special issues related to elite athletes. Needless to say, for other sports medicine practitioners, the first step may be to make a referral to a psychiatrist so that a diagnosis can be made.

### The Process of Clinical Evaluation
To help connect with the athlete, the clinician's initial task is to evaluate the individual; that is, the athlete's personality and coping mechanisms. Psychological status has been found to be associated with performance events [14]. It may be difficult to differentiate the "person" from the athletic "persona." Although it is not common, emotional maturity may be delayed in professional athletes due to their iconization—placing athletes on a pedestal and having others insulate them from the stresses and problems of daily life [12–15]. Adolescent or childlike attitudes and behaviors (eg, inappropriate anger, inability to follow team rules, and so on) may be prominent despite chronological adult age [1,6,15].

Secondly, to the extent that personal relationships affect athletic performance, interpersonal issues must be considered. For example, coaches play a large role in determining the impact sports may have on an athlete's mental health [16]. The impact of the coach as a father figure versus punitive authority figure versus buddy is important. Family and significant others may also be relevant [16].

Third, phenomenological issues, the signs and symptoms defining a psychiatric diagnosis (for example, major depressive disorder or alcohol abuse), should be explored in the context of the work-up. Denial of both psychological difficulty and of pain associated with enhancing performance is common among successful athletes [17]. On the other hand, some elite athletes, being keenly aware of the capabilities (and limitations) of their bodies, are less likely to ignore pain and discomfort stemming from physical exertion. If such issues are not addressed, the clinician will have increasing difficulty developing and maintaining a therapeutic alliance.

## Methods and Goals of Evaluation

Methods of evaluation include a clinical interview with the athlete, significant others (including agents, teammates, and so on), or the family. Laboratory tests, such as a toxicology screen for illegal substances or a fasting blood sugar for medical illnesses that can cause psychiatric problems, or psychological testing may be indicated [1,5,6,8].

The primary goal is to differentiate the cause of the athlete's difficulties from its effects. Daily functioning and athletic performance go hand-in-hand, and consequently may affect interpersonal relationships. By way of example, some suggest that the professional sports climate may increase the likelihood of athlete violence [18–20]. Poor performance may result in aggressive behavior toward a significant other, usually the spouse. Conversely, an interpersonal relationship may temporarily improve from a good performance. Monitoring the athlete's problem-coping cycle will lead to appropriate interventions and subsequent resolution of the relational difficulties. Therefore, when trying to get a history, the sports psychiatrist must exercise judgment and maintain confidentiality when contacting others (including coaches, players, agents, and family members). The authors have much more to say about confidentiality later. In some cases (depending on the treatment), written informed consent must be obtained [5].

## Special Issues

Athletes have problems and psychiatric illness like anyone else. These include societal problems, such as violence, substance abuse, and the like, that have a high secular prevalence independently of athletes. Those issues are highly scrutinized by the media and athletes as a group tend to get "tarred by the same brush." The authors' point here is to cover the range of possibilities and emphasize that treatment is often necessary. And of course, a major factor directly affecting the interview process is whether the athlete is coming voluntarily or involuntarily, under pressure from third parties.

## CASE 2

Mr. Y was a professional baseball player in his mid-20s. He had a lifelong history of lowered mood, and also had one family member who had what was probably a major depressive disorder. During spring training, he noted the onset of irritability, anhedonia, and lowered mood. His wife encouraged him to seek treatment. He felt that there was "nothing wrong." He became more isolated from his teammates and less motivated to go to the ball park. A discussion with his manager resulted in the patient being blamed for his illness (he wasn't "trying hard enough"). On the urging of his agent, he sought help from the psychiatrist working with his team. He was started on an antidepressant, a selective serotonin reuptake inhibitor (SSRI), and within 6 weeks felt better. He was still not well enough to pitch, and returned only in the latter part of the season. He continued medication the following season and returned to prior form.

## RANGE OF PSYCHIATRIC PROBLEMS IN ATHLETES

The range of problems or illness in the elite athlete is broad. These problems and symptoms (eg, a drinking or other substance-abuse problem) usually do not present like a fracture presents to an orthopedist—most commonly they present either via referral from a third party such as the family or team in confidence, or emerge after the athlete's complaints or problems with others in his life are discussed. Substance abuse and antisocial behavior are among the most common issues treated in this population [21,22], but elite athletes may also present with mood, anxiety, and adjustment disorders [5,19,23,24]. So-called "character-ological issues," including narcissistic ("big ego") and antisocial personality traits (eg, stealing, cheating, and so on) may also occur in the athlete population, despite large incomes [23]. Other issues include individual issues (eg, deciding when and how to quit) as well as transition issues (eg, being out of the spotlight), family issues (eg, marriage, spouse abuse, fidelity concerns), and sports- relationship issues (eg, difficulties with the team, owners, league, agents, or fans). Having said that, there is literature suggesting that athletes in general show better emotional health compared with nonathletes [2,25], and the same is true for elite athletes compared with nonelite athletes [26]. At the very least, athletes do not have any worse emotional health than others, but they are subject to different stressors and their difficulties may be amplified. Likewise, changes in mental health over time have been associated with performance [14].

In addition, there are issues relating to evaluation that are unique to athletes. First, as we mentioned above, clinicians must decide when and under what circumstances to contact other sources of history (coaches and team). Understanding the individual's sports environment can increase the success of psychiatric intervention outcome [27]. Second, cross-cultural, ethnic, or racial issues may underlie the athlete's difficulties. For example, a player from one country may misinterpret (or may be misunderstood) by other players who represent the majority of the team because of culturally dictated behaviors or traditions. An example is an American on an Italian basketball team. Therapist sensitivity to these issues and awareness of personal biases (that is, countertransference) is paramount [28]. Third, the sports physician must consider "organicity" in the search for etiology of the athlete's problems. Boxers, football players, or soccer players may experience mild head trauma (ie, concussions), due to high-impact actions [29]. For example, Matser and coworkers [30] found that among soccer players, heading the ball may impair performance in memory, planning, and visual-perceptual processing. Furthermore, severe organic disorders (eg, dementia pugilistica) should be ruled out before psychotherapy is suggested, because therapy would be ineffective if they exist. Substance abusers may also present with neurologic difficulties that may or may not subside after detoxification and rehabilitation. These athletes may benefit from neuropsychological testing before entering treatment. Lastly, developmental level or characterological functioning should be evaluated. Athletes presenting with narcissistic, grandiose, or antisocial character traits may use denial as a defense (among other diffuse mechanisms), resulting in failure to form an effective therapeutic alliance [1].

Especially in males, the pampered, highly paid, professional athlete may be developmentally immature, that is, have a childlike personality in contrast to a "macho adult" presentation to the public. Exactly how common this is remains unknown because systematic studies have not been done.

## INDUCING ATHLETES TO UNDERGO TREATMENT

Unfortunately, college and professional athletes are often very reluctant to use psychiatric treatment [2,25,31]. As previously mentioned, the athletes' tendency to deny weakness and assume a macho posture is characterological (ie, part of the personality), resulting in denial of an illness and fear of social stigma [5]. Constant pressures of competition and performance may lead to the development of dysfunctional coping skills in what is thought to be a small percentage of athletes. Problematic mechanisms include driving too fast (as in the 1999 death of a basketball player racing his car with a teammate), sexual promiscuity, using recreational drugs, or using performance-enhancing drugs. The psychology underlying these behaviors is outside the scope of this article, but involves a variety of mechanisms, some involved with athletic skills and performance (eg, the need to win) and others involved with identity (eg, using drugs with their peers). Provision of psychiatric services is paramount for rehabilitation and improvement of quality of life for both the athletes and their families. Most sports psychiatry clinicians believe that unless the athlete presents with overt disabling psychiatric symptoms or societal issues (psychomotor retardation, mania, rapid weight loss, agitation, marital difficulties, or legal troubles), traditional referral to a psychiatrist and development of a therapeutic alliance is unlikely. The recent (1999) case of a Chicago high school basketball player who attempted to move directly to professional sports and presented at training camp with bizarre aggressive symptoms and suicidal behavior, makes this point clear. In the authors' view, the player (or their families or teams) must work in conjunction with a psychiatrist and an "intermediate person/league liaison" such as a peer, former player or agent to facilitate treatment (L. Baccus, personal communication, 1999). The idea of treatment may be reframed as "performance help" (similar to individual coaching for improvement of athletic skills) to encourage active participation in the process. In addition, the rationale for intervention should appeal to the athlete's self-interest in increasing skills, money, or quality of life, rather than focusing on a "mental illness" (elite athletes usually have great resistance to accepting the diagnosis, especially in the early stages). Lastly, substance abuse problems almost always require collaboration with a support organization such as Alcoholics Anonymous or Narcotics Anonymous.

Most problems of living and many depressive or anxiety disorders can be managed by the nonpsychiatric clinician. In some cases, the nuances of modern psychopharmacology or complicated interpersonal issues may require referral to a psychiatrist, who is capable of delivering psychopharmacologic intervention or combined medication-psychotherapy treatment.

Most important is to understand how the athletes perceive the clinicians. One former Olympic swimmer believes that athletes have great difficulty in finding a doctor who they "can feel connected to, in part due to the "stigma they attach to doctors," and especially if they haven't worked with athletes." More often than not, the athlete only wants to hear one answer, "that they can perform" (K. Radke, personal communication, 2000). In order for treatment to succeed, the connection and trust built between clinician and athlete will be major determining factors in outcome of treatment.

## CASE 3

Mr. Z was a jockey in his mid-40s. He had been highly successful throughout his career. During one of his races, he was thrown from his horse and severely injured, with multiple fractures to his face and body that required extensive surgery. Following the injury, he developed signs and symptoms of post-traumatic stress disorder (PTSD), and subsequently a major depressive episode. He was unable to ride. He was reluctant to try psychotherapy, but tried it briefly and then quit. After 2 years of being unable to work, he was approached by a friend who convinced him to consult a psychiatrist. He tried individual psychiatry, which helped a little regarding self-esteem issues, but he still felt depressed. For 2 years while in therapy he refused medication. He finally (in desperation) agreed. He was started on an SSRI and made a "miraculous recovery." He returned to riding and was able to get back to his previous form. He felt better than he ever had in his life, because he had suffered from a low-grade mood disorder for many years.

## PRINCIPLES OF TREATMENT

### Step 1: Make an Accurate Diagnosis

As outlined in the previous section, making an accurate diagnosis includes identifying individual, family, and other interpersonal dynamics, as well as DSM phenomenology.

### Step 2: Set Realistic Goals

The primary goal is to differentiate the person from the athlete. The person comes before the sport. The aim is to strengthen the therapeutic alliance, aid with problem or illness resolution, and maintain or enhance sports performance.

### Step 3: Deliver Psycho-Education

Routinely, psycho-education is delivered to the patient as well as to the family following the initial evaluation. Psycho-education entails defining the problem for the family, identifying the causes of the problem, explaining the treatment plan, and delivering the prognosis with and without treatment.

Issues of transference (the athlete's feelings about the clinician) and countertransference must be addressed at this stage of intervention. It is common for the athlete to experience a strong initial transference reaction, usually negative (eg, "you don't understand the pressures I'm under"), or when contemplating getting help, the athlete is "scared and believes he cannot trust anyone" (Cooney, personal communication, 1999). Likewise, "athlete-envy" can trigger counter-transference issues for the psychiatrist. It is crucial for the physician to follow existing well-accepted guidelines for treating celebrated individuals and to avoid hero worship. Exceptions may result in inappropriate treatment and poor outcome [1].

### Step 4: Involve the Family and Significant-Others

Integration of interpersonal issues into the therapeutic process is usually important for successful treatment outcome. The family members may help to guide treatment and provide insight into the background and history of presenting issues. During this phase, the context in which the athlete lives and functions may also be explored [27]. Involving the coaches, agents, and team members in the process may be important for the athlete's full recovery, but varies greatly depending on the personalities involved. Again, the sport psychiatrist must use this technique judiciously and must obtain informed consent [5].

### Step 5: "Do the Right Thing"

"Doing the right thing" entails delivering appropriate and adequate treatment, including both pharmacotherapy and psychotherapy as indicated [32]. Typically, the athlete will attempt to define his or her own treatment. The guideline that the physician directs the treatment and does not acquiesce to an athlete's inappropriate requests is often ignored.. For example, if medicine is prescribed, the athlete may suggest a homeopathic dose. Although treatment must be dictated by the therapist, the athlete's input should always be respected [33]. The sports psychiatrist must continuously work to maintain the therapeutic alliance in order to avoid premature dropout and noncompliance.

### Step 6: Refer

Refer the patient to a sport psychiatrist or consulting psychologist for consultation or management as the needs (ie, medications or psychotherapy) of the case dictate. New strategies and medications for all the psychiatric illnesses are beyond the scope of this article, but are detailed in psychiatric texts [34], consensus guidelines [35], and in a recent overview paper Dr. Glick and coauthors have written [36]. The issue of psychiatric medications and their effects on performance is the key therapeutic dilemma for most psychiatrists and their patients. As a rule of thumb, most Axis I disorders require medications for at least 6 to 12 months to achieve effectiveness (ie, full remission). The usual problem is lack of compliance when experiencing side effects, especially in the early phase of treatment. For example, in cases of bipolar mania or most depressive illness that interfere with function, mood stabilizers or antidepressants are required. These medications can produce weight gain, ataxia, and other undesirable side effects that may adversely affect performance. As a generalization, most athletes will take medication if they believe (or discover) it will improve their psychiatric disorder (and function) regardless of side effects ( J. Khron, personal communication, May, 2000).

## OTHER TREATMENT ISSUES

Although extremely difficult, confidentiality (especially with psychotherapeutic issues) must be maintained during contact with significant others. Written informed consent must be obtained for most psychiatric treatments needed [5]. In other cases, informed consent is used to disclose information (crucial to treatment compliance) to the coach, other members of the coaching staff, or to the team physician. Coercion must be avoided–psychiatric information usually should not be provided to the coach when the patient is being compelled to provide it and does not want to provide it. Obviously, it should not be provided for the purposes of selecting membership or starting status on a team; however, sometimes team goals contradict the goals of the patient, and coaches and team members may ignore the individual needs of the athlete. If the athlete is suffering from increased stress (eg, a close pennant race) or an Axis I disorder, however, inducing him into treatment may be difficult. The authors suggest a technique common to forensic psychiatry. One physician focuses on the patient-athlete treatment, and a second may act as liaison with coaches and team to address the need of the team member-athlete [19]. Involving the second therapist separates out the issue of team-needs versus individual-needs.

Within the evaluation and treatment phases, one must distinguish the symptoms of the illness from the pressures of competing. For example, anxiety before or associated with a game is normal and requires no treatment; however, severe anxiety that persists and prevents functioning may be indicative of an anxiety disorder and requires intervention [1]. It is important for the sports psychiatrist to treat the illness and psychiatric issues while the team focuses on performance [37]. That the patient always comes before the sport is a principle worth reiterating.

Finally, the sports psychiatrist must avoid collusion in denial–agreeing with the athlete that there is no problem when one clearly exists. This most commonly occurs when the athlete or team attempts to rationalize antisocial behavior and substance abuse. Axis I and II disorders–disorders of personality–must be clearly defined for appropriate treatment, and the psychiatrist must maintain boundaries to ensure successful outcome.

## SUMMARY

The authors have reviewed diagnostic and treatment issues related to treating athletes involved in individual as well as team sports on college and professional levels. We have described guidelines to maximize not only the quality of the athletes' lives, but their performance. We believe that these principles may maximize individual talent and improve life function by treating the illness or problem, with the ultimate aim of improving individual health. The usual mistake is to undertreat [35]. Therefore, to achieve maximal efficacy, we recommend that the office physician err on the side of providing at least the minimal effective dose and duration of medication and psychotherapeutic intervention as dictated by the needs of the patient. Further reports of psychiatric intervention for athletes are needed, as are scientific studies of different strategies of treatment.

References

[1] Begel D. An overview of sport psychiatry. Am J Psychiatry 1992;149:606–14.
[2] Carmen LR, Zerman L, Blaine B. Use of the Harvard Psychiatric Service by athletes and non-athletes. Ment Hyg 1968;52:134–7.
[3] Petrie T, Diehl N, Watkins C. Sport psychology: an emerging domain in the counseling psychology profession? Couns Psychol 1995;23:535–45.
[4] Linder D, Brewer B, Van Raalte J, et al. A negative halo for athletes who consult sport psychologists: replication and extension. Journal of Sport and Exercise Psychology 1991; 13:133–48.
[5] Begel D. Occupational, psychopathologic, and therapeutic aspects of sport psychiatry. Dir Psychiatry 1994;14:1–8.
[6] Macleod AD. Sport psychiatry. Aust N Z J Psychiatry 1998;32:860–6.
[7] Nicholi A. Psychiatric consultation in professional football. N Engl J Med 1986;31: 1095–100.
[8] Begel D, Burton R. Sport psychiatry theory and practice. New York: Norton; 2000.
[9] Tofler I, editor. Sport psychiatry. Child Adolesc Psychiatr Clin N Am 1998.
[10] Vaughn J, Emener W. Rehabilitation counseling with college athletes: a hypothesis generating study. Journal of Applied Rehabilitation Counseling 1994;25:30–5.
[11] Stryer BK, Tofler IR, Lapchick R. A developmental overview of child and youth sports in society. Child Adolesc Psychiatr Clin N Am 1998;7:697–724.
[12] Eppright TD, Sanfacon JA, Beck NC, et al. Sport psychiatry in childhood and adolescence: an overview. Child Psychiatry Hum Dev 1997;28:71–88.
[13] Meyers AW, Whelan JP, Murphy SM. Cognitive behavioral strategies in athletic performance enhancement. Prog Behav Modif 1996;30:137–64.
[14] May JR, Veach TL, Reed MW, et al. A psychological study of health, injury, and performance in athletes on the US Alpine Ski Team. Phys Sportsmed 1985;13:111–5.
[15] Glick ID, Marcotte DB. Psychiatric aspects of basketball. J Sports Med Phys Fitness 1989;29:104–12.
[16] Bell C. Promotion of mental health through coaching competitive sports. J Natl Med Assoc 1997;89:517–20.
[17] Pavelski R, Kryden A, Steiner H, et al. Adaptive styles in elite collegiate athletes [abstract]. Presented at the 45th Annual Meeting of The American Academy of Child and Adolescent Psychiatry. Anaheim, CA, November 1998.
[18] Benedict J, Klein A. Arrest and conviction rates for athletes accused of sexual assault. In: Bergen R, editor. Issues in intimate violence. Thousand Oaks (CA): Sage Publications; 1998. p. 169–75.
[19] Calhoun J, Ogilvie B, Hendrickson T, et al. The psychiatric consultant in professional team sports. Child Adolesc Psychiatr Clin N Am 1998;7:791–802.
[20] Pipe A. Sport, science, and society: ethics in sports medicine. Med Sci Sports Exerc 1993; 25:888–900.
[21] Martin H, Thrasher D. Chemical dependence and treatment of the professional athlete. In: Lawson G, Lawson A, editors. Alcoholism and substance abuse in special populations. New York: Aspen Publishers; 1998. p. 315–39.
[22] Stainback R. Alcohol and sport. Champaign (IL): Human Kinetics; 1997.
[23] Anderson M, Denson E, Brewer B, et al. Disorders of personality and mood in athletes: recognition and referral. J Appl Sport Psychol 1994;6:168–84.
[24] Cogan K. Putting the "clinical" into sport psychology counseling. In: Hays K, editor. Integrating exercise, sports, movement, and mind: therapeutic unity. New York: The Haworth Press; 1998. p. 131–43.

[25] Pierce RA. Athletes in psychotherapy: how many, how come? J Am Coll Health Assoc 1969;17:244–9.

[26] Morgan WP. Selected psychological factors limiting performance: a mental health model. In: Clarke DH, Eckert HM, editors. Limits of human performance. Champaign (IL): Human Kinetics; 1985. p. 70–80.

[27] Van Raalte J. Working in competitive sport: what coaches and athletes want psychologists to know. In: Hays K, editor. Integrating exercise, sports, movement, and mind: therapeutic unity. New York: The Haworth Press; 1998. p. 101–10.

[28] Lee C, Rotella R. Special concerns and considerations for sport psychology consulting with black student athletes. Sport Psychologist 1991;5:365–9.

[29] Hinton-Bayre A, Geffen G, McFarland K. Mild head injury and speed of information processing: a prospective study of professional rugby league players. J Clin Exp Neuropsychol 1997;19:275–89.

[30] Matser E, Kessels A, Jordan B, et al. Chronic traumatic brain injury in professional soccer players. Neurology 1998;51:791–6.

[31] Little JC. The athlete's neurosis—a deprivation crisis. Acta Psychiatr Scand 1969;45: 187–96.

[32] Glick ID. Adding psychotherapy to pharmacotherapy: data, benefits and guidelines for integration. Am J Psychotherapy 2004;58:186–208.

[33] Orlick T. Reflections on sport psych consulting with individual and team sport athletes at Summer and Winter Olympic Games. Sport Psychologist 1989;3:358–65.

[34] Schatzberg AF, Nemeroff CB, editors. Textbook of psychopharmacology. 3rd edition. Washington (DC): American Psychiatric Press; 2004.

[35] Practice guideline for the treatment of patients with major depressive disorder. Am J Psychiatry 2000;157(Suppl):1–45.

[36] Glick ID, Suppes T, DeBattista C, et al. Clinical update: psychopharmacological treatment strategies for depression, bipolar disorder and schizophrenia. Ann Intern Med 2001; 134:47–60.

[37] Massimino J. Sport psychiatry. Annals of Sports Medicine 1987;3:55–8.

Clin Sports Med 24 (2005) 783–804

# CLINICS IN SPORTS MEDICINE

# Developmental Overview of Child and Youth Sports for the Twenty-first Century

Ian R. Tofler, MB, BS[a],*, Grant J. Butterbaugh, PhD[b]

[a]*Charles R. Drew University of Medicine and Science/University of California, Los Angeles, 1731 East 120th Street, Los Angeles, CA 90059, USA*
[b]*Departments of Clinical Psychiatry and Neuropsychology, Louisiana State University 1542 Tulane Avenue, Room 358, New Orleans, LA 70112, USA*

nvolvement in sports is important throughout the life cycle, but may be more critical in children, adolescents, and young adults for the potential enhancement of health, disease prevention, and psychological well-being. This is especially so at a time when sedentary lifestyle and obesity are such problems among our youth [1]. Sports participation can make a critical contribution in the development of personal and social identity. In childhood and adolescence, sports are the most prevalent organized extracurricular activity.

Each year an increasing number of youngsters participate in organized sports. In the United States at least 7 million children between the ages of 5 and 17 participate in school athletic programs. Another 22 million between the ages of 5 and 17 are involved in organized athletic programs, and 14 million more are involved in less structured sports, including weekend skiing and neighborhood kickball. Newer sports such as in-line skating and snowboarding claim 23 and 1.5 million participants, respectively [2]. Virtually all children, at some time during their development, have some experience with organized sports. Although intensity of involvement varies, many children have already participated in intensive sports training and competition for several years by early adolescence.

This article presents an overview of sporting participation for children and adolescents from psychological, physical, social, developmental, and historical perspectives. The following areas are reviewed: (1) normal developmental readiness and sporting participation; (2) benefits and risks of athletic participation for the child and adolescent; (3) self concept and sporting participation; (4) adverse psychophysiological and somatoform effects of sports; (5) interactional and systemic contributions to adverse physical and psychological effects; (6) a historical/social perspective of sport in the United States; (7) the current and future role of psychiatrists in conjunction with sports medicine physicians;

* Corresponding author. *E-mail address:* robertoff@aol.com (I.R. Tofler).

0278-5919/05/$ – see front matter
doi:10.1016/j.csm.2005.05.006

(8) the sports psychiatry interview of the child, family, and coach; and (9) summary and future challenges.

## NORMAL DEVELOPMENTAL READINESS AND SPORTING PARTICIPATION

During the preschool and early grade school years, children may lack the physical, emotional, and cognitive maturity necessary to play many sports. They are not physically capable of mastering the necessary skills, emotionally mature enough for competition, or cognitively able to understand and follow the rules. For children younger than 10, adult feedback and validation are extremely important; however, maturation is associated with peer comparison, reliance on one's own conscience, and the ability to follow rules.

During early adolescence, peer-to-peer evaluation becomes a more valued measure [3]. There is a further shift toward the nonparental adult role modeling in later adolescence. Adolescence is characterized by the development of abstract thinking, an increased desire for autonomy, conflict between independence and dependence, and the struggle to find a social niche in which to express and delineate one's identity. Meeting the demands of increased new interests and responsibilities such as applying for college and taking Scholastic Aptitude Tests (SATs) can be overwhelming. These normally stressful developmental demands conflict with adolescent yearnings for greater independence, control, and autonomy. The hierarchical, goal-oriented, coach-controlled culture of structured and competitive sports can provide both panacea and poison for these adolescents. Adult nurturing, support, balanced parental encouragement, consistency, and understanding of the child athlete as a person are vital to this aspect of development.

### Physical and Physiological Readiness

Children develop according to different physical trajectories. The earlier physical development of girls can give them a relative edge over boys during latency, but this changes after puberty. On the other hand, in sports such as female gymnastics and figure skating, in which small size conveys great advantage, there is great pressure for girls to short-circuit the process of normal physical trajectory and to maintain a prepubertal mesomorphic body habitus.

In early childhood, taller children—boys and girls—may excel, and may have better motor skills, such as rapid hand-eye coordination. They may experience a relative decline and a consequent dip in self-esteem as others catch up [4].

The developing skeleton in the preteen is flexible and primarily cartilaginous. Competitive sports such as gymnastics can subject the immature spine to considerable physical stress [5]. This predisposes a child to potential deformity, stress fractures, chronic injury, and growth retardation. Little League baseball more appropriately restricts the number of pitches used, because of an appreciation of the great risk of injury to the immature, unstable shoulder girdle.

Eyesight does not fully mature until age 6 or 7. Before that time, farsighted children may exhibit more difficulty tracking and catching or hitting moving objects such as baseballs.

## Neuropsychological Readiness

### Attention

A developing child should have mastered the ability to take turns and attend to the game without undue distractibility. These attentional milestones often do not fully kick in until age 6 to 10, and later, if at all, in attention deficit/hyperactivity disorder (ADHD) youngsters. They mediate a child's ability to focus on a game, as well as to follow and understand the rules, strategies, and teamwork required in team sports. Children who have attentional impairments may excel at games because of their improved motivation when facing novel situations. Impulsivity may also be an adaptive attribute in some circumstances. These children may actually have superior ability to deal with novel situations that can present themselves in a game setting. Exercise also increases blood flow to areas of the brain involved in decision-making and judgment, such as the prefrontal cortex. Thus children who are prone to distractibility on the field may pay more attention to beetles on the ground than to continuously changing events on the action at the other end of the playing field, perhaps not unusual for many 7 year olds.

### Cognitive development and its effect on sporting performance

With the emergence of late concrete operational thinking, many children are able to differentiate between their effort and perception of performance outcome. Simply understanding the rules and process of a game may itself not come easily. Children under the age of 9 may believe that greater effort should always predict more positive outcomes irrespective of the task difficulty or challenge. The tendency of some children to get "stuck" at this level of thinking may impair their ability to perform in cooperative team sports. The ability of many adolescents to reason at a higher abstract level during adolescence should transfer to the sporting arena, but does not necessarily do so. The playing out of autonomy and Oedipal struggles may frequently involve the coach, all too often the only available male parental transferential figure. An adolescent's ability to juggle and master greater social and academic activities and responsibilities, in addition to any sporting or extracurricular involvement, may be critical for development and balance of a strong multidimensional personality. It may also diminish an adolescent's dedication to a particular sporting activity.

### Self-evaluative thinking

The ability to self-attribute and compare oneself to others develops throughout latency. For example, "I am the best at dribbling!," or "I am always picked last, so I must be the absolute worst" become increasingly sophisticated during the latency age. This may impact upon self-esteem and the requisite motivation and confidence to participate and compete in or abstain from sporting activities. This exquisite sensitivity to the primarily adult and peer judgment of self and others needs to be taken very seriously. Coaches are commonly the major role model beyond parents and teachers. Negative coaching is exemplified by US Olympics women's coaches such as Bela Karolyi, with his comment "little girls are like scorpions in a bottle, only the strongest can survive" [6]. Especially for younger children, it is critical to give positive feedback for their efforts, regardless of the win/loss outcome. Likewise, it is crucial to recognize the impact of negative feedback and outcome-driven parenting and coaching. In early adolescence, primary validation tends to be derived more from the group. Social isolation from the peer group through professional training is problematic, and can easily distort "normal" development.

*Process versus outcome thinking*

Younger children tend to be process- rather than outcome-oriented [7]. They take their cues from adult role models at a very young age, however, and are keen to please, particularly to please their often achievement-driven parents. With maturation, females are more likely to maintain a more process-oriented outlook, but males can, with perhaps more help, be educated in the benefits of process and micro-goal orientation, as opposed to a more macro win-lose mentality.

## Social Readiness

The developmental ability to switch roles and to play cooperatively and imaginatively is one in which all children have their own individual trajectories, with females sometimes appearing more advanced than males. Increasing sophistication through latency brings with it a greater ability for children to empathize with and tolerate another point of view.

For example, in Little League baseball, everyone wants to be pitcher, perceived as the most important role in a team. Rotating positions and education regarding the importance of every position in a team sport is helpful. Reassuring and including those who are temporarily on the bench is vital as well.

## Moral Developmental Readiness

Kohlberg's stages of moral development [8], Bandura's social learning theory [9], and Rest's model of moral action [10] have all proved helpful. The Rest model consists of the four steps of: (1) interpreting a situation and its moral possibilities; (2) forming a moral opinion as to what should be done; (2) choosing a value, either moral or nonmoral, which can be put into action; and (3) carrying out the intended action. Shields and Bredemeier's [11] research on moral practice in sport has been helpful in understanding the readiness skills required to effectively take part in competitive sports. Three areas of morality that Shields and Bredemeier address include fair play, sportsmanship, and character, as evidenced by integrity and compassion. The ability to integrate or differentiate between the sometimes very serious world of game playing and other aspects of life is critical. Acquisition of this developmental step is one that many sporting professional adults, let alone children, have difficulty with. "It's only a game" rings somewhat hollow in the world of millionaire professional athletes.

Lessons in morality and hard work to achieve goals while maintaining ethical standards can be a major teaching goal in sports. Coaches and parents have the opportunity to model pro-social behaviors. In many sports, however, the more adept child will quickly learn the opposite behaviors, often with adult encouragement. That is, an antisocial approach to bending or exploiting the rules to the point where "it's OK to cheat or deliberately hurt the opposition as long as you don't get caught." The implication here is that a form of sport-associated moral regression is acceptable, even tacitly encouraged. This may be a lesson that is transferred to and from other aspects of life [12].

Although an admirable and often achieved goal, the moral fiber that many children's sporting pioneers and current parents are seeking, through Little League participation for example, is not necessarily the final outcome. Bruce Ogilvie, one of the fathers of sport psychology, stated in an article written with Tutko [13], "If you want to build character, try something else besides sport." This is a cautionary if somewhat pessimistic aphorism that all parents, coaches, and sports medicine professionals should keep in mind [1,13]. This assertion is countered by research supporting a decline in delinquency, pregnancy, and substance abuse, accompanied by higher self-esteem and educational attainment, with involvement in organized sporting activities, especially in lower socioeconomic groups and adolescent females [14,15]. Decreased "downtime," delegitimization of delinquent behavior, and dependence on male peers for self-esteem are thought to be important mediators of this process [14,16–20].

The adolescent is developing more sophisticated methods and rationales for comprehending the complex moral world, and this will certainly influence his actions in the sporting arena as well. Ideally, the playing field should facilitate if not define the development of these more mature developmental goals and rationales for interpreting life.

Parental developmental parallels for all these readiness skills should also be considered by the clinician. Parents' or coaches' ability to cope with winning or losing, how they themselves manage aggression and regression during a game, how they interact in a crowd, how they handle violence, how they perform as referees, and how they may rationalize certain behaviors, are all absorbed and internalized by the developing child [21].

## ATHLETIC PARTICIPATION: BENEFITS AND RISKS FOR THE CHILD AND ADOLESCENT

### Benefits of Youth Sports

Within the sporting arena, children in both individual and team sports encounter challenges that reflect other life experiences.

Children develop leadership skills, teamwork, self-discipline, coping skills and cooperation in times of success and adversity. Competitiveness, sportsmanship, self-confidence, and resilience, in addition to exposure to and a respect for authority, are instilled. Sports also provide the opportunity for the testing of self, peer comparison, and healthy competition, which helps to facilitate the development of positive, realistic self-esteem, self-concept, and mental toughness [4,17,22–24].

Youth sports can also provide a healthy outlet for energy and expression, and are potentially rewarding in multiple domains. They encourage socialization, social competence, and family bonding, and facilitate the development of friendships and peer respect beyond narrow demographics and across racial and ethnic groups. In addition to promoting individual physical and psychological growth and lifelong healthy behavioral patterns, there is also exposure to unique future adult career choices.

A child's sometimes fragile sense of positive self-esteem and belonging is often reinforced by adults. Children's perceived levels of accomplishments and self-efficacy are evidenced by self statements such as "I am a tennis player," or "I am bad at math." Participation in sports can have a therapeutic effect on self-efficacy for fragile, emotionally disturbed, and developmentally disabled youngsters, not unlike the benefits seen with exercise in postinfarct adult patients. Peer, parental, teacher, and community support promote a belief in oneself. Encouraging sport participation can help children to optimize their capabilities across many domains [20].

In 1992 Kapp-Simon and colleagues [25] looked at self-perception, social skills, overall adjustment, and social inhibition in 10 to 16 year olds who had craniofacial anomalies. The best predictors of emotional adjustment were social skills and athletic competence. This further supports the idea that the psychiatrists should not only take a careful athletic and sporting history as a part of the normal evaluation, but should encourage athletic participation as part of any multimodal treatment approach.

In addition, children believed they were more socially accepted when their parents felt they had better sporting skills. Brook and Heim [26] evaluated 16 asthmatic children whose participation in sports, in comparison with nonparticipation, led to improved self-image, less anxiety, and improved coping with their chronic illness. It is noteworthy and often inspirational that every illness seems to have its own successful role model in sports. Swimmer Amy Van Dykens has asthma, baseball player Jim Eisenreich has Tourette's syndrome, and hall of fame jockey Julie Krone has post-traumatic stress disorder. Children and adolescents who have psychiatric disorders, for example, ADHD, Tourette's syndrome, learning disorders, and mood disorders, similarly often benefit greatly from athletic participation. For those youngsters who have impaired social skills, difficulty modulating behavior, affect, anxiety, or impulse control, or problems with coordination, individual sports such as martial arts [15,22] provide structure and a sense of accomplishment and success. These are all critically important factors in the development of physical well-being, self-esteem, and psychological growth.

The Special Olympics has allowed handicapped children who are so impaired mentally and physically that they cannot participate in the usual competitive leagues to also experience feelings of mastery, healthy competition, and a sense of community. This competitive involvement within the larger society enables members of the disabled population to optimize their physical and psychological development and coping skills [27].

Most recently Jacobs Lehman and coworkers [16] assessed the link between organized sports involvement during high school and sexual behavior and health among 176 adolescent women, and demonstrated that involvement in organized team sports was positively correlated with improved sexual reproductive health, sexual/reproductive health-seeking behavior and, perhaps most importantly, negatively correlated with sexual risk-taking behavior itself. The authors posited that changing the traditional female cultural script was central to this beneficial effect of sports involvement, because participation in sports promoted self-reliance over traditional passivity, and moving beyond dependence on looks and attention from boys for self-worth. They used the cultural resource theory to assess functional body orientation and levels of self-empowerment, efficacy, and assertiveness [28].

### Risks of Sports Participation

The athletic experience, as beneficial as it may be, can prove equally devastating under some circumstances. Repeated failures; criticism; poor role models; negative peer interactions, including ostracism; and overambitious internal and external pressures to perform are all risk factors for the development of psychological disability and low self-esteem. Care must be taken to find a fulfilling place in sports and physical recreation for the "athletically challenged" child. Inappropriate expectations for success of parents, coaches, and teammates can all negatively affect an individual's functioning. This not only impairs a child's ability to reach his or her potential, but promotes behaviors detrimental to the athlete's physical and psychological well-being. These behaviors can border on exploitation, and even potentially abusive behaviors, described as the "achievement by proxy distortion (ABPD)" spectrum of behaviors in sports [29]. See the article on that topic by Tofler and Knapp elsewhere in this issue for more information.

The seductive fantasy of stardom causes many adults to lose sight of reality, and to emphasize sports to the detriment of other important developmental activities. The unfortunate reality for most is that only an extremely small percentage of involved children will ever compete athletically at the elite or professional level.

Economically and culturally deprived inner-city youth have seen sports as their passport to the American dream of financial and social success. The drive to achieve this dream often supports a sole focus on one's sport, leaving little time for education, socialization, and the development of other necessary life skills. This presents the risk for a distorted, unidimensional development [4,30].

When the careers of athletes of any social class are terminated, be it by natural attrition, injury, or not being chosen for the exponentially more difficult next tier, these athletes must contend with a major life change. Without their sport, they often feel ill-equipped to function in and contribute to adult society. The closure of an intense athletic career is often fraught with adjustment-related depression, identity difficulties, and an unrealistic sense of failure and lack of purpose. Well-rounded education and preparation for these inevitable transitions is critical to all athletes. Most young athletes are unaware of or resistant to the message of how few persons actually become successful professional or elite amateur athletes [31–34].

Of every 2300 high school senior basketball players, only 40 will play college basketball, and only 1 will play in the National Basketball Association (NBA). Fewer than 4% of varsity high school football players play college football, and fewer than 1% of college players are offered a professional contract. Even for those who are talented enough and fortunate enough to play at the professional level, careers are typically short-lived. The average active tenure in the National Football League (NFL) is 3.2 years, yet one must be in the NFL for 4.5 years (3 seasons after 1992) to qualify for a pension, and be 55 years old to draw on it. Unfortunately, the average career of a professional football player is only 5.4 years [35]. In the United States, 2 million children and adolescents participate in competitive gymnastics per year, and only 7 or 8 participate in the Olympic Games every 4 years. These findings illustrate why we have an obligation to attempt to ensure that even children who have superior athletic talent have a well-rounded developmental experience. No matter how much they achieve in sports, they must be fully prepared for life [17,18].

## THE EFFECTS OF SPORTING PARTICIPATION ON SELF-CONCEPT

Self-concept is multifaceted, and is shaped by one's internal and external experiences throughout development. Primary to this development of a sense of self through self-regulation, or ontogenesis, is early reciprocal stable attachment in the first months and years of life. Self-esteem is enhanced by a sense of accomplishment, a sense of belonging, and a perceived sense of normality; that is, being able to perform and achieve like one's peers. Athletic participation allows people to not only experience social interaction and group membership, but also to experience varying degrees of success and achievement [16,18,20,22,36–38].

According to Coopersmith [37] and others, successful mastering of developmental milestones and skills fosters both positive self-esteem and self-concept. Normally developing children and adolescents are able to use positive and negative feedback from peers, adults, and role models to define themselves, their abilities, competencies, self-worth, and sense of their own limitations. The most powerful influences for a developing child's self-esteem are the relationships formed during interactive experiences with one's family, school, and extracurricular activities.

## ADVERSE PSYCHOPHYSIOLOGICAL AND SOMATOFORM EFFECTS OF SPORTS

Some youngsters are involved in their sport almost to the exclusion of all else. This potentially eliminates some crucial developmental experiences and exacerbates social isolation. Spartan training may breed an adaptive resilience to other life demands; however, this pressured existence is also often traumatic. Young children and adolescents may work out 4 to 6 hours daily, travel without their families, and have a coach regulate their activities in a surrogate parental role. These children may have compromised social, school, and family contact.

Excessive stress, the anxiety-provoking pressure from coaches, parents, and athletes themselves associated with suboptimal performance, and injuries that limit participation all have a potential role in the genesis of dysthymic disorder, depression, chronic fatigue, substance abuse, conversion, and eating disorders [17,18,33,39–48].

The desire, conscious or unconscious, of young athletes to avoid the stress and trauma of competition or intense participation may be sometimes evident in attempts to malinger, or to engage in purposeful , partially purposeful, or even unconscious psychosomatic, conversion-related, self-injury [32,49].

Finally, overtraining can lead to medical and emotional problems, sometimes called burnout, staleness, or overtraining syndrome. The burnout syndrome can be defined as "the sequelae of working too hard, under too much pressure for too long, coincident with progressive loss of idealism, energy and purpose" [50]. The physical and psychological markers of this syndrome may mimic and overlap with other medical and psychiatric disorders. Many proficient athletes leave their sports before reaching their potential because of this burnout. Overtraining is the primary cause of chronic fatigue and depression in both high school and college athletes [51].

Stress can manifest in athletes in a plethora of ways. It can present as weakness, pain, or injury, with or without any clear physiological etiology. Pain and injury can be an acceptable way for a young athlete to quit, decrease or evade expectations, or escape high-pressured competition without loss of pride or honor to either self or highly motivated parent or mentor. An injured teammate can still be a valued part of the team [32,52].

As cited in Stryer's review [17], Marks and Goldberg evaluated 25 athletes who presented to them for a second opinion regarding severe, incapacitating pain subsequent to orthopedic injuries, which are usually self-limited and minimally distressing. All were diagnosed by family practitioners, pediatricians, or orthopedists as having relatively minor or common orthopedic problems that are usually self-limited. Intensive medical and imaging workups confirmed the original somatoform diagnosis, as well as an adjustment disorder with disproportionate pain unconsciously motivated by the need to escape the pressure associated with sporting involvement.

Micheli (L. Micheli, personal communication, 1996) and others [52,53] have reported seeing more than 100 cases of reflex sympathetic dystrophy in children and adolescents between 1982 and 1995. This is an abnormal response of the sympathetic nervous system to a minor trauma in which the athlete develops severe, recurrent, chronic pain affecting an entire extremity, accompanied by autonomic nervous system changes and subsequent bone, skin, and soft tissue dystrophic changes. This condition, rarely documented in children, is notable for its presence in a population of children and adolescents intensively involved in athletic training and stressful competition, generally in individual sports [32,52,53]. Dvonch and coworkers [49] reported five cases of conversion reaction in response to the stress of athletic competition.

In the area of risk, safety, and lifestyle, Nattiv and Puffer [54] compared college athletes with age-matched peers. Behaviors compared included alcohol use, driving under the influence of drugs and alcohol; getting into a car with an impaired driver; nonuse of seat belts in cars, nonuse of helmets on bikes, mopeds, or motorcycles; nonuse of contraception; and increased number of sexual partners and sexually transmitted diseases. Thus, college athletes, primarily male, tend to have a significantly higher proportion of risky lifestyle behaviors, perhaps peer-pressure related.

## INTERACTIONAL AND SYSTEMIC CONTRIBUTION TO POTENTIAL ADVERSE PHYSICAL AND PSYCHOLOGICAL SYMPTOMS
### Parents as Both Role Models and Active Stress Inducers

"My dad really never paid much attention to me … . We didn't talk that much … . All those quotes, those now famous sayings—I had to read them or hear them on TV." What hurt Vince Lombardi Jr was his dad's disinterest in the sport as far as his son was concerned. "My freshman year in high school, he had his friend take me to my first practice … . It really hurt at the time … . He'd tear you down to build you up" [55].

A 12-year-old girl was offered the decision by her parents to make to move her family to a different state so she could pursue her gymnastics career. She chose not to, perhaps sensing their ambivalence, and 10 years later, feels great regret at this decision, the "opportunity of a lifetime gone begging."

A 6-year-old struck out and his coach, trying to console him, tells him that Pete Rose, who had the most hits in all of baseball history, struck out more than 1000 times. The child said, "Yeah but Pete doesn't have to ride home with my dad" [17].

An organizer of a private youth soccer league says, "I used to have all the games be competitive and the parents sometimes would actually fight each other, and of course they would always be yelling at the referees and mad at their kids. Now we don't keep score, everyone has a good time, everyone gets a trophy and some of the parents complain it's not competitive enough … but there are no fights any more and the parents seem to be nicer to the kids, the coaches and each other as well."

The drive to be outstanding, high achieving, and successful, and perhaps a revisionist backlash against the self-esteem movement, is represented in the animated movie *The Incredibles*, when a character states that something is wrong with a society where being the best is no longer valued. "Let him compete, he would be great," says Mr. Incredible of his super-talented son Dash.

Parents are the primary role models for a child's development. Children internalize their attitudes and values—constructive, less adaptive, and even maladaptive ones. They thrive on and need the approval of nurturing parents with whom they can identify. This modeling of parental and other influential role figures is a good predictor of a child's behavior.

An athlete's attitudes, participation, enjoyment, values, beliefs, perception of achievement, expectations, and capabilities are all shaped and molded by the attitudes and behavior of parents and, to a lesser extent, coaches. Parents sometimes only acknowledge their children for their athletic achievements [29]. These not infrequent strategic choices place a child's athletic success above his or her psychological and physical health and needs. Some examples of this behavior include not encouraging one's child to rest when he or she is injured, holding a child back a year in school to give him or her a physical advantage in sports to enhance opportunities for college scholarships, and requesting surgical procedures or even hormonal interventions on healthy children in an effort to somehow improve their performance or appearance, or to artificially decrease or increase their growth or height [32,56,57]. In addition, parents may react with enraged hostility when child athletes make mistakes, or may want to change or discontinue their children's involvement in sports [29].

In such cases, a parent's self-worth and even financial well-being can become so dependent on the successes and failures of the child in sports that the pressure the parent places on the child becomes far and away his or her primary stressor. This vicarious living through the child is addressed elsewhere in this in this issue in the article by Tofler and Knapp on ABPD behavior.

## Coaches

Coaches also play a critical role in an athlete's development. Social behavior and self perception are both directly affected by the coach [3]. Most community-based coaches have no formal training. The training of school coaches remains variable at best. Typically, coaches have minimal knowledge of physiological and psychological development or healthy ways of instructing and motivating children, although some improvement in training has been occurring. Likewise, they may not possess the skills necessary for tactful communication and parent education about the complex developmental issues that arise in sport participation [12,21,39,41,58–60].

At the junior high school level and higher, the primary coaching style has tended to be one of high expectations for performance, with a decreasing emphasis on socially mature behavior, warmth, communication, and nurturance. This approach continues to be reinforced by "winners" [3]. Coaches who emphasize this verbally and sometimes physically tough punitive style favor the outcome over the process of sporting participation. They often use aversive motivational methods, and model inappropriate poor-sportsmanship behaviors to players, officials, parents, and spectators alike [17]. Like parents, ambitious coaches are vulnerable to ABPD pressures as they become increasingly unable to differentiate the needs and goals of their athletes from their own [29].

## Program Coordinators

Formal sports program are organized by adult program coordinators who may not always place the developmental needs of children and adolescents as their highest priority. The modeling after college and professional sports can foster goals of providing entertainment and financial profit, in addition to an emphasis on a winning outcome. Training the program coordinators may be just as important as training the coaching staff about the developmental aspects of child and youth sports. The recent book and film *Friday Night Lights* demonstrates both positive and negative aspects of all of these issues in abundance.

## A SOCIAL-HISTORICAL PERSPECTIVE ON SPORT IN THE UNITED STATES

### Social Roles of Sports

Throughout the last century, sports have provided an escape vehicle from poverty and the ghetto for some talented athletes; Pelé and Diego Maradona, the Brazilian and Argentine soccer stars, are good international examples. Pioneering such opportunities was the breakthrough of Jack Johnson, the audacious African-American world heavyweight boxing champion who reigned from 1908 to 1916. Immigrant Irish, Jewish, and Italian-American youths followed this path. Later, as racial barriers decreased after the Second World War, African-American and Latino athletes and audiences rose to prominence. The celebration of the 50th anniversary of Jackie Robinson's debut in major league baseball marked a significant American milestone.

Sport has always played a significant role in international politics and prestige. Hitler's pompously staged anti-Semitic and racism-charged 1936 Olympics is perhaps the best example. The black power salutes of 1968 made a huge impact in the United States. Olympic boycotts of the United States and the Union of Soviet Socialist Republics in the 1980s were a sporting stalemate. An extended sporting boycott played an important role in the disintegration of apartheid in South Africa. Government-controlled, medically supervised, systemic abuse of steroids by East German and more recently Chinese swimmers has given way to private sector performance enhancement drug use in the United States, in Olympic athletes and baseball players in particular. The re-emergence of Iran on the world stage with its 1998 World Cup soccer team playing the United States and the involvement of Palestine in the 2004 Olympics were diplomatic signals to the world.

Sport by its very nature easily transcends physical, cultural, socioeconomic, ethnic, gender, and racial boundaries. Several national organizations play prominent roles in extending this potential power of sport to improve society. The National Consortium for Academics in Sport (NCAS) [61], founded in 1985, is one of these. It now has over 220 affiliated tertiary institutions. NCAS athletes were able to work with almost a million at-risk young people, using sport participation to indirectly address issues such as drug and alcohol abuse, conflict resolution skills, violence against women, and racism. Student-athletes and coaches are in a unique and powerful position to positively impact the lives of our children [61].

### The Racial and Gender Report Card

The racial report card has been published annually since 1989 by R. Lapchick of the Northeastern University Center for the Study of Sport in Society and, more recently, at the University of Central Florida [18,62,63]. The initial goal of this report card was to raise awareness among professional sports organizations and, since 1998, in college sports where significant integration problems remain, particularly in the administrative front office and coaching opportunities on the playing field. The report card may prove valuable in progress in addressing these ongoing challenges. The release of this report occurred during the National Collegiate Athletic Association (NCAA) tournaments of 2005, and provided information on graduation rates of Division I basketball teams. Fifty-one percent of white male players have graduated, as compared with 59% of general white male college students; but only 38% of African-American players have graduated, as compared with 34% of general African-American college males [63].

Positional segregation or "stacking" remains an issue requiring close monitoring, particularly at the college level, despite generally enlightened leadership. Although approximately 90% of positions, including running back, wide receiver, cornerback, and safety, were held by African-Americans in the NFL, it is interesting that despite such an improvement, only 24% of quarterbacks and 17% of centers are African-American [62].

Similarly, in athletic positions such as pitching and catching that major league baseball managers have characterized as requiring "intelligence, quick thinking, and decision-making," the numbers of African-Americans were 3% and 1% respectively [62].

Latino players have made significant gains in major league baseball over the past decade, now accounting for 22% of pitchers, 37% of catchers, and 60% of shortstops [62]. The NBA continues to lead other sports in terms of greater player opportunities for African-Americans, with 79% of players being black. The NBA has instituted a plan for providing league-wide diversity workshops. The professional player associations have generally excellent records for providing equal opportunity in terms of both racial and gender diversity.

In the NBA, the percentage of white physicians was 98%, with the remaining 2% being Asian-American. Only 1% of all NFL physicians are African-American [62].

## THE INTERFACE BETWEEN SPORTS PSYCHIATRY AND SPORTS MEDICINE SPECIALISTS

Primary health care and sports medicine specialists are in an unique position to educate athletes, parents, and coaches regarding the benefits of healthy, safe, and balanced athletic participation. The preseason physical, which can sometimes be undertaken by a multidisciplinary team of sports physicians, offers a format and forum for parents and children to discuss general information about healthy participation in sports, including related mental health, substance abuse prevention, and stress management issues. Increased awareness and early identification of psychiatric disorders, such as ADHD, depression, eating disorders, substance abuse, and risk-taking behaviors, should be another goal of preseason physicals, which should include screening for treatable disorders as well as problematic parent-child and coach-child disorders. Referral to a psychiatrist who has interest and training in sport psychiatry could be helpful at this stage [18,64].

The psychiatrist also has an opportunity to be involved in this multidisciplinary health education process by promoting the well-known benefits of youth sports while helping to minimize and prevent its potential deleterious effects. At the same time, we can help the pediatricians and orthopedists screen for the warning signs of psychiatric disorders in order to promote early referral, diagnosis, and treatment. In the general practice of psychiatry, we should pay careful attention to the role of sports and physical exercise, as well as all other major developmental activities in our patient's lives.

Psychiatrists can play a useful role in the management of adjustment issues in athletes during rehabilitation after injury, and when medical recommendations involve no longer playing or retiring from a sport. These can be extremely stressful and traumatic passages for many athletes. The benefit of exercise as a treatment modality for depression remains a powerful intervention, and its value is noted by both the American Psychological and Psychiatric Associations [65].

Comorbid psychiatric illness can be treated in a sport-aware fashion with psychopharmacological interventions carefully tailored with knowledge of the specific needs and requirements of the patient within the rules related to medication use in a particular sport. The Olympic sports, for example, allow the antidepressant venlafaxine, but disallow bupropion (M. Larden, personal communication, 2005). Professionals should be vigilant for psychiatric illnesses that are associated with sporting participation, such as eating disorders (anorexia athletica) [56], performance enhancement-related substance abuse, and the systemic risks for ABPD [5,29,66]. Though rare, the potential for emotional, physical, and sexual abuse of vulnerable youth is high. The sport psychiatrist can contribute to performance enhancement of individual athletes working within a consultation liaison framework. At higher competitive levels, athletes should receive anticipatory counseling to prepare for the time when they will withdraw from participation because of natural attrition, injury, or other causes.

Sports participation in some form is readily available to most school-aged children. It can provide opportunities to communicate by "speaking the child's language" and to facilitate insight about a whole host of developmental concepts related to self-esteem, influences of role models, body image, autonomy, self-efficacy, leadership skills, and moral development. Psychiatrists are increasingly incorporating a sport component into their formal clinical evaluations. This can accomplished through the history and as part of individual assessment of actual play or social recreation. Presenting psychological and psychosomatic symptoms that may be related to sports participation or performance difficulties may often mask other significant mental health concerns. The psychotherapy framework can be integrated with sports participation and exploration of other significant developmental issues, starting from this relatively safe base. Serious performance problems may signal underlying psychological concerns. In addition to the customary comprehensive psychiatric history, a sport-focused developmental and family history should be undertaken for patients heavily involved with athletics. The issues listed in Box 1 should be focused upon in a psychiatric interview of a child athlete and his or her family [67].

## BOX 1: THE SPORT PSYCHIATRY INTERVIEW FOR CHILDREN, YOUTH AND YOUNG ADULTS

General Guidelines

1. The initial interview focuses on parameters of consultation, including fee, timing, general overview of identifying information, referral process, presenting difficulties, and confidentiality issues, with full psychiatric assessment. Subsequent interviews review history, collateral history if permission is obtained, and individual, family, and perhaps coach interviews, with the goal of developing an initial formulation with which to approach treatment.

2. Review general psychiatric assessment with focus on issues such as neurovegetative symptoms of mood disorder, any severe psychiatric or medical symptoms that may be sport-related, and refer for further assessment elsewhere as required.

3. Determine if there were any acute stressors at the time any symptoms may have started to appear.

4. Assess developmental readiness skills for sport in physical, neuropsychological, social, and moral domains with child and parents, interviewed separately. Coaches may also need to be interviewed separately.

Questions to the Child Athlete

1. What is your first sports memory?

2. How and when did you first participate in sports, and in the specific sport?

3. What or who led to your involvement in that sport?

4. Do you have a history of involvement in child-organized or spontaneous games?

5. Are you involved in more than one sport?

6. What is the relevance of sports to you and your family?

7. What are the needs, expectations, and ambitions for athletic achievement for you, your family, and coach? Example: is your parent's first question likely to be "did you win?" or "did you have fun?"

8. How does your family handle achievement and success by one child compared with other siblings or peers?

9. What is your relationship with your coach like?

10. What is the relationship between your parents and the coach like?

11. Does your consider your parents (rate each parent)

    Underinvolved?

    Moderately involved?

    Overinvolved?

12. Are you asked to work to help defray athletic expenses?

13. Do you have any role models in your sport?

14. How important are role models for you in your sport, and in what ways do you think they influence your life?

15. How much television do you watch each week, and how much of this is sport-related?

16. Do you have a major sporting role model who is regularly on television or in other media?

17. What is your sports participation schedule and how has it changed to date?

18. How many days and hours per week throughout the year do you practice?

19. When does the season begin and end?

20. Describe your school schedule, hours of unstructured time, how athletics involvement enhances or interferes with your other activities.

21. How do you feel about competition, practice schedules, coaches, and parental involvement?

22. How are family relationships, peer and age-appropriate relationships, and school performance impacted upon, either negatively or positively, by sport involvement?

23. Are you using, considering the use of, or being encouraged to use performance-enhancing substances, or expedient health endangering behaviors such as rapid weight loss, or fluid and food restrictions to achieve an advantage in your sport?

24. What are the attitudes of family members to these substances and techniques?

25. If the answer to question 23 is yes, are the other family members aware of this, and what has been their reaction? Do they try to influence you to discontinue use, to get you involved in counseling or therapy? Do they ignore or pretend not to know about any potential negative behavior.

26. What are the attitudes and practices of you and your family members to alcohol and drug use in general, as part of the "enjoyment" of the athletic process?

27. Have you been subjected to boundary violation, exploitation, or physical or sexual abuse by adults or peers within the context of your sporting activities?

28. If the answer to 27 is yes, are parents or other important adults aware of this, and what was their reaction and response to being informed?

29. What has been your comfort level with aggression since early childhood?

30. What was your level of aggression in sports when you were younger and what is it now?

31. Do you have a history of disordered behavior, including physical or sexual assault, promiscuity, or legal infractions such as curfew violation, truancy, shoplifting, substance possession, underage drinking, or drug dealing?

32. Is any of this disordered behavior focused on sporting or sporting spectator activities?

33. What are your social and peer relationships inside and outside the sporting arena?

34. Are you dating? Sexually active? if so, what form of birth control, if any, are you using?

35. How do you perceive your involvement in sport affecting your peer relations?

36. How you perceive your sporting involvement affecting your academic or life goal progress?

37. How do you perceive sporting involvement affecting your mood?

38. How do you feel about your own femininity or masculinity?

39. Is this sense of your gender or sexual identity affected by your sporting involvement?

40. What has been the high point of your life so far?

41. What has been the high point of your athletic life?

42. What has been the low point of your life so far?

43. What has been the low point of your athletic life?

44. Do you experience performance anxiety over tests or examinations in school?

45. Does this performance anxiety extend to the sporting situation?

46. Do you have any sleep-related symptoms, such as recurrent dreams, insomnia at any stage, or sport-related sleep difficulties?

47. If you have a medical or psychiatric condition, does it influence your athletic involvement and performance, or is it affected by your athletic involvement and performance?

48. Does medication you are taking for a medical or psychiatric condition (for example, asthma or ADHD) affect your performance in a positive or negative fashion?

49. Do you have any comorbid psychiatric illness in which the sporting involvement may directly impact the illness; for example, learning disability, ADHD, eating disorder, or substance abuse ?

50. Do you have any specific performance-related issues?

51. Do you have any symptoms of pain, or chronic injuries impairing performance, and how are these being managed?

52. How do you cope with stress?

53. Do you have a history of:

    "Choking"?

    Slumps?

    Conflicts with teammates?

    Conflicts with coaches?

54. Do you have any transitional adjustment issues such as planning on quitting or recently quitting a sport because of medical, psychiatric, injury, academic, or sporting performance reasons (for example, "being cut" or lack of interest)?

55. If you are "high profile" as an athlete, how do you manage your fame?

Parents often have a different perspective on all the children's questions as well, so all of the questions above can also be reviewed with the parents in separate interviews.

Questions to the Parents (Each Parent Should Respond)

1. Do you consider the child

   Underinvolved?

   Moderately involved?

   Overinvolved?

2. What are the athlete's and family's levels of involvement in the sport; for example, as spectators, coaches, referees?

3. How do you model behavior for your children within your specific roles; for example, as spectators when your child's team loses?

4. What is the sporting participation of family members, currently and previously?

5. What do each of you do for fun and relaxation?

6. Is the child using, considering use of, or being encouraged to use performance-enhancing substances, or expedient health-threatening behaviors such as rapid weight loss, or fluid and food restrictions, to achieve an advantage in his or her chosen field?

7. What are the attitudes of family members to these substances and techniques?

8. If the answer to question 6 is positive, are the other family members aware of this, and what has been their reaction? For example, do they attempt to influence the child to discontinue use; attempt to get the child involved in counseling or therapy; provide support or "plausible deniability" with attempts to ignore any potential negative behavior?

9. What are the attitudes and practices of the child and family members to alcohol and drug use in general, as part of the "enjoyment" of the athletic process?

10. Are you aware of our child having been subjected to boundary violation, exploitation, or physical or sexual abuse by adults or peers within the context of his or her sporting activities?

11. If the answer to 10 is yes, what was the reaction and response of you and other important adults to being informed?

Questions to Coaches

1. How do you rate the child's and each parent's level of involvement in the sport?

   Child:

   Underinvolved?

   Moderately involved?

   Overinvolved?

Mother:

    Underinvolved?

    Moderately involved?

    Overinvolved?

Father:

    Underinvolved?

    Moderately involved?

    Overinvolved?

2. Do you believe the child is using, considering use of, or being encouraged to use performance-enhancing substances, or expedient health threatening behaviors such as rapid weight loss, or fluid and food restrictions, to achieve an advantage in his or her chosen field?

3. What are your attitudes and those of your coaching staff to these substances and techniques?

4. If the answer to question 19 is positive, are the coaching staff aware of this, and what has been their reaction? Are you attempting to influence the child to discontinue use, attempting to get the child involved in counseling or therapy, or providing supportive or "plausible deniability," with attempts to ignore any potential negative behavior?

5. What are the attitudes and practices of you and your coaching staff to alcohol and drug use in general, as part of the "enjoyment" of the athletic process?

6. Has the child been subjected to boundary violation, exploitation, or physical or sexual abuse by adults or peers within the context of his or her sporting activities?

7. If the answer to 6 is yes, what were the reactions and responses of you, parents, and other important adults to being informed?

*Adapted from* Tofler IR, Katz Stryer B, Kamm R. The sport psychiatry interview for children, youth and young adults. In: Stryker BK, Tofler IR, Lapchick R, editors. A developmental overview of child and youth sports in society. Child Adolesc Psychiatr Clin N Am 1998. p. 697–725; with permission.

## SUMMARY AND FUTURE CHALLENGES

Sports participation plays an important role in the development of most young-sters, regardless of natural ability or level of athletic competition. At any level of participation, their sports experience can be rewarding and positive; however, their athletic experience may also negatively distort their psychological and physical development. Thus, we could, in the final analysis, perform a disservice to a child, even those who have superior sporting prowess, notwithstanding the outstanding success of "stars from conception" such as the Manning quarterback dynasty, the Williams sisters, and Tiger Woods [68].

We as a society should not lose sight of our children's and youths' needs to develop psychological resilience and confidence, accompanied by realistic positive self-esteem based on emotional and physical health; and we should allow them to meet the challenges of adult life. Competition and its attendant stresses are integral to development in our modern lifestyle. This exposure to, and developmental mastery of, competitive stress can contribute to the primary goals of youth sports, which should be to have fun while building developmental motor, social, and emotional competence, and enhancing social or team relationships. Long-term positive health and educational behaviors resulting from participation in sports may include minimizing adolescent problems such as delinquency, school dropout, substance abuse, and teen pregnancy. Providing positive, developmentally appropriate legal and coaching guidelines for youth athletes as well as safeguarding youth protection against exploitation and abuse are priorities.

Psychiatrists have become more active in the new field of sport psychiatry. By working with sports medicine specialists, we have the professional opportunity to advocate and promote greater understanding of the developing emotional, social, and physical worlds of the child, adolescent, and young adult.

## References

[1] Olshansky SJ, Passaro DJ, Hershaw RC, et al. A potential decline in life expectancy in the united states in the 21st century. NEJM 2005;352:1138–45.

[2] Children in youth sports in the United States. USA Today June 18, 1997;section 3C.

[3] Weiss MR, Bredemeier BJ. Moral development in sport. Exerc Sport Sci Rev 1990;18:331–77.

[4] Malina R. The young athlete: biological growth and maturation in a biosocial context. In: Smoll F, Smith R, editors. Children and youth in sports: a biosocial perspective. Dubuque (IA): Brown and Benchmark; 1996. p. 161–86.

[5] Tofler IR, Katz Stryer B, Micheli L, et al. Letters to the editor re: Physical and emotional problems of elite female gymnasts. N Engl J Med 1997;336(2):140–1.

[6] Ryan J. Little girls in pretty boxes: the making and breaking of elite gymnasts and figure skaters. New York: Doubleday; 1995.

[7] Nicholls JG. Achievement motivation: conceptions of ability, subjective experience, task choice and performance. Psychol Rev 1984;91:328–46.

[8] Colby A, Kohlberg L, Gibbs J, et al. A longitudinal study of moral judgement. Monogr Soc Res Child Dev 1983;48(200):1–96.

[9] Bandura A. Social learning theory. Englewood Cliffs (NJ): Prentice-Hall; 1977.

[10] Rest JR. The major components of morality. In: Kurtines W, Gewirtz J, editors. Morality, moral behavior, and moral development. New York: Wiley; 1984. p. 356–429.

[11] Shields DL, Bredemeier BJ. Character development and physical activity. Champaign (IL): Human Kinetics; 1995.

[12] Smith RE, Zane NWS, Smoll FL, et al. Behavioral assessment in youth sports: coaching behaviors and children's attitudes. Med Sci Sports Exerc 1983;15(3):208–14.

[13] Ogilvie BC, Tutko TA. Sport: if you want to build character, try something else. Psychol Today 1971;5:60–3.

[14] Hastad DN, Segrave JO, Pangrazi R, et al. Youth sport participation and deviant behavior. Sociol Sport J 1984;1:366–73.

[15] Trulson ME. Martial arts training: a novel "cure" for juvenile delinquency. Hum Relat 1986; 39:1131–40.

[16] Jacobs Lehman S, Silverberg Koerner S. Adolescent women's sports involvement and sexual behavior/health: a process-level investigation. J Youth Adolesc 2004;33:443–55.

[17] Stryer BK, Katz S, Cantwell D. Youth sports and adolescent development. In: Noshpitz J, editor. Handbook of child and adolescent psychiatry. Adolescence: development and syndromes, vol. 3. New York: Wiley; 1997. p. 209–24.

[18] Stryer BK, Tofler IR, Lapchick R. A developmental overview of child and youth sports in society. Child Adolesc Psychiatr Clin N Am 1998;7:697–724.

[19] Kimm SYS, Glynn NW, Kriska AM, et al. Decline in physical activity in black girls and white girls during adolescence. NEJM 2002;347:709–15.

[20] Steptoe A, Butler N. Sports participation and emotional wellbeing in adolescents. University of London; City University, London. Lancet 1996;347:1789–92.

[21] Seefeldt V. Coaching certification: an essential step for the revival of a faltering profession. Journal of Physical Education, Recreation & Dance 1992;63:29–30.

[22] Bell C, Suggs H. Using sports to strengthen resiliency in children: training heart. Child Adolesc Psychiatr Clin N Am 1998;7:859–96.

[23] Magill RA, Ash MJ, Smoll FC, editors. Children in sport. 2nd editon. Champaign (IL): Human Kinetics; 1982.

[24] Weiss MR. Psychological effects of intensive sport participation on children and youth: self-esteem and motivation. In: Cahill BR, Pearl AJ, editors. Intensive participation in children's sports. Champaign (IL): Human Kinetics; 1993. p. 39–70.

[25] Kapp-Simon KA, Simon DJ, Kristovich S. Self-perception, social skills, adjustment and inhibition in young adolescents with craniofacial anomalies. Cleft Palate Craniofac J 1992;29(4):352–6.

[26] Brook U, Heim M. A pilot study to investigate whether sport influences psychological parameters in personality of asthmatic children. Fam Pract 1991;8(3):213–5.

[27] Super JT, Block JR. Self-concept and need for achievement of men with physical disabilities. Journal of General Psychology 1992;119(1):73–80.

[28] Miller K, Sabo D, Farrell M, et al. Sports, sexual behavior, contraception use, and pregnancy among female and male high school students: testing cultural resource theory. Sociol Sport J 1999;16:366–87.

[29] Tofler IR, Knapp P, Drell M. The "achievement by proxy" spectrum: historical perspective and clinical approach to pressured and high achieving children and adolescents. Child Adolesc Psychiatr Clin N Am 1998;7:803–20.

[30] Engel G. The need for a new medical model: a challenge for biomedicine. Science 1977; 196.129 06.

[31] Gould D, Feltz D, Horn T, et al. Reasons for attrition in competitive youth swimming. Journal of Sport Behavior 1982;5:155–65.

[32] Nash HL. Elite child athletes: how much does victory cost? Phys Sportsmed 1987;15(8): 129–33.

[33] Scanlan TK, Passer MW. Factors influencing the competitive performance expectancies of young female athletes. Journal of Sport Psychology 1979;1:212–20.

[34] Taylor A. Chrysler hoop dreams challenge. Boston: Center for the Study of Sport in Society, Northeastern University; 1994.

[35] Poole D. Pension issue should at least be examined. Charlotte Observer August 5, 2005.

[36] Bradley E. Survey: sports foster racial unity. USA Today November 9, 1993.

[37] Coopersmith S. The antecedents of self-esteem. San Francisco (CA): W.H. Freemen; 1967.

[38] Smoll FL, Smith RE. Leadership behaviors in sport: a theoretical model and research paradigm. J Appl Soc Psychol 1989;19:1522–51.

[39] Barnett NP, Smoll FL, Smith RE. Effects of enhancing coach-athlete relationships on youth sport attrition. The Sport Psychologist 1992;6:111–27.

[40] Feigley D. Psychological burnout in high level athletes. Phys Sportsmed 1984;12(10): 109–19.

[41] Horn TS. Coaches' feedback and changes in children's perceptions of their physical competence. J Educ Psychol 1985;77:174–86.

[42] Passer MW. Fear of failure, fear of evaluation, perceived competence and self-esteem in competitive trait anxious children. Journal of Sport Psychology 1983;5:172–88.

[43] Poinsett A. Barriers to participation in youth sports. The role of organized sport in the education and health of American children and youth. Carnegie Corporation Meeting. 3.18.1996. p. 21.

[44] Robinson T, Carron A. Personal and situational factors associated with dropping out versus maintaining participation in competitive sport. Journal Sport Psychology 1982;4:364–78.

[45] Ruibal S. Looking for a sharper edge. USA Today June 18, 1997;section 3C.
[46] Scanlan TK, Lewthwaite R. Social aspects of competition for male youth sport participants. IV. Predictor of enjoyment. Journal of Sport Psychology 1986;8:25–35.
[47] Scanlan TK, Passer MW. Factors related to competitive stress among male youth sport participants. Med Sci Sports 1978;10(2):103–8.
[48] Simon JA, Martens R. Children's anxiety in sport and nonsport evaluative activities. Journal of Sport Psychology 1979;1:100–69.
[49] Dvonch VM, Bunch WH, Sigler AH. Conversion reactions in pediatric athletes. J Pediatr Orthop 1991;11:770–2.
[50] Maslach C. Understanding burnout: definitional issues in analyzing a complex phenomenon. In: Paine WS, editor. Job stress and burnout: research, theory, and intervention perspectives. Beverly Hills (CA): Sage; 1982. p. 29–40.
[51] Lidstone JE, Amundson ML, Amundson LH. Depression and chronic fatigue in the high school student and athlete. Prim Care 1991;18(2):283–96.
[52] Pillemer FG, Micheli LJ. Psychological consideration in youth sports. Clin Sports Med 1988;7(3):679–89.
[53] Fermaglick DR. Reflex sympathetic dystrophy in children. Pediatrics 1977;60(6):881–3.
[54] Nattiv A, Puffer J. Lifestyles and health risks of collegiate athletes. J Fam Pract 1991;33(6): 585–90.
[55] Horovitz B. In the name of the father. USA Today January 28, 1997; section 4C.
[56] Nattiv A, Agostini R, Drinkwater B, et al. The female athlete triad: the interrelatedness of disordered eating, amenorrhea, and osteoporosis. Clin Sports Med 1994;13(2):405–18.
[57] Theintz GE, Howard H, Weiss U, et al. Evidence for a reduction of growth potential in adolescent female gymnasts. J Pediatr 1996;122:306–13.
[58] Gould D. Intensive sport participation and the prepubescent athlete. Competitive stress and burnout. In: Cahill BR, Pearl AJ, editors. Intensive participation in children's sports. Champaign (IL): Human Kinetics; 1993. p. 19–38.
[59] McPherson B, Marteniuk R, Tihany J, et al. The social system of age group swimmers: the perception of swimmers, parents and coaches. Can J Appl Sport Sci 1980;4:142–5.
[60] Smith RE, Smoll FL, Curtis B. Coaches effectiveness training: a cognitive-behavioral approach to enhancing relationship skill in youth sport coaches. Journal of Sport Psychology 1979;1:59–75.
[61] National Consortium for Academics in Sport (NCAS). 2002–2003 annual report. Available at: http://ncasports.org/2003-04%/20Annual%20Report/50502.htm. Accessed August 11, 2005.
[62] Lapchick RE. 2003 racial and gender report card. Northeastern University Center for the Study of Sport in Society; University of Central Florida. Available at: http://www.bus.ucf. edu/sport/public/downloads/media/ides/release_05.pdf. Accessed August 11, 2005.
[63] University of Central Florida. De Vos Sport Business Management. Available at: http://www.bus.ucf.edu/sport/cgi-bin/site/sitew.cgi?page=/index.htx. Accessed August 11, 2005.
[64] Rosen LW, Hough DO. Pathogenic weight control behaviors of female college gymnasts. Phys Sportsmed 1988;16(9):140–6.
[65] Dunn AL, Trivedi MH, Kampert JB, et al. Exercise treatment for depression: efficacy and dose response. American Journal of Preventive Medicine 2005;1–8.
[66] Tofler IR, Katz Stryer B, Micheli L, et al. Physical and emotional problems of elite female gymnasts. N Engl J Med 1996;335(4):281–3.
[67] Katz Stryer B, Tofler IR, Lapchick RA. A developmental overview of child and youth sports in society. Child Adolesc Psychiatr Clin N Am 1998;7:697–724.
[68] Woods E, McDaniel P. Training a tiger. New York: Harper Collins; 1997.

Clin Sports Med 24 (2005) 805–828

# CLINICS IN SPORTS MEDICINE

ELSEVIER
SAUNDERS

# Achievement by Proxy Distortion in Sports: A Distorted Mentoring of High-Achieving Youth. Historical Perspectives and Clinical Intervention with Children, Adolescents, and their Families

Ian R. Tofler, MB, BS[a],*, Penelope Krener Knapp, MD[b], Michael Larden, MD[c]

[a]Charles R. Drew University of Medicine and Science/University of California, Los Angeles, 1731 East 120th Street, Los Angeles, CA 90059, USA
[b]Department of Psychiatry, University of California, Davis, 2230 Stockton Boulevard, Sacramento, CA 95817, USA
[c]Department of Psychiatry, School of Medicine, University of California, Alvarado Parkway Institute, 399 Camino Elevado, Bonito, CA 92103, USA

Pediatricians, psychologists, and child psychiatrists have long been aware of the dangers of child abuse. There has been a tendency to expect neglect and abuse among lower socioeconomic groups, although children, adolescents, and even adults in any demographic group are potentially at risk [1–4] (Table 1).

In regarding children who have talent and promise, health professionals, including sports medicine physicians, have had a blind spot to possible emotional neglect, physical abuse, and the potential harm of "by proxy" ambitions.

In the last 2 decades, pressures on high-achieving children in sports and other forms of artistic and academic endeavor have been recognized [1,5–16]. This special population is at significant potential risk for a broad range of neglect, boundary violation, and potential abuse in the push to achieve extraordinary success. Sports medicine physicians may be the first to recognize situations in which parents have gone beyond normal ambition for their child's success. They may play a major role in protecting children from the reciprocal pressures of athletic organizations, which may influence and be influenced by coaches and parents to pressure children in ways that are pathogenic and even frankly abusive.

* Corresponding author. E-mail address: robertoff@aol.com (I.R. Tofler).

0278-5919/05/$ – see front matter
doi:10.1016/j.csm.2005.06.007

**Table 1**
Stabilization/re-equilibration for ABPD families

|  | Normal, healthy pattern | Danger signals | Therapeutic indicators for positive change |
|---|---|---|---|
| Child development | Parents are sensitive to child's stages, provide opportunities that are challenging but not impossible or unfair. | ABPD parents see child as an economic asset or as an impaired adult who needs to be forced to work harder. | Child's interests are foremost. Parents can describe child's reactions and empathize with child's point of view. |
| Parent-child relationship | Mutually responsive, joyful, appreciative of each other's strengths and challenges. | ABPD parents can be exploitative, domineering, critical, nonreciprocal, abusive, etc. | Parents can visualize and anticipate the effects of their own actions on the child and vice-versa. |
| Balance of child's role within family system | Child's needs are considered in relationship to those of siblings, both parents. | Other family members' needs subordinated to the goal of training child and enrolling him in competitive situations. | Input of other siblings and both parents are taken into account. The parents can both articulate this input, and seek compromise. |
| Balance of family within community | Community experiences enhance positive parenting. Parents can support child's efforts in school or sporting context. Model, ensure child sees and experiences mutually respectful interactions with other adults and children. | Family is isolated, adversarial, migratory, financially struggling, and dependent on child's potential career, performance. | Parents appreciate and encourage the contributions and involvement of spouse, other adults, and other children in the child's life. |

The extraordinary achievements by child stars attract breathless tabloid headlines and television specials. What actually, we wonder, are the requisite developmental hurdles in producing a 4-year-old golfing prodigy, a 6-year-old beauty queen, a 7-year-old pilot, a 12-year-old movie actor, a 14-year-old Olympic gold medalist gymnast, a 15-year-old champion ice hockey player, a 16-year-old Rachmaninoff virtuoso, or an 18-year-old National Basketball Association (NBA) phenom? Voyeuristic publicity invites the inevitable questions: why can't our own children be like the star?, and should any child be like this?

Talented, driven children and their driven parents may excite and engender open or grudging admiration, wonder, or envy. They may stimulate others to competitively emulate their child-rearing examples. They may also evoke some appropriate concerns and caveats about the methods used to foster and market these precocious talents. Were risks taken and corners cut in the development of those skills, actions that have jeopardized these children? Should the physician evaluate morbidity and mortality risks? Or is this infringement on a subgroup of parents a paternalistic imposition of medical opinion upon their constitution-ally protected child-rearing practices [17–19]?

Are parents who push their children to excel in sports any different from those who push children to excel academically? The recent shooting of a coach by a disgruntled, frustrated parent or the beating death with a baseball bat of a Pony League player by a friend do seem to suggest otherwise [20,21].

This article describes a typology of high-achieving children and their parents, and formulates a multidimensional response to these questions. First the authors present a brief historical view of childhood and of the development of psychiatric approaches to the problems encountered by talented children. Second, we hope to enhance understanding of the risks for talented children caused by adult distortions of perception and parenting, at the individual, family, systemic, and societal levels. These adult behavioral patterns may in fact be integral to the process of developing talented, successful children. The authors have chosen to use a psychiatric model, with the behaviors understood within a construct similar to the *Diagnostic and Statistical Manual of Mental Disorders, 4th edition* (DSMIV) [22] diagnosis of "factitious disorder by proxy." Parental behavior ranges from normal to achievement by proxy distortion (ABPD), a distorted, potentially pathogenic behavioral zone, the extreme of which is frank, reportable abuse [13,15,16,23].

Third, the authors seek to broaden understanding of the dynamic, inter-active process between children, both normal and gifted, with their equally talented, ambitious parents and mentors that enables them to achieve such degrees of success in sports at such an early age.

Finally, we review possible responses, interventions, and management ap-proaches that psychiatrists, sports medicine physicians, pediatricians, social workers and others interested in promoting the child's welfare may use to address the ABP concerns of highly pressured, high-achieving children and adolescents. It should be emphasized that with all their nurturing and support, they remain, from a psychosocial, if not a biological perspective, a paradoxically underprotected group.

## AN EVOLUTIONARY HISTORICAL PERSPECTIVE

The fields of evolutionary psychology, genetics, and anthropology evaluate behavior within the context of at least 2 million years of hominid evolution. They represent complex human behavior as phenotypically similar to other traits [24–27]. A seemingly cruel pattern of exploitative behavior may actually conceal an evolutionary, adaptive form of "chromosomal empathy" for the future offspring [28]. Dawkins has moved beyond kin preference and reciprocal altruism in his book *The Selfish Gene* [24]. He coined the term "meme"( derived from the Latin root for imitation) to describe culturally beneficial, altruistic propagation of ideas, including those related to achievement for our children [24]. Our much more recently derived moral, religious, and ethical imperatives appear to stand in dramatic contradistinction with our cutthroat biological, psychological, and behavioral evolutionary past.

Six thousand years of recorded human history confirms a somewhat dismal role for childhood. Children have been generally of inferior status, essentially property and raw material belonging to their parents or their parents' masters. They were objects to be sacrificed and circumcised, goods to be bartered, slaves for work and sex, and fetishes to be venerated or discarded. This form of objectification was normative behavior from the lowest to the highest level [29–31]. Monotheistic moral and ethical tradition traces now-outlawed child sacrifice back some 4000 years, with Abraham's divinely aborted sacrifice of Isaac [32]. The killing of infants, generally female, not necessarily as a form of sacrifice, but rather as a crude form of "fourth-trimester abortion," continues routinely in China, India, and to a lesser degree all over the world, including the United States, where infanticide has actually increased over the past 30 years [33,34]. This also reflects an evolutionary gender differential preference, with the perceived advantages and greater economic importance attached to male offspring still being a prime factor.

It was not until 1842 [31] that child labor was outlawed in British mines. Building on pioneering 1924 League of Nations support for the international rights of the child, the United Nations developed edicts on child labor laws in 1973. These were revamped in 2002 by the International Labor Organization (ILO), but remain essentially unenforceable in most countries, with 210 million children worldwide working full time. Controversy over the last decade regarding American dependence on imports using exploitive child labor by Nike, Disney, and Kathy Lee Gifford has also highlighted this issue [35].

Overall then, despite dramatic increases in freedom, particularly in Western countries, the child has remained an instrument for the implementation of parental agendas, often for economic reasons, within an approving social context. In the United States, the fourteenth amendment due process clause essentially gives parents carte blanche as far as their child's upbringing is concerned [17,36,37]. Inculcating the parental religious, educational, nationalistic, cultural, or sporting imperatives continues to be an inalienable right.

Children have long been regarded as offering a second chance to achieve lifelong dreams and unfulfilled parental goals. An early Biblical example replete with ABP spectrum behavior is the story of the infertile Hannah praying in the temple to have a child. She bargains with God that if she is blessed with a male child, that his, the future prophet Samuel's, entire life would be devoted to the higher cause of God, in effect repaying Hannah's debt [38].

The Greek Olympics began according to tradition in 776 BCE in Greece as an amalgam of religion, war, sacrifice, sex, death, and celebration [39,40]. The association of the athlete as a glorified and objectified warrior consolidated the Homeric agonistic ideal, still held today. that there is no second place on the battlefield. This "victory or death" motto (often "victory and death") summed up Phidippides' first marathon run and is still venerated today. When given a hypothetical challenge by G. Mirkin in a 1983 questionnaire, 80% of top US athletes would have taken a magic pill that would assure them of Olympic gold but cause their death within 1 year [41]. It should come as no surprise or coincidence that such powerful and seductive beliefs are often inculcated in our children.

Is there anything wrong with this? Implementation of parental agendas and goals opens the door for possible exploitation and abuse at many levels and degrees. That these abuses can occur in the name of love, support, or altruistic parenting, is at the very least ironic. When, one might ask, is a "good enough child," to invert a Winnicott concept about parenting [42], simply not good enough for hard-driving parents?

## PRIOR PSYCHOLOGICAL AND PSYCHIATRIC RESEARCH

Since Freud, psychiatrists have been cognizant of the risks of projection of adult goals onto unborn and young children [43–45]. At the time of our birth we may be invested with all the pluripotential properties of a bone-marrow stem cell, but our limitations, defects, and total dependence, as well as our potentials, are never more obvious than at that moment [46].

Motivation theory delineated "the need to achieve"–the normal range of behaviors that propel humans and their offspring to succeed at the highest levels. Beginning with Hull's drive theory based on habits strengthened by positive reinforcement, there are multiple approaches. Murray developed a classification in 1938 that was further refined by Atkinson, in which among 20 basic human needs he described the needs to accomplish something difficult; to master, manipulate or organize physical objects, human beings or ideas; to achieve this as rapidly and independently as possible; to overcome obstacles and to attain and aspire to a high standard; to excel one's self; to rival and surpass others; and to increase self regard by the successful exercise of talent. Reiss and Havercamp [47] developed a useful standardized measure of 15 core motivational traits that have been used to explore athleticism and sports motivation. They found athleticism to be significantly associated with motivational traits for social contact, family life, physical exercise, competition/vengeance, and power/achievement, as well as with low curiosity levels [36,47].

Further developing the ideas inherent in Lewin's resultant valence theory, Thibault and Kelly presented a differential satisfaction/dissatisfaction comparison level between parents and their children. They evaluated changes in the "need to achieve" to be ambitious or aspire to success, defining a "neutral point," which may vary over time during development. McLelland developed this idea in discussion of early independence training and growth of achievement motivation. A gender bias, described by Horner, toward male achievement has traditionally been associated with a mirror image–a concurrent female need to underachieve, not to achieve, or to fear success that has changed significantly in some but not all societies over the past century. Cloninger discusses differential responses to harm avoidance, reward dependence, and novelty seeking, among other genetically influenced traits that can affect drive for success and are associated with involvement in risk-taking extreme sports such as rock climbing that require high novelty-seeking and low harm-avoidance. Motivational approaches to achievement may differ among groups of people, different cultures, and indeed entire countries. These differences, not surprisingly, affect responses and results in areas as disparate as geopolitics, economics, financial success, education, and of course national and international sports achievement and success [48].

Murray Bowen [49], psychiatrist and family therapist coined the term "family projection" to describe the spoken and unspoken goals and roles assigned by families, that affect an individuals' ability to "differentiate" as an adult.

The Swiss psychologist Alice Miller, drawing from sources such as self psychologist Heinz Kohut, pediatrician/analyst D.W. Winnicott, and analyst Margaret Mahler, further developed understanding of this important dilemma in child rearing, which she described as "the drama of the gifted child" [50]. According to Miller, the most appropriate objects for narcissistic gratification are a parent's own children. She stated that "from the very first day onward, he [the newborn baby] will muster all his resources to this end, like a small plant that turns towards the sun to survive" [50]. The intuitive understanding, reciprocity, and attachment a child has for his parents and what he can do to please them is central to these ideas. She states that "in spite of excellent performance, the [specially gifted] child's own true self cannot develop" [50].

This conditional love that objectified, highly successful children, the products of "poisonous pedagogy," can experience often comes at a high price—the very authenticity of that individual.

Miller's many books since have used famous case examples to further develop her ideas, particularly those about early abuse, pathogenic parenting, and its effects on the developed high-achieving adult [50].

Meadow [51] included "Victa Ludorum by proxy" in more recent discussions on variations of Munchausen's syndrome by proxy in the pediatric literature. This reference to the academic prize of excellence rewarded at British schools reflected his concern that ambitious parents could potentially damage their children by overstressing or pushing them toward apparently laudable goals.

## THE DEVELOPMENTAL TASKS OF RELATIONSHIP BETWEEN HIGH-ACHIEVING CHILDREN AND THEIR ADULT CAREGIVERS

Children do not develop in a vacuum, whether they are normal or talented and gifted. Their development is a highly interactive process between child, adult, and adult systems. Trainable, genetically able, talented, and resilient children have sufficient "right stuff" of suitable temperament, the right body habitus, psychological malleability, and obedience to excel. In the twenty-first century gender remains a major cultural variable in international parental attitudes, reflecting a bias toward a perceived need for higher male achievement. Marsh and colleagues [52–54] have elucidated the "big fish, little pond" and

**BOX 1: HIGH POTENTIAL FOR ACHIEVEMENT BY PROXY DISTORTION: SYSTEMS INVOLVEMENT FOR ASPIRING PROFESSIONAL CHILD GOLFERS**

Child

1. The child has a clear ability for golf, nurtured from a very early age by ambitious parents.
2. Golf aptitude is developed by strenuous daily practicing for 2–10 hours per day (up to 70 hours per week!).
3. Psychological "toughening up" for resiliency under pressure
4. Social isolation and sacrifice, delayed gratification for normal psychosocial development—a large part of the early training for junior professional golfers
5. Unidimensional identity if isolated from school and peers. Home schooling can be potentially problematic.
6. Stressful relationships with parents and less talented siblings in which the child's performance and level of success are clear factors in a realistic sense of "contingent" love
7. "Contingent Love" is a good model for later opportunistic "fair weather" relationships when on adult tour. "I don't know who to trust" is a normal reaction to involvement with professional friends, family, sponsors, and agents.
8. The young professional golfer can begin to objectify and distance from himself as well. Like his parents, entourage, and the larger systems, he may begin to view and accept himself as a commodity or product.

Family

1. Reciprocal positive, noncontingent support from parents and siblings for emotional and attachment needs is ideal.
2. Financial support for the child's career may be upwards of $100,000 per year.
3. Parents may depend on their child's financial contract for their own lavish lifestyle and support. Role reversal and diffuse boundary situations can be dangerous.
4. Parents can take on roles of both the child's entourage and larger systems to save money or provide a shortcut to success. Father may continue to be primary golfing coach, personal trainer, and tutor combined.
5. A business relationship with the child rather than a parent–child relationship is possible and often problematic; it may lead to later "divorce."
6. Parents may want to keep confidential information about the child from their agent, a "part owner" with the parents of the child. For example, psychological or physical injuries such as overuse injuries (eg, stress fractures) can be deliberately ignored. Parents may medicate the child without medical supervision for performance enhancement and other purposes.

Entourage

1. Personal trainer/coach: spends most of the time with the child; a highly influential paid "friend."

2. Agent: a very powerful influence, often in surrogate parent position, with sometimes an even greater influence than parents, because parents have in effect "outsourced" the child's ownership to the agency.

3. Tutors/academic trainers: important but peripheral. No teaching qualifications are necessary, and academics are not considered important to the child's development.

4. Travel agent: very important when traveling on a "shoestring" in early career.

5. Social relationships: fellow golfers primarily; initially peers, friends and competitors. When the child joins the tour, friends and adult competitors are now business rivals, with varying degrees of social isolation possible for the young golfer.

6. Performance enhancing "guru," sports "psychologist": unlikely to protect the child's confidentiality; tend to use name recognition for advertising purposes.

Larger Systems

1. Golfing schools: for example, a Florida golf academy where "good isn't good enough" is the motto. Minimum age for enrollment is 8.

2. US Children's Golf Association; American Junior Golf

3. Swing and stroke coaches/teachers

4. Agencies: owners of schools, therefore running professional player development "nurseries," controlling the flow and shaping the education and values of juniors funneling into the tour. They run their own tournaments.

5. Tour/qualification school: no age limit at this stage.

6. College/National Collegiate Athletic Association (NCAA) golf circuit: involves scholarships from high school level. Also involves "delayed gratification" in terms of temporarily delayed access to large contracts from the professional tour. Allows for more normal adolescent social development and access to higher education and degrees, with potential careers outside of or after golf, peer relationships—buffers against the unidimensional identity quality of the professional child.

7. Multinational companies and other sponsors: golf equipment (eg, Calloway, Rossignol, Telem, Nike); have their own career-long demands.

8. Advertising agencies: in conjunction with agents. Goal is to "build a brand product," whether through lifestyle or sexuality, particularly for teenage females, but also "cool" males. Tend to create a "false self," about which the young golfers are often ambivalent.

9. Media: special deals with TV companies through an agency may promote the young player by pairing with contracted "stars" from the same agency, for example. Importance of "marketable personality"

and advertising brand clear here as well. Enhance objectification of the youngster.

10. Medical systems: internist, orthopedist, psychologist, psychiatrist, hospitals and health maintenance organizations (HMOs). Rarely work in concert to enhance the child's overall physical and psychological development, and may have their own agendas to promote.

"reflected glory" effects. Their research addresses the sense of relative achievement, self concept in different cultural environments, through different frames of reference. Children and their families often realize that their abilities are not quite as great as they initially believed; for example, when a child moves to a school for gifted children and realizes he is now only average or even below average in a more challenging context.

To excel, optimal interaction with experienced, ambitious, inspirational, and charismatic adults keenly adept at interfacing with the systems is critical. That interaction may focus training and develop the child's skills to a sufficiently high level to achieve success. The child and his adult mentors combine their talents in a relationship that, given opportunity, luck, and other intangibles, culminates when that potential is brought to fruition, rendering the talent a career-worthy, marketable commodity. The relationships that occur in the sport of junior golf, detailed in Box 1, provide an excellent illustration of how multiple individuals and systems may interact in the process of producing a champion (Fig. 1) [14–16,55,56].

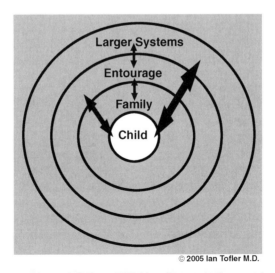

© 2005 Ian Tofler M.D.

**Fig. 1.** Systems involvement for aspiring child golfers and other "professional" children.

## ACHIEVEMENT BY PROXY DISTORTION AND FACTITIOUS DISORDER BY PROXY

There is an evolutionary adaptive element with widespread social and cultural acceptance and sanction for highly focused and sometimes distorted, even abusive, parenting behaviors described in this article. By selecting the term APBD [13–15], the authors have placed them within the range of behaviors known as the psychopathology of everyday life. Factitious and factitious by proxy disorders [22] from the psychiatric nosology of DSMIV, and *Diagnostic and Statistical Manual IV Text Revision* (DSMIVTR) have also been employed as models for describing these behaviors.

In 1977, English pediatrician Roy Meadow [10] noted that highly engageable, intelligent, and apparently caring mothers could induce illness and even death in their children while themselves seeking to be nurtured in the sick role by proxy. This nurturance was often of a systemic nature, the result of the care and support of doctors, nurses, social workers, support staff, and even the institution itself, which provided a form of support and identification [18]. Meadow placed this behavior within "the hinterland of child abuse" [10], which he called "Munchausen's syndrome by proxy," named factitious by proxy (FBP) disorder in psychiatry nomenclature [22].

Meadow [51] and Schreier [57] affirmed that "it was expected that professionals other than doctors would be involved." Jones [58] opposed this diagnostic broadening, suggesting that to include a wider umbrella of diagnoses and interactions beyond DSMIV criteria that "external incentives for a behavior such as economic gain are absent" would dilute any meaning from the diagnosis [22,58].

It remains difficult to ever be sure of the internal motivation of a person. Attention-seeking behaviors or financial gain at the expense of the child's normal developmental needs may be just as potentially pathogenic. Externally motivated behaviors, those of a by-proxy sense of achievement and other collateral benefits such as fame, are also present in accepted cases of FBP [22,38,57]. These incentives may not be the primary motivation, but they may still be vital and significant factors in the pathogenesis and perpetuation of FBP cases.

This model explains interfamily social processes and motivations leading adults to place their children in potentially risky, even dangerous and abusive, situations. Parents, teams, sports, and even Olympic committees may use children to pursue "a higher goal" such as national or Olympic-level sports promotion, entertainment, or the arts. Consideration for short- and long-term potential consequences to the child may be lacking. For example, the Australian government paid 32 million dollars per gold medal in the recent Athens Olympics, a price well worth it to the population of that country, judging by the lack of negative reaction [59].

Just as parents' response to their child's physical illness may range from normally supportive and help-seeking, through anxious doctor shopping, to the creation of factitious illness, so may parents' encouragement of their children's achievements range from normal support to overzealous pressure. The authors describe this continuum below, delineating the normal supportive range, defining the disorder, and clarifying the four levels of ABPD.

## NORMAL SUPPORTIVE RANGE OF ACHIEVEMENT BY PROXY BEHAVIOR

Normal supportive range of achievement by proxy behavior refers to adult pride and satisfaction experienced in supporting a child's development while also nurturing that child's abilities, special talents, and performances.

Although the parents and family may benefit financially and socially from their child's success, these are not the primary goals; rather, they are collateral benefits of more general altruistic behavior. The individuality of the child or adolescent is acknowledged, and the involved adults have the ability to distinguish the child's needs and goals from their own. Normal adult pride in a child's performance includes parents sharing the triumph of a child scoring a goal in a youth soccer game despite the team's loss, with which they are able to empathize on both an individual and team level. Sometimes a parent may insist that a child decrease or even quit an activity cherished by both, if the overall impact is deleterious to that child's developmental progress. Good parents should be able to monitor their own reactions, and to differentiate their own from their child's goals. A child must never feel that the love of her parents is contingent on success in one field or endeavor, be it an educational, sporting, career, or social goal.

A community's pride in their children's success is illustrated in the 1991 book *Friday Night Lights* [60], later a film, which vividly portrays reactions of highly ambitious families in the small Texan town of Odessa. Adult behaviors both in the normal range and in severely distorted and pathogenic ranges of ABPD are also depicted in *Hoop Dreams* [61], the book and later the superb documentary by the director of *Friday Night Lights* that follows two teenage basketball players in the inner-city Chicago Cabrini Green housing project as they pursue their National Basketball Association (NBA) dream.

The normal range of parent support for children's success also includes an element of "normal sacrifice." Parents want to and are expected to make reasonable sacrifices in their attempts to provide opportunities for their children. Children, in turn, are expected to behave in a responsible fashion, striving for success at the highest manageable level that they are capable of. This does not imply giving carte blanche to adults to place inappropriate and unacceptable pressures endangering their youngsters' physical or mental health to achieve success in any area.

## MAINTENANCE OF SUPPORTIVE ACHIEVEMENT BY PROXY BEHAVIOR IN FAMILIES: ACHIEVEMENT BY PROXY DISTORTION—DEFINITION AND SPECTRUM DESCRIPTION

ABPD can be defined as occurring when a child is placed, with his collusion, volitional or otherwise, in a potentially exploitative situation in order for a perpetrating adult or adult system to gratify conscious and unconscious adult needs and ambitions for the attainment of certain goals or achievements.

ABPD could be considered as pathogenic and potentially problematic parenting. Much of this behavior lies in a "gray zone"; however, at its most severe, when unacceptable physical or psychological harm is inflicted, it can be a variant of child abuse [1,13–15]. Children are intentionally placed in situations in which they must focus on a single activity to the exclusion of all others. In such cases, most or all other childhood activities may be subordinated to goals such as attaining sporting, entertainment, music, or educational success. The goal may be pursued to the detriment of the child's physical and psychological well-being, and may put overall developmental progress at risk.

The adult's vicarious experience of the child's success may gratify a desire to derive collateral benefits from that success. These benefits may be manifold and may parallel the child's clear benefits. They include fame, financial gain, career advancement, peer recognition and respect, stronger relationships with the child, social acceptance, and improved socioeconomic status. The vicarious success may benefit an individual adult, a system, a company, or a local or national entity. Just as in FBP, a role reversal occurs in which the child nurtures the adult. Thus the adult's vicarious achievement of success hints at an underlying dynamic motivation for ABP: the adult gets the child to provide emotional and sometimes economic nurturance [37].

The authors describe five stages of ABP. The first stage falls within the normal range of ABP behavior. The next four stages progress through potentially pathogenic range of ABP distortion. There may of course be significant overlap between normal ABP behavior and all ABP distortion components. The general trend, however, is from benign to abusive.

## Risky Sacrifice

Risky sacrifice is a mild loss of an adult's ability to differentiate his own needs for success and achievement from a child's developmental needs and goals.

At this level of behavior, a family or a system may construct conditions for a child or adolescent whereby there is increasing pressure, of a subtle but easily comprehended nature, that the child must "perform." Parents may take a second or even a third job to support a child's career. Families may move closer to a gym or training facility, or may allow a 13-year-old to make the decision to travel to a different state to live at a training facility, or even to be adopted into the custody of a coach. Plausibly deniable rationalizations that may be emotionally compelling become major conscious and unconscious defensive strategies at this stage. Parents may appear helpless and even passive with comments such as "I want my child to train less, but she loves it. If she insists on training 8 hours a day, 6 days a week, how can I say no? I love my child." Children and adolescents collude with their parents and coaches goals, as shown by comments of encouraged pseudoautonomy such as, "It is my decision to play injured; no one forces me to." When the child gets injured, neither the parent nor the coach need feel responsible. An adult's and particularly a parent's role to protect the safety of the child may be abrogated. The level of sacrifice demanded from a child surpasses defensible, safe levels.

Re-establishing normal parental autonomy—as for example when parents insist that a child miss practice to complete a school assignment—may produce unpleasant situations in which a respected, charismatic coach threatens to remove the child from his roster, saying "there are others who are more serious and may be more worthy." The sacrifice is now not only expected, it is demanded. To resist this external and internal pressure requires not only insight but also painful parental courage.

## Objectification

Objectification is the moderate loss of the ability of adults to differentiate their own needs and goals for success and achievement from those of the child.

At this stage, the child begins to become an object rather than a person. The intensity of the pressure on a child is further increased. With increasing social isolation, a child or adolescent becomes increasingly defined by one activity in which she is able to perform well, and begins to develop a "unidimensional identity" [15]. Excessive focus on the sport or other achievement necessarily isolates the child from social interactions, and potentially hinders her developmental possibilities, limiting many social, physical, and emotional experiences. Objectification of the child is associated with the adult caretakers' loss of the ability to distinguish their own needs and goals from those of the child [62].

This leads to rationalizing routine risk-taking, which also occurs in states of abusive neglect, such as when a mother severely burns her child to teach him that he should not play with matches. A child may be encouraged or even forced to train at levels that are potentially health-endangering. A young athlete may be advised to use pathogenic forms of weight control that may lead to life-endangering eating disorders. Parents, coaches, and sometimes entire systems, such as the media and governments, turn a blind eye to pathogenic behaviors or actively and passively encourage and support them.

To involved adults, the end justifies the means. Winning is the end, and the objectified child becomes the means. It is much more difficult to empathize with an adolescent's pain or experience once the youngster has become objectified. Emerging malleable, talented young entertainers, actors, musicians, and sports stars understand what is expected of them and may actively accept it. They may cope by emotionally distancing themselves from their own feelings, colluding in this objectification of themselves, a process resembling Anna Freud's concept of "identification with the aggressor" [63]. The 14-year-old gymnast who assumes full responsibility for training with a broken wrist, with the full knowledge of coach and parents, is a good example. The child prodigy's body and mind become, even to herself, machines to be driven and exploited in the pursuit of a "worthy" goal. "She can leave at any time" is a frequently heard statement from parents and coaches, echoing the claim of cult leaders, but not as obviously exploitative.

A recent Sports Illustrated article [64], quoting an agent closely involved with a family, exemplifies the rationalizing employed to justify this adult behavior: "I know how this looks. I know you are going to say that what is going on here is weird. People are going to say it looks bad, like I'm manipulating this kid. Like I'm trying to take advantage. But I'm not going to get a thing out of this. My only hope is that maybe, one day, when D is in the NBA, he can come back and sponsor my team. We'll call it the Demetrius Walker All-Stars. If he wants to do that, great. If not, that's fine. I'm doing everything that's right for the kid, and right now, what he wants, what I want, what his mom wants—we all want the same thing, and that's for D to succeed and grow and graduate and do all those things he is supposed to do."

## Potential Abuse

Potential abuse is a severe or complete loss of the ability of adults to differentiate their own needs and goals for success and achievement from those of the involved child.

At this level, the child is at risk of becoming chiefly an objectified and exploited instrument of the involved adult's goals. These goals are pursued without regard for short- and long-term potential physical and emotional morbidity or mortality in the child.

Adults, whether they be parents, mentors, coaches, or sponsors, may often appear to be perfectly attuned with the child—"She is my best friend"— but all the features of risky sacrifice and objectification may still be present. A child may become, in essence, an adult's meal ticket. If badly injured in practice, it is because "She is a daredevil" (conditioned from age 4 to ignore pain and to take risks). If injured representing her country, team doctors may have colluded with her competing with potentially catastrophic injuries. Here, the national team system is an important component of a potentially abusive process. The media and its spectators and consumers, ourselves, are also part of this cascade. If an adolescent boy is sexually abused by a guardian or coach, such as occurred recently in the Canadian junior hockey league, he may remain silent, fearing he will not be believed. If he reports the abuser, in all likelihood his future career will be terminated, his character besmirched as an ungrateful liar, and his emerging sexual identity questioned by others, and perhaps by himself as well.

## Distinct Abuse

The loss of ability to differentiate one's own adult needs from those of the child has led to damaging behaviors toward to the child that can be life-threatening or can cause severe lifelong emotional and physical scars for the child.

### Physical abuse

Performance-related results lead adults and sometimes other children to assault a child, or to encourage the child to take severe physical risks on a repeated

**Table 2**
Parental typologies in ABPD

| Parent type | Strengths | Motivation: positive/negative | Parent behavior: positive/negative | Parent-child relationships | Adaptation of child, not type-specific |
|---|---|---|---|---|---|
| Autocratic controller | Sets limits; offers discipline, guidance. | Shapes behavior/abuses, bullies | Structured/micro-manages, controls, dominates. | Dominating, critical. Child wishes to please, but never good enough | Dutiful, successful escape from parent for autonomy. |
| Narcissistic | High, usually external ideals and standards | Holds child to highest potential/parent, child self-esteem performance-contingent | Forces child to do things to make parent feel or look good. | Parental love contingent on child success. Child senses superficiality, emotional abandonment. | Estranged from parent. Role reversal: caring for needy parents. |
| Greedy | May seek financial benefits for self or the whole family. | Win-win situation/child objectified; business asset and investment. | Child develops a marketable skill/long Service to parental goal | Child is used and may be abused; may collude with abuse of self. | Child may feel guilt if insufficient success for family expectations. |
| Competitive | Consistent with US culture | Instills self belief in child for success/belittles child if unsuccessful. | Encourage resilience/ shames child if he loses. | Child feels driven to succeed to please parent, but loses validation of self if fails. | Child can embrace competitive pattern, avoid it, or actively seek failure. |
| Frustrated | Believes child can do better due to learning from own experience/ mistakes. | Higher chance of success/ parent's own thwarted early life ambition | May try to compete with child. Child pushed into areas of parent's interest. | Child experiences parent's frustration, but not pride in his own achievements. | Child distanced from own success or failure. Fighting another's battles. |
| Rationalizer (parent not actively perpetrating ABPD) | Peace-maker | Avoid conflict by passive collusion with partner. | Allows dangerous situation to perpetuate itself. | Child sacrificed by both parents; sense of loss. | Confused, angry at collusion; may join parent goals. |

basis to improve performance. This can also be demonstrated by tacit encouragement to use potentially risky performance-enhancement drugs.

*Emotional abuse*

Denigration, belittlement, and verbal abuse in the service of "toughening up" the child and motivating him may lead to the child's improved performance, but also to his increased dependence, his isolation from peers, his missing developmentally important experiences, and to his emotional constriction.

*Sexual abuse*

Sexual feelings may arise in the protracted and intense closeness of a training relationship. It is the mentor/coach's responsibility to contain and manage these feelings. If a mentor takes advantage of the power differential between himself and a young student, this constitutes sexual exploitation and is reportable. This power differential and the vulnerability of a child is most palpable when on the verge of success [1]. Inappropriate sexual relationships may occur over time, and may reflect a form of favoritism, and if terminated when a younger, more talented or more beautiful replacement is found, may lead to a subsequent loss of status for the victim.

Parents may be aware of physical, emotional, or sexual abuse by coaches or other mentors but allow it to continue because of the potential rewards of success.

Parents, coaches, mentors, teachers, and systems are all at risk of perpetrating distinct abuse.

Although it remains difficult to prove and prosecute this abuse, it is beyond dispute that this behavior occurs and is not uncommon (Table 2) (Fig. 2).

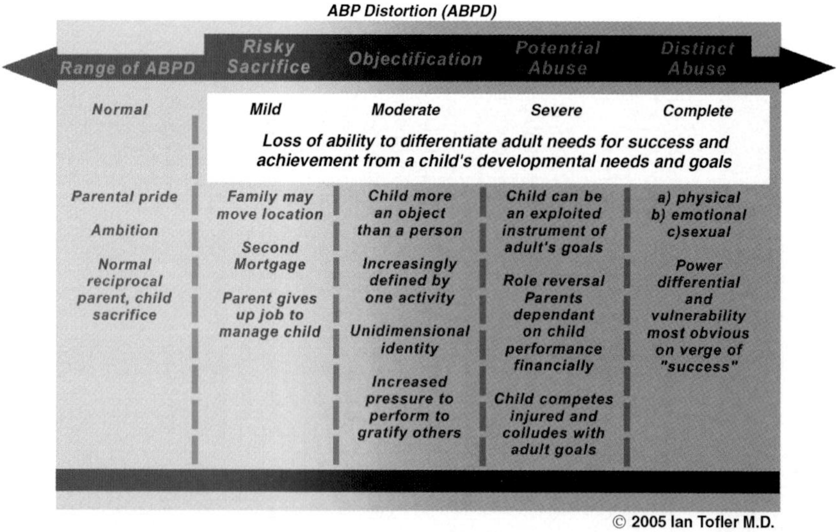

**ABP Distortion (ABPD)**

| Range of ABPD | Risky Sacrifice | Objectification | Potential Abuse | Distinct Abuse |
|---|---|---|---|---|
| Normal | Mild | Moderate | Severe | Complete |
| | Loss of ability to differentiate adult needs for success and achievement from a child's developmental needs and goals | | | |
| Parental pride | Family may move location | Child more an object than a person | Child can be an exploited instrument of adult's goals | a) physical b) emotional c) sexual |
| Ambition | Second Mortgage | Increasingly defined by one activity | Role reversal Parents dependant on child performance financially | Power differential and vulnerability most obvious on verge of "success" |
| Normal reciprocal parent, child sacrifice | Parent gives up job to manage child | Unidimensional identity | | |
| | | Increased pressure to perform to gratify others | Child competes injured and colludes with adult goals | |

© 2005 Ian Tofler M.D.

**Fig. 2.** The ABP distortion spectrum.

## PARENTAL TYPOLOGIES IN ACHIEVEMENT BY PROXY DISORDER
### Response to Achievement by Proxy Disorder: Management, Recommendations, and Interventions

A critical first step in the management of ABPD situations is to recognize the potential risks to professional children and adolescents in sports.

Psycho-education of parents, mentors, and coaches will refocus attention on the child's developmental needs, the importance of supportive adult relationships, and the motives of adults and children in a particular situation. Adults must be encouraged to frequently and honestly re-evaluate their own and other interested adults' goals, motives, and agendas in the professional development of a child.

### Recognize the "Red Flags" of Achievement by Proxy Disorder

Examples illustrating when adults are being overdirective and too goal-oriented with children include:

1. Parents making life decisions based on a child's activity; for example, selling their home and moving to another city, getting a second or third job so that their child can work full time as a gymnast, or removing the child from regular school.
2. Parents may allow the coach to make all decisions in their child's life. They may even suggest that the coach take custody of the child, so that the child can "live and breathe the sport."
3. The parents, the 13-year-old competitor, the coach, the orthopedic surgeon, and the team manager are all aware of an injury, but all agree that the decision to compete with a broken wrist is the child's to make.
4. The child develops psychosomatic illnesses from malingering: factitious, hypochondriac, conversion, and pain disorders that can help to consciously or unconsciously escape from or avoid training or competition. Psychiatric illnesses such as depression, anxiety, and substance abuse may also be unmasked by the stresses of competition.

Providing self-help tips to parents, educators, and coaches assists them to fulfill their obligations to children. It is necessary to recognize and respect the child's individuality and age-appropriate differentiation from the involved adult. This can be accomplished without denying outstanding children and adolescents the opportunity to succeed at any level. Some examples include:

1. Balancing career goals with developmental goals and requirements. If an adolescent takes a summer vacation with friends and family, and misses coaching or classes, this may go against both the child's wishes and the acting coach's orders. Being able to be a parent and to sometimes resist pressures from the child as well as internal ambitions and external professional pressures is an important skill. The ability to say "no" is a vital if disagreeable part of being a parent.
2. Parents must be able to objectively examine their own motivations for encouraging or pushing a child to develop a skill or talent. Help the parent to ask, "Am I doing this for my child or myself? If I am doing this a little for myself, where does my child fit into this equation?"

3. The parent or involved primary care physician must know when to consult with or refer to a psychiatrist or other therapist or counselor. Parents often need an outside specialist to help them better comprehend the "big picture." A more objective view of the child and other family members, including siblings, when the risks and benefits of a child's involvement in an activity are great can be very helpful. For example, when parents feels themselves trusting a charismatic coach over their own instincts, getting a second opinion is crucial.
4. Parents and physicians must learn to recognize risky rationalizations such as "plausible deniability."

## ROLE OF THE MENTAL HEALTH CONSULTANT

Using a flexible, developmental biological/psycho-social/systemic and cultural model, therapists may guide involved adults to support the progress of a child. Such a model allows for gauging developmental progress against an ethical or moral risk/benefit analysis of the child's involvement in professional activities such as acting or in sports training. It provides a context of the child's overall development from which to view possible developmental risks of over-specialization and social isolation from peers, as well as other physical and psychological morbidity. It assists in judging whether that child's continued involvement is justified by the trauma or illness induced in the service of a professional goal.

The mental health professional, whether a therapist for the child or family or a consultant to the coach or sports physician, must rapidly establish boundaries clarifying his primary role. The therapist must recognize and avoid the interference of personal ulterior motives or obligations that may interfere with protecting the child from abuse or unnecessary risk taking. If the client is a famous child or family, this be even more difficult. Only if the therapist can recognize such issues will he be able to avoid collusion with exploitive patterns. It is important to confront or detoxify rationalizations emanating from parents, governing bodies, or the children themselves that endanger children.

All parts of the system need to be aware that, as in the case of a suicidal adolescent, confidentiality is inappropriate when the child is at significant risk. Any abuse must be reported to appropriate authorities. The risks of systemic collusion by omission or of not communicating important information are greatest when the stakes are high.

An example is if a national gymnastics organization encourages, hides, or turns a blind eye to chronic injuries, eating disorders, analgesic abuse, or sexual or physical abuse of minors in the run-up to the Olympic Games. National pride and patriotism are invoked to justify any expediency. For a minor, to represent one's country seems to confer honorary adult status. But the minor is still a minor, and coaches and team physicians are responsible for protecting children from situations such as competing with a severe injury.

Because of the potential for exploitation and abuse, a rigorous history must be taken from the child and others involved in the situation. As in all mental health evaluations, history must be accompanied by a thorough mental status examination, and by indicated investigations such as physical and psychological testing, blood work, cardiac work-ups, and other physical, physiological, and radiological investigations. Toxic screens for substances abuse and use of performance enhancement drugs may be necessary. Forensic assessments may sometimes be required. Mandated reporting is required in situations when abuse is suspected. ABPD standardized interviews and risk/benefit scales can contribute to our understanding of these conditions.

The role of psychiatrist as physician advocating for the safety of children at all levels of endeavor in society includes advocating for high-achieving children and adolescents in sports.

Because of the potential risks for exploitation, there is a growing need for legal protection of the rights of professional children, and development of enforceable laws to limit hours of training. Removal of loopholes that suggest that these working professionals are "simply enjoying themselves and having fun" will be useful. Changes in the rules of Olympic competitions to eliminate dangerous routines and to minimize the unrealistic and health-risk–taking aesthetic demands of judging, and age limitations favoring, or at the very least not sabotaging, adult participation are examples of useful child psychiatric interventions at the general societal level, and have been presented elsewhere.

## VIGNETTE WITH SUGGESTED CLINICAL STRATEGIES

G.D., a 14-year-old Asian American female, is badly injured in a vaulting routine, sustaining spinal cord injuries at the C6–7 level. Father A.D., a 40-year-old professional soldier, has been instrumental in her involvement in gymnastics despite having no training himself, and was her first coach. It was his ambition initially that she become an Olympic gymnast.

Mother, M.D., a 39-year-old executive, is only minimally involved in her daughter's gymnastics. She seems to be somewhat absent during G.D.'s recovery. D.C., a 35-year-old coach, has been working with G.D. almost daily since age 8, and was her major role model, confidante, and "big sister," a mother figure traveling with her to all competitions. D.C. believed that G.D. would reach the elite level, and possibly the Olympic level. She attends all therapy sessions during the hospitalization, giving advice to staff members.

### Some Quotes

14-year-old: " I don't feel sorry for me, and I don't expect others to be either, I don't feel sorry for them [coach and family]."

Father: "Of course I was in shock at the beginning, but you've got to adapt … . I guess I was ready for something like this, having my mother in a wheelchair most of her life … you've got to adapt and adapt quickly. I am certain my daughter will improve and I won't be surprised if she returns to gymnastics at a competitive level. If not, she will be a success at whatever she puts her mind to."

Coach: "As soon as it happened I felt, and I know this sounds selfish, that this was the end of my chance to coach a champion. I was upset about the loss of her and my own future. It doesn't matter any more … all I care about now is will she be able to walk again, will she have a functional life? Everyone wants me back coaching, but I'm not ready yet. None of the other children have quit … ."

## Possible Therapeutic Strategies Illustrated by the Vignette

1. The importance of anticipatory case finding methods. In this case a psychiatrist had not been consulted beyond initial trauma issues, but was able to be of benefit in immediate and longer-term management. Establishing credibility within school systems and sports medicine facilities and with parents and teams can only occur over time.
2. Be flexible in providing therapy, including face-to-face, family involvement, and intermittent long distance telephone involvement.
3. Build on the child's and the family's strengths. Recognize adaptive "positive denial" strategies, as well as maladaptive coping strategies.
4. Do not prematurely interpret child or parental behaviors. This may result in the family fleeing therapy. In this vignette, the father's striving and goal directedness may actually facilitate this child's resilience during her long, slow, painful recovery toward a fuller physical life; however, his emotional distance and the pressure he places on her may limit her tolerance and ability to express her own affect. This may lead to masked and unrecognized psychopathology in both the short and long term, with potentially severe consequences, including major depression and suicide.
5. The importance of establishing rapport and alliances with all members of the extended family. This may include custodial and noncustodial parents, and a coach and even the coach's family in surrogate parental or family roles, after full permission has been obtained. If the child's biological parents refuse or are reluctant to engage in therapy themselves, the surrogate parent/coach may be the best person to work with for ongoing contact with the child or adolescent and the parents. It is crucial to include the adults who are closest to the child.
6. The child's injury is traumatic. Trauma should be anticipated and dealt with when it occurs. A parent or coach's reaction to the trauma of witnessing and supervising an athlete during a life-threatening and altering event cannot be minimized. Short- or long-term trauma-related psychotherapy may be helpful. The adult may be able to model her own fairly adaptive coping skills for this child recovering from and dealing with ongoing lifelong physical impairment.
7. Broadening the alliance with the child, parents, and coach. Being able to empathically approach the reasons a parent may be covertly or overtly creating extra and possibly unacceptable ABPD pressure on a child. In the vignette, both the father and the coach appear to be straddling the risky sacrifice and objectification levels of ABPD, with mother apparently less attached to the child in all respects.
8. Understanding the child, parents, and the coach's needs and goals is critical. To do this, the therapist must be able to deal with her own possibly negative judgments about the situation. Attempt to take each person's perspectives into

account. This may help the clients accept the existence of problems and to consider the benefits of psychotherapeutic intervention. Unfortunately, many individuals disparage the "weakness" of any involvement with psychosocial supports. If parents are covertly creating ABPD pressure, trying to empathize as much as possible with them helps them toward alternatives and different strategies to fulfill their own needs for the vicarious pride, success, and achievement currently funneled through their child.

## SUMMARY

When there is the possibility of reaping financial reward or other collateral advantage, children have historically been exposed to the risks of exploitation and abuse. There may be an evolutionary behavioral basis to the need to have children succeed and achieve, but "enlightened times" have not altered this social phenomenon. Primary prevention of this exploitation through outlawing the most flagrant abuses; secondary preventive strategies through minimizing risks; anticipatory guidance; and tertiary preventions including psycho-education will minimize the pathogenic dangers of ABPD.

The authors define ABPD as a condition that occurs when children are placed, with or without their collusion, in a potentially exploitive situation in order for a perpetrating adult or adult system to gratify their own needs and ambitions for the attainment of certain goals or achievements. We have provided definitions, descriptions and examples of four stages of ABPD behavior: (1) pathogenic risk/sacrifice, (2) pathogenic objectification, (3) potential abuse, and (4) distinct abuse. This typology will increase awareness of this phenomenon, especially in the practice of sports medicine. It should facilitate communication, enabling sports psychiatrists and other sports medicine professionals to identify the "red flags" that can lead to exploitation and potentially to abuse of children and adolescents in sports. It can further contribute toward psycho-education of ABP self-help skills, especially in the understanding of parental and other adult motivations; it can help young athletes in understanding their colluding roles for their behavior and risky rationalizations; and it can enhance prevention strategies.

References

[1] Brackenridge CH. Spoilsports. Understanding and preventing sexual exploitation in sport. London: Routledge; 2001. p. 116–7.
[2] Cicchetti D, Rogosch F. The toll of child maltreatment on the developing child. Insights from developmental psychopathology. Child Adolesc Psychiatr Clin N Am 1994;13:759–76.
[3] Kempe C, Silverman F, Steele B, et al. The battered child syndrome. JAMA 1962;181: 17–24.
[4] Radbill SX. Children in a world of violence: a history of child abuse. In: Kempe ME, Helfer RS, editors. The battered child. Chicago: University of Chicago Press; 1980. p. 3–20.
[5] Beamish R, Borowy JQ. What do you do for a living? I'm an athlete. Kingston (ON): The sports Research Group, Queen's University; 1988.
[6] Cantelon H. High performance sport and the child athlete: learning to labor. In: Ingham AG, Broom EF, editors. Career patterns and career contingencies in sport. Vancouver (Canada): University of British Columbia; 1981. p. 258–86.
[7] Donnelly P. Problems associated with youth involvement in high performance sports. In:

Cahill B, Pearl A, editors. Intensive participation in children's sports. Champaign (IL): American Orthopedic Society for Sports Medicine. Human Kinetics; 1993. p. 95–126.

[8] Elkind D. The hurried child, growing up too fast too soon. Reading (MA): Addison-Wesley; 1981.

[9] Ewing ME, Seefeldt VD, Brown TP. Role of organized sport in the education and health of American children and youth. New York: Carnegie Corporation Papers. Institute for the Study of Youth Sports, Michigan State University; 1996.

[10] Meadow R. Munchausen syndrome by proxy: the hinterland of child abuse. Lancet 1977; ii:343–5.

[11] Miller A. The drama of the gifted child. New York: Basic Books; 1981.

[12] Tofler IR. Parental and adult professional gain from exceptional children. In: Eminson M, Postlethwaite E, editors. Munchausen Syndrome by proxy, a practical approach. Woburn (MA): Elsevier; 2000. p. 215–30.

[13] Tofler IR, Stryer BK, Micheli LJ, et al. Physical and emotional problems of elite female gymnasts. N Engl J Med 1996;335:281–3.

[14] Tofler IR, Di Geronimo T. Keeping your kids out front without kicking them from behind. San Francisco: Jossey Bass; 2000.

[15] Tofler IR, Knapp PK, Drell MJ. The "achievement by proxy" spectrum in youth sports: historical perspective and clinical approach to pressured and high achieving children and adolescents. Child Adolesc Psychiatr Clin N Am 1998;7(4):803–20.

[16] Tofler IR, Knapp PK, Drell MJ. Clinical perspectives. The "achievement by proxy" spectrum: recognition and clinical response to pressured and high achieving children and adolescents. J Am Acad Child Adolesc Psychiatry 1999;38:213–6.

[17] Bell v City of Milwaukee, 746 F2d 1205: US Ct App (7th Cir WI 1984).

[18] Santosky v Kramer, 102 S.Ct 1388; 455 US, 745 (1982).

[19] Stanley v Illinois, 405 US 645, 652;92 S.Ct.1208 (1972).

[20] Boy convicted of murder in Palmdale baseball bat beating death. Associated Press July 8, 2005. Available at: http://sfgate.com/cgi-bin/article.cgi?file-/n/a/2005/07/08/ state/n143605D86.DTL. Accessed August 5, 2005.

[21] Falkenberg L. Texas man charged with shooting coach. Associated Press April 8, 2005. Available at: http://www.wjla.com/news/stories/0405/219314.html. Accessed August 5, 2005.

[22] Diagnostic and statistical manual of mental disorders. 4th edition. Washington, DC: APA; 1994.

[23] Tofler IR. Interview on "achievement by proxy". Penn State Sports Medicine Newsletter 1996;5(2):4.

[24] Dawkins R. The selfish gene. Oxford (UK): Oxford University Press; 1976.

[25] Hamilton W. The genetic evolution of social behavior. I, II. J Theor Biol 1964;7:7–52.

[26] Lancaster J, Lancaster C. The watershed: change in parental investment and family formation strategies in the course of human evolution. In: Lancaster J, Altmann J, Rossi AS, et al, editors. Parenting across the life span: biosocial dimensions. New York: Aldine de Gruyter; 1987. p. 187–205.

[27] Noonan KM. Evolution: a primer for psychologists. In: Crawford C, Smith M, Krebs D, editors. Sociobiology and psychology. Hillsdale (NJ): Erlbaum Associates; 1987. p. 31–60.

[28] Popenoe D. Life without father. New York: The Free Press; 1996. p. 166–7.

[29] Greenacre P. The fetish and the transitional object. Psychoanal Study Child 1969;24: 144–64.

[30] King RA, Noshpitz J, Joseph D. Pathways of growth: essentials of child psychiatry, vol. 2. Psychopathology. New York: Wiley; 1987.

[31] Kroll J, Bachrach B. Child care and child abuse in early medieval Europe. J Am Acad Child Adolesc Psychiatry 1986;25:562–8.

[32] Genesis 22:1–19.

[33] Bureau of Justice statistics. Available at: www.ojp.usdoj.gov/bjs/homicide/children.htm. Accessed August 4, 2005.

[34] US Department of Health and Human Services. Administration for Children and Families, Children's Bureau; 2003. National Clearinghouse on child abuse and neglect. Available at: http://cbexpress.acf.hhs.gov/index.cfm. Accessed August 4, 2005.

[35] BBC news. Exploitation of child labor by US labels. Available at: http://bbc.co.uk. Accessed August 5, 2005.

[36] Reiss S, Wiltz J, Sherman M. Trait motivational correlates of athleticism. Pers Individ Dif 2001;30:1139–45.

[37] Schreier H, Libow J. Hurting for love: Munchausen by proxy syndrome. The perversion of mothering. New York: Guilford Press; 1993.

[38] 1 Samuel 1:11.

[39] Finley MI, Pleket HW. The Olympic Games: the first thousand years. London: Chatto and Windus; 1976.

[40] Mathias MB. The competing demands of sport and health: an essay on the history of ethics in sports medicine. Clin Sports Med 2004;23:195–214.

[41] Ardell DB. Human growth hormone (HGH) and other Faustian promises of aging prevention. Available at: http://www.seekwellness.com/reports/2003-05-27.htm. Accessed August 5, 2005.

[42] Winnicott DW. Collected papers: through pediatrics to psycho-analysis. New York: Basic Books; 1958.

[43] Freud S. On narcissism: an introduction, vol. XIV.3. Standard edition, XIV. London: Hogarth Press; 1957.

[44] Freud S. 1917, mourning and melancholia, vol. XIV.4. Standard edition. London: Hogarth Press; 1957.

[45] Freud S. 1923, the ego and the id. Standard edition. London: Hogarth Press; 1987.

[46] Solnit A, Stark M. Mourning and the birth of a defective child. Psychoanal Study Child 1961;16:523–37.

[47] Reiss S, Havercamp SM. Toward a comprehensive assessment of fundamental motivation: factor structure of the Reiss profiles. Psychol Assess 1998;10:97–106.

[48] Weiner B. Human motivation, metaphors, theories and research. Newbury Park (CA): Sage Publications; 1992.

[49] Bowen M. Family therapy in clinical practice. New York: Jason Aronson; 1978.

[50] Miller A. For your own good: hidden cruelty in child rearing and the roots of violence. New York: Farrar, Strauss and Giroux; 1983.

[51] Meadow R. Arch Dis Child 1995;72(6):534–9.

[52] Marsh HW, Craven RG. The pivotal role of frames of reference in academic self-concept formation: the big fish little pond effect. Greenwich (CT): Information Age Publishing; 2002.

[53] Marsh HW, Kong CK, Hau KT. Longitudinal multilevel modeling of the big fish little pond effect on academic self concept. Counterbalancing social comparison and reflected glory effects in Hong Kong High schools. J Pers Soc Psychol 2000;78:337–49.

[54] Marsh HW, Hau KT. Big-fish-little pond effect on academic self concept. A cross cultural (26 country) test of the negative effects of academically selective schools. Am Psychol 2003;58:364–76.

[55] Elling S. Golf World. 1.26.2005. What price success? Available at: http://www.golfdigest.com/newsandtour/index.ssf?/gwmag/2005/0121/index.htm. Accessed August 5, 2005.

[56] Reilly R. Fear factor. Sports Illustrated January 24, 2005.

[57] Schreier H. Repeated false allegations of sexual abuse presenting to a sheriff. When is it Munchausen's syndrome by proxy? Child Abuse Neg 1996;20(10):985–91.

[58] Jones DPH. Commentary: Munchausen's syndrome by proxy: Is expansion justified? Child Abuse Neg 1996;20(10):983–4.

[59] Savulescu J, Foddy B, Clayton M. Why we should allow performance enhancing drugs in sports. Br J Sports Med 2004;38:666–70.

[60] Bissinger HG. Friday night lights: a town, a team and a dream. New York: Harper Collins; 1991.

[61] Joravsky B. Hoop dreams: a true story of hardship and triumph. New York: Harper Perennial; 1995.
[62] Eminson DM, Postlethwaite RJ. Factitious illness: recognition and management. Arch Dis Child 1992;67:1510–6.
[63] Freud A. Identification with the aggressor. Writings, vol. 2. 109–21.
[64] Lawrence A. Demetrius Walker. Sports Illustrated January 24, 2005;58–69.

Clin Sports Med 24 (2005) 829–843

# CLINICS IN SPORTS MEDICINE

ELSEVIER
SAUNDERS

# Attention Deficit/Hyperactivity Disorder and Psychopharmacologic Treatments in the Athlete

David O. Conant-Norville, MD[a],*, Ian R. Tofler, MB, BS[b]

[a]Division of Child and Adolescent Psychiatry, Oregon Health and Sciences University, 15050 SW Koll Parkway, Suite 2A, Beaverton, OR 97006, USA
[b]Charles R. Drew University of Medicine and Science/University of California, Los Angeles, 8835 Key Street, Los Angeles, CA 90035, USA

Attention deficit/hyperactivity disorder (ADHD) is a very common and chronic heterogeneous neuropsychiatric disorder affecting 8% to 10% of school-aged children [1] that often persists into adulthood [2]. The disorder has been defined diagnostically [3] and studied extensively. Using the phrase "review of ADHD," a search of the National Library of Medicine database reveals a total of 1617 articles on ADHD. In 1996, one literature review [4] noted 155 controlled treatment studies of ADHD that included 5768 children, adolescents, and adults. Research into ADHD has continued. ADHD is a common topic in the popular media. A meta-analysis of research in ADHD treatment with methylphenidate over 4 decades has demonstrated that despite differences in study design, subject selection, and methodology, findings have been very consistent regarding the successful treatment of core ADHD symptoms [5]. Despite the convergence of research results, ADHD and treatment interventions in special populations such as the elite athlete are not well-studied. Surprisingly, even the impact of ADHD on youth wishing to participate in sport is not specifically studied.

It is reasonable to conjecture that ADHD symptoms that adversely impact performance in academics, family functioning, social relationships, and vocational performance might also negatively affect athletic and sport performance and enjoyment; this is a complex issue that warrants further scientific inquiry. Children, adolescents, and adults participate in sport activities that are both organized and impromptu, and that are both team and individually oriented. With the increased national concern about an epidemic of obesity in the United States, barriers to participation in sport and exercise, such as common psychiatric disorders like ADHD, need to be better understood. This article approaches ADHD in sports by first providing a brief introduction to ADHD,

* Corresponding author. E-mail address: drdocn@hotmail.com (D.O. Conant-Norville).

0278-5919/05/$ – see front matter
doi:10.1016/j.csm.2005.05.007
sportsmed.theclinics.com

with a review of general clinical findings. The subject is then divided into sections pertaining to recreational youth sports and psychopharmacological treatment risks and benefits for the elite athlete.

## CHARACTERISTICS OF ATTENTION DEFICIT/HYPERACTIVITY DISORDER

ADHD is characterized by the inability to maintain attention span and focus concentration ability at a normal developmental level. In addition, symptoms of increased motor activity, restlessness, and lack of developmentally appropriate impulse control are often present. The current 4th edition of the *Diagnostic and Statistical Manual of Mental Disorders* [3] diagnostic criteria require that some of these symptoms must be observed before age 7, and that symptoms may evolve and change with age and developmental level. Symptoms are present in at least two or more settings, such as home, school, work, or social activities. Therefore, symptoms may also be observed during athletic endeavors and may affect sport participation. To make a diagnosis of ADHD, there needs to be clear clinical evidence of impairment in functioning, and yet these symptoms may not always be evident or noteworthy in every setting. Unlike most psychiatric disorders that are first described in adults and later observed in children and adolescents, ADHD is a disorder that was first identified in children, but is now observed to persist into adulthood. To diagnose ADHD, six of nine symptoms of inattention or six of nine symptoms of impulsivity/hyperactivity must be present and must have persisted for greater than 6 months. Inattentive symptoms include difficulty paying close attention to details or making careless mistakes in schoolwork or other activities, difficulty in sustaining attention in tasks or play activities, not seeming to listen when spoken to directly, not following through on instructions and failing to finish tasks (not clearly due to oppositional behavior or a failure to understand), difficulty organizing tasks, tendency to avoid and procrastinate, tendency to lose things necessary for tasks or activities, distractibility to extraneous stimuli, and poor time management and forgetfulness in daily activities. Hyperactive/impulsive symptoms include a tendency to fidget with hands and feet or squirm in seat; failure to remain seated when such behavior is expected; running and climbing excessively in situations where this is inappropriate (or feelings of restlessness in adolescents and adults); difficulty in engaging in leisure activities quietly; seeming as if "always on the go"; or talking excessively. Socially, symptoms may include a tendency to blurt out answers before questions are completed, difficulty waiting ones turn, and interruptions and disruptions in social interactions [3].

The diagnosis of ADHD is still made by clinical history and direct observation in multiple settings. There are no consistent or pathognomonic psychological tests, computerized continuous performance tests, or brain imaging studies that can make a diagnosis of ADHD [1]. Persons who have ADHD often have difficulty with either initiating or completing tasks, or with activities that they find boring or nonengaging. On the other hand, they may do very well in activities that they find interesting and positively reinforcing. For example, a child who may struggle with paying attention to a science teacher in a classroom may easily maintain focus on a video game for long periods of time. The interactive nature, structure, and positive reinforcement of the video game, as well as the constant need for vigilance in identifying changes, seem to capture the child's interest and keep the child's attention span. At times, ADHD does not seem to be a diagnosis of lack of attention, but more specifically a diagnosis of "too much attention to novel situations." Oftentimes these children are seen as disruptive and impatient by adults, especially when they are in a group and not being dealt with individually. Frequently, a diagnosis of ADHD is found to co-occur with other psychiatric disorders, such as disruptive behavioral disorders, anxiety disorders, depressive disorders, psychotic disorders, pervasive developmental disorders, substance abuse disorders, and learning disorders [6].

The identification of symptoms is often made in the school classroom, where the child is demonstrating either academic or behavioral difficulties. The child will also often show difficulties in unstructured school activities such as lunch-time activities and recess activities. With age, symptoms of ADHD tend to change. Adolescents may have less difficulty with hyperactivity, but may show more risk-taking behavior and inability to manage their own time. Adults who have ADHD often show disturbance in executive functioning, such as time management, prioritization, and completion of tasks.

## CASE VIGNETTE

Ben, a 15 year old tenth grader, was referred by his school psychologist for psychiatric evaluation because of school failure. Ben came to the office with his parents. The first impression of Ben and his family was that they were all very large. Ben was 250 pounds and 6 feet 4 inches tall. The entire family was professionally dressed. Ben was quiet and his father started describing Ben's problems. Ben had struggled in school through middle school but always put in good effort. As a ninth grader he received special help on school work from teachers and parents, but still could only earn Cs and Ds. The school psychologist evaluated Ben for learning disorders with a standard psychoeducational testing battery. Intelligence was above average and academic achievement was at grade level. The psychologist noted that Ben had difficulty maintaining his attention span.

Ben's parents were very concerned that he would fail his classes and would not be able to go to college or even participate in high school sports. They noted that Ben was an exceptional athlete. As a freshman he was dominant on the offensive and defensive line for the varsity football team. Ben's real love was track and field, where he was one of the top performers in the shot put and discus. Ben had decided to focus his efforts on the throwing events full time, and had given up all other sports (his father was a former running back at a major Midwestern university). Ben's father, now an architect, became very involved in Ben's training and worried that if Ben did not pass his classes he would be ineligible for the spring track and field season.

Ben acknowledged that he tried in school but was easily distracted in class. He tended to daydream and often misunderstood directions to assignments.

Both at home and in school he would start a task, but easily find himself off task. He insisted he always finished important tasks, though he always did them at the last minute and they were often late. Reading school books was particularly boring, but he enjoyed reading historical fiction. Organization was always a problem for Ben, so both of his parents were frequently reminding him or picking up after him. Ben reported that he was always the last in class to finish a test because his mind kept wandering. Socially Ben was quiet and shy. He had a good sense of humor and was well-liked. He had no history of impulsivity or hyperactivity. Ben, his school teachers, and his parents scored Ben as moderately inattentive on standardized ADHD checklists. Ben completed two different computerized continuous performance tests. Each test demonstrated errors of inattention (omission errors) and inconsistency of reaction time, findings consistent with ADHD inattentive type. Ben did not report symptoms of other psychiatric or medical problems, and had recently had a normal sports physical examination.

Ben was given a diagnosis of ADHD, primarily inattentive type. After a lengthy discussion of treatment, Ben and his parents decided to try a stimulant medication trial. Ben was started on dextroamphetamine, 5 mg morning and noon. Ben's improvement was immediate, and within a week teachers were commenting on the improvement. His English grade improved from F to B, and his grade point average (GPA) improved from 1.5 to 2.5. Increasing Ben's dose made Ben feel restless and uncomfortable. On higher doses he complained that he "lost [his] personality," and was overfocused. Ben found that he was less shy and more confident as his attention span improved. He was given a methylphenidate trial but reported that he felt more "normal" on the dextroamphetamine. Trials of dextroamphetamine spansule at 5 and 10 mg doses were tried with hope of skipping the noon dose at school (administered in the school office). Again, Ben preferred the dextroamphetamine tablets. Ben continued to do well in school, taking advanced classes and earning a GPA of 3.0 or better. Athletically, he continued to develop under the watchful eye of his father. As a eleventh grader he was nationally ranked and traveling to meets outside of his region. He began to be informally recruited by college coaches. Using dextroamphetamine during competition never was noticed to be a benefit or detriment to his throwing. Ben did note that the medication was helpful during coaching sessions, when he needed to listen carefully to his coach.

As a senior, he was recruited to major universities and received a "full-ride" scholarship. He set the state high school record in the shot put and was invited to compete in the national Junior Olympics. Ben's father was uncertain about medication rules for Junior Olympic competition and contacted USA Track and Field and the US Olympic Committee. At that time (mid 1990s), there was no US Anti-Doping Agency and information was scant. He got a list of asthma drugs that had been banned, but surprisingly, there was no listing for amphetamine. Ben decided that he wanted to use his medication because he was traveling across the country and would be meeting many people. He opined that he would have better social interactions if he continued his medication. He was warned about the risk of disqualification, but his psychiatrist, parents, and coach were all unaware of the rules regarding banned drugs for Junior Olympics participation. Before competing he showed his prescription to the field judge, who reviewed the list of banned drugs and told Ben that because "Dexedrine" was not on his list it was permitted. Ben competed and did very well, qualifying for international competition at the Junior Pan American Games. A few weeks later, he was contacted by track officials informing him that his drug test was positive for amphetamines, and that he was disqualified and facing a 2-year suspension. Ben was very disheartened, because he had a dream of competing in the Olympics.

Ben went to college and continued to take dextroamphetamine because it was essential for academic success. As an athlete he had additional academic support. His coach and university were well aware of his ADHD, and the National Collegiate Athletic Association (NCAA) was officially informed. A therapeutic drug exception was granted, yet he never again took dextroamphetamine within 24 hours of a competition. Ben worked hard but never regained his dominance. He suffered a few injuries that impaired his performance. Ben graduated from his university in 4.5 years and stopped his medication. Ben joined the Navy and had to be off his ADHD treatment for 6 months before enlistment, due to perhaps archaic US service rules.

## ATTENTION DEFICIT HYPERACTIVITY DISORDER AND THE YOUTH ATHLETE

Although there is often much speculation on the effect that ADHD plays on a child's participation in sporting activities, there is very little published research in this area. To generate hypotheses for later, more directed, study, 22 child psychiatrists interested in sports psychiatry were surveyed [7]. Eighty-six percent of the participating child psychiatrists reported that children and adolescents who had ADHD benefited either "always" or "often" when participating in organized youth sports. In the same survey, most child psychiatrists did not show any preference for individual or team sports. Sixty-four percent specifically indicated "no preference between individual and team sports" when advising participation by children who have ADHD. These child psychiatrists were then asked to rate the suitability for 37 specific sports (such as tennis or golf) or sport positions (such as basketball guard or baseball pitcher) on a five-point scale for youth who have untreated ADHD. The average scores were calculated and sport or sport position was rank-ordered for "suitability" for the untreated ADHD-affected athlete. The untreated athlete is an athlete who has ADHD and who is not given a pharmacologic treatment to diminish the ADHD symptoms. Even though these athletes are not receiving medication for their ADHD, they may be receiving educational and psychosocial treatments and support. The "most suitable sport" was thought to be swimming, followed in order by wrestling, track/sprints, track/field events, ski/snowboarding, dance, and distance running/cross country. The least suitable sport or position was considered to be baseball catcher, followed in rank order by football quarterback, equestrian events, hockey goalie, soccer goalie, golf, and gymnastics. Participants were not polled on their opinions about sport participation for ADHD-affected athletes once the ADHD symptoms have been successfully treated with medications. Participants were also not surveyed on their expert opinions as to whether ADHD symptoms actually impart some advantage to young athletes. These are important and complex issues for the sports medicine physician and primary care physician, and may warrant a referral to a sport psychiatrist when initially advising and treating young athletes.

A general impression from the study of the group of child psychiatrists was that different sports or sport positions demonstrated different suitability for the untreated ADHD-affected athlete. More specific and careful study needs to be done to help more accurately assess whether there is any validity to this preliminary survey. Surveying groups of coaches, parents, and athletes may be the next step in gathering validating data. Subsequently, a more careful assessment of an ADHD affected athlete's specific cognitive and behavioral strengths and challenges will be of value in working to match the athlete to the most suitable sport.

More study is necessary to determine how the specific symptoms noted in ADHD affect participation in a specific sport or sporting position. Because the diagnosis of ADHD may include symptoms of inattention, hyperactivity, and impulsivity, presentation of symptoms may be very different, depending on which of the three subtypes is present: ADHD, combined type; ADHD, inattentive type; or ADHD, hyperactive/impulsive type. With such information, children and their parents can be advised as to which sports may give the athlete the greatest likelihood for sporting enjoyment and success, given the athlete's temperament and psychiatric disorder. Physical attributes such as height, build, or running speed are often used to help guide children in their choice of sporting activities. A greater understanding of a child's neuropsychiatric functioning should also be an important consideration in guiding young athletes, their families, and their sports medicine physicians.

In treating ADHD, key tenets for successful care are providing education to the patient and family about the disorder—clarifying with the family the affected individual's strengths as well as challenges—and the development of a treatment plan that modifies the environment so that the individual is more likely to be successful in chosen activities. Key interventions include the establishment of a structured and predictable schedule and clear behavioral expectations. Positive reinforcement and experience of success are critical in helping the child or adolescent maintain interest. "Time out" (or sitting on the bench) can be a helpful intervention by temporarily removing the positive experience of playing when one is playing with poor impulse control. Adding a token incentive program to reinforce positive behavior can be quite helpful. Often this may be judiciously combined with a consistent plan to briefly remove privileges if unwanted behavior occurs (response-cost technique). Five ADHD-affected children were studied using various behavioral interventions on and off medication in a summer program to determine which interventions increased "sportsmanlike behavior" [8]. Although a delayed reward had little effect of sportsmanship, the addition of tokens (praise) significantly increased the sportsmanlike behavior in all subjects. The effect of medication was studied in three subjects and found to have very little influence on sportsmanship behavior.

In the study of 22 child psychiatrists noted previously [7], 77% felt that special training was necessary for coaches of youths who have ADHD. Eighty-six percent of the same child psychiatric respondents believed that parents of ADHD-affected athletes needed special information to help their children successfully participate in youth sports. Such training would give the coach or parent greater understanding of ADHD symptoms, the challenges and opportunities involved, and behavioral interventions that work well. Just as the skilled teacher must employ different teaching techniques with different students, so too the successful youth coach must have a repertoire of different coaching techniques. The awareness of developmentally appropriate youth coaching has led to several efforts to train youth coaches. Recently a small and easy-to-read introductory book has been written to educate coaches and parents about the ADHD affected athlete [9].

Coaching skill and adaptation becomes even more of a challenge when symptoms of ADHD occur comorbidly with another psychiatric disorder, as is commonly the case. Fifty percent of children who have ADHD simultaneously meet criteria for either oppositional defiant disorder or conduct disorder [3]. These children are particularly difficult to parent, teach, or coach because of their hostile and reactive attitudes and impulsive, aggressive behaviors. These are also the children who need the most structure and adult supervision, experiences often provided by participation in youth sporting activities. The behavioral training strategies employed in sport can help children develop greater mastery in controlling their behavior and developing respect for authority figures. These youths are likely to view the sporting outcome, such as winning or losing, as much more important than the process, such as playing by the rules or showing good sportsmanship. The general psychiatric literature suggests that the presence of aggressive behavior and conduct disorder with ADHD increases the risk of substance abuse [10]. There is no research studying the incidence of substance abuse in the young athletic population affected by ADHD.

In the Multimodal Treatment Study of Children with Attention Deficit/ Hyperactivity Disorder (MTA) study [11], a large multicenter random controlled trial of ADHD treatment efficacy, anxiety disorders were found to co-occur in 34% of subjects who had ADHD. These anxious and inattentive children also present special challenges to the youth coach. Often they can be avoidant and aversive to risk taking. The sensitive, experienced, and well-trained coach can play a significant role in helping these children desensitize and overcome their fears and anxieties. These children are often very sensitive to criticism and perceived failure. Loud or threatening coaching behavior is only likely to increase the young athletes' anxiety. The likely outcome is that these children, who may be fairly noncompetitive to begin with, will actively avoid later sporting opportunities.

Depressive disorders usually develop after the symptoms of ADHD have already been noted. Commonly, children struggling with school and social relationships because of ADHD symptoms will show signs of discouragement and demoralization, especially as they enter puberty. Rates of depressive disorders in children who have ADHD vary considerably from the general population rate of about 3% to a rate as high as 75%, depending upon the criteria and source of information [12]. The MTA study [13] found a rate of 6% of depressive disorders in the study subjects who had ADHD. Exercise at public health recommended rates is helpful in overcoming symptoms of depression in adults [14], yet there are no such studies in children. Presumably, the somatic symptoms of depressive disorders and anhedonia with low motivation impair athletic performance. An understanding and encouraging coach interested in the well-being and development of a young athlete can help set realistic goals, and keep the depressed athlete engaged in the sport and engaged with the social support of the team. Coaches that tend to be critical and rejecting of athletes that do not perform well (perhaps secondary to depression) tend to drive the young person away from the sport. Once young athletes quit a sport, usually due to lack of enjoyment, they are unlikely to return to that sport.

## MEDICATION TREATMENT OF ATHLETES WHO HAVE ATTENTION DEFICIT HYPERACTIVITY DISORDER

In addition to environmental and behavioral interventions, the use of psychopharmacologic agents has been the primary element in successful treatment of ADHD. The most established treatment for ADHD symptoms is the use of psychostimulants. The use of these medications has been validated as very helpful in the school setting and the less structured home setting. Similar studies have not yet been done to justify use of these agents during sporting activities. Enhancing a person's ability to maintain concentration on a fairly tedious and boring intellectual exercise may be of value in the classroom, but it may not be of the same value on the practice field or in competition. A quiet and less impulsive child may be helpful in a classroom setting, because such behavior optimizes the potential for learning and decreases disruption to other students. Such behavior, however, may not be beneficial in the sporting context.

The 22 child psychiatrists polled [7] regarding their expert opinions were evenly divided on whether or not young athletes should be treated with medication for ADHD during sports, practice, or competition. Approximately half of the respondents indicated that they always or often treat young athletes with medication during sporting activities, whereas a nearly equal number indicated they only sometimes or rarely treat young athletes with medication during competition. Clearly more study is needed to address this lack of consensus among clinicians. It probably emphasizes, however, an underlying reality for the competitive athlete who has ADHD. Some athletes actually perform better in some sports when their ADHD symptoms are treated with medication, whereas they may not do as well in other sports, depending upon the demand of the sport or the specific traits of the person. For example, basketball point guards or wrestlers who have ADHD may actually have an advantage if their symptoms allow them to be more spontaneous or unpredictable to their opponent. The ADHD-affected basketball center who has a hard time disciplining himself to stay near the basket may find that he is out of position frequently unless ADHD symptoms are treated with medication. One double-blind, placebo-controlled crossover study of methylphenidate effect on 17 boys aged 8 to 10 playing baseball [15] revealed that methylphenidate at doses of 0.3 and 0.6 mg/kg had a beneficial effect on attention span during the game.

Psychostimulants, as a medication class, are primarily represented in the United States by various amphetamine and amphetamine-like methylphenidate preparations. Commonly used short-acting amphetamine preparations with the duration of action of approximately 3 to 4 hours include dextroamphetamine. Dextroamphetamine also comes as time-released spansules, which may provide 6 to 8 hours of effective action. Amphetamine salts may also work for 5 to 7 hours. There is a dual-release beaded time capsule that often provides 10 or more hours of medication effect.

Methylphenidate preparations also come in short-acting, intermediate-acting, and long-acting preparations. Short-acting preparations include generic methylphenidate. Dexmethylphenidate, the purified right-handed (dextro) optical isomer of methylphenidate, is available in short-acting tablets and soon will be available in long-acting capsules. Intermediate-acting preparations, usually working or 7 to 8 hours, are available in various forms and with various levels of efficacy. There is one long-acting methylphenidate preparation that last approximately 12 hours. It is designed to release methylphenidate gradually over a 12-hour period using an osmotic release (OROS) drug delivery system. Magnesium pemoline is another stimulant with a long half-life that has been used for treating ADHD. Its advantages include its long half-life, low psychiatric side-effect profile, and low abuse potential. Since it is not a Drug Enforcement Administration Class II controlled substance, Pemoline is more convenient to prescribe. Pemoline, however, is now considered a third-line agent because of concern that it might induce serious liver disease (the Food and Drug Administration [FDA] has placed a black box warning on this medication).

In addition to the psychostimulants, there is one nonstimulant medication approved in 2003 by the FDA for treatment of ADHD, despite its equivocal results in clinical practice. Atomoxetine is a selective norepinephrine reuptake inhibiter. It has up to a 24-hour effect. Other reported treatments for ADHD that are not approved by the FDA but have been found to be effective by psychiatrists for ADHD include bupropion, tricyclic antidepressants, and alpha 2 adrenergic agonists such as clonidine and guanfacine.

When judging whether or not the use of a psychopharmacologic agent will be beneficial for the young athlete in sport (either practice or competition) the physician needs to have data demonstrating that symptoms of ADHD are actively impairing sport performance. In addition, the attending physician must have some understanding about the potential adverse effects that the athlete may experience from the treating agent. A careful clinical trial then needs to be orchestrated with the support of the athlete, parents, and coaches.

Possible adverse effects of psychostimulants in the general psychiatric literature include appetite suppression, sleep disturbance, irritability, motor tics, gastrointestinal complaints, palpitations, tachycardia, hypertension, anxiety, tremor, and possibly risk of serious cardiovascular event. Because there is no stimulant study in the athlete population, the 22 child psychiatrists were polled about their adverse experiences derived from the use of psychostimulants in their young athletic patients during competition [7]. They were asked to respond in a three-point scale indicating whether the adverse outcome was often, sometimes, or never. Adverse outcomes were then tallied, given an average score, and rank-ordered. The most common adverse complaint was "over focus" followed by "decline in athletic performance," "decreased enjoyment," "lack of creativity," and "irritability," much different than the medication side effects in the general population.

In the general psychiatric literature the most common adverse effects of atomoxetine are sedation and gastrointestinal discomfort such as nausea and vomiting, which often limit its usefulness. Of 19 child psychiatric respondents, only 5 indicated experience with adverse effects from atomoxetine [7]. The reported side effects in athletes included nausea, lethargy, palpitations, tremulousness, and sweating. Clearly more systematic research in this area needs to be done to be able to provide more adequate direction to treating physicians of athletes.

The goal in treating the young and developing athletes' ADHD symptoms is often to improve the young people's attention spans to a developmentally appropriate level so that they can listen and learn from coaching instructions, persist in skill building drills, and play with a team. Often the objective for the parent or coach is to ensure that the child athlete is "in the game" by making sure the medication effects persist through the athletic competition or practice. With older high school and college athletes, there is often a desire to be off the medication during competition, while continuing to use the medication to help with academic and sometimes with social functioning. One distance runner described that he could not run "in the zone" while on stimulant medications for ADHD, but on medications he could concentrate on his race plan. He felt that the medication effect made each run seem harder, but his times were better off the stimulants. Basketball point guards almost universally find that their performance falters when on medication. They complain of lack of spontaneity and too much predictability in their play. Soccer goalies, on the other hand, often report that their discipline to stay in position is improved when their ADHD is treated during competition, and that they make fewer mental errors (greater self awareness). Although there are many such anecdotal reports, no systematic study has assessed their validity.

One strategy often used is to time the medication effect by using medications with different durations of action. For example, a collegiate athlete might use a short acting preparation (3–4 hour effect) for attending classes and for a study period, but time the medication so that it wears off for practice and competition. Another athlete and his coach may see value in medication use for taking in coaching instruction or activities such as learning new plays or watching films, but prefer to practice and compete off medications. High school athletes might desire an intermediate-acting stimulant for the school hours, with expectation that the effects will wear off in 7 or 8 hours, in time for sport practice or competition. They may then require a later short-acting preparation for evening studying. Combinations of atomoxetine and stimulants have been used to get the desired effect in controlling ADHD symptoms outside of competition, while avoiding adverse stimulant effects during sporting activity.

The subelite and elite adolescent and adult athlete may have a very different motivation to seek treatment for ADHD. For these athletes, stimulant treatment may not be used to overcome ADHD symptoms, but to gain an advantage over the competition and enhance their sport performance. During the early years of athlete drug testing in the United States, most athletes were using supplements that contained some sort of stimulant (often ephedrine or caffeine), hoping to mimic the training regimen of the most successful elite athletes in the sport (David Baron, MD, personal communication, 2005). Some athletes abuse stimulants with hope that they will suppress appetite and lead to weight loss. Athletes competing in sports in which aesthetics are judged highly (ie, gymnastics, diving, ice skating) and athletes competing in sports with specific weight classes (boxing, wrestling) may be particularly vulnerable to misuse and abuse of stimulants as a weight loss agent.

The World Anti Doping Agency (WADA), the US Anti-Doping Agency (USADA), and the NCAA ban use of stimulants during competition [16–21]. Athletes testing positive for stimulants (the specific list is long) face suspension from competition. The NCAA requires athletes affected by ADHD to inform the school of their medical need to use a banned stimulant for ADHD treatment when no alternative exists. The college then can respond to an NCAA inquiry with medical justification that treatment is necessary for the student-athlete [22]. There is no such appeals process in the Olympic movement, and the athlete is declared responsible for assuring that supplements and medications taken do not include any forbidden substances. The only medication indicated for ADHD that is approved during competition is atomoxetine [23], and it has not yet been studied in athletes. Anecdotal reports that some athletes experience mental quietness on atomoxetine, and are thus able to comprehend coaching directions in practice and apply those lessons to a game situation (David Baron MD, personal communication, 2005) suggest that for some athletes an atomoxetine trial may be warranted as a permitted treatment to impairing ADHD.

## HISTORY OF STIMULANT USE IN SPORTS

But is there scientific proof that stimulants actually enhance sport performance? Various substances have been used throughout history to enhance athletic performance. Gladiators were reported to use stimulants as far back as 600 BCE [24]. These athletes were expected to be victorious, and the price for defeat was often death. Athletes during the Greek and Roman games used opioids and mushrooms to enhance their athletic performance [25]. In the 1800s marathon runners and cyclists were using ethanol and strychnine to give them a competitive edge [24]. In the 1930s the German military was using amphetamines to enhance troop endurance, and by the 1940s professional football players in the National Football League (NFL) were beginning to use amphetamines to improve strength and speed [24]. In 1957 two Olympic athletes admitted to using amphetemine in competition, leading the American Medical Association (AMA) to create an ad-hoc committee to study the use of amphetamine in sport [26]. The AMA commissioned two studies.

Smith and Beecher [27] used a double-blind, placebo controlled design to study performance enhancement from amphetamines. The study measured performance on six experiments, and used 18 swimmers, 26 runners, and 13 weight throwers. Amphetamines were dosed at 14 mg/70 kg administered 2 to 3 hours before each exercise experiment. Testing was done in both the rested and fatigued state. Their results showed that 73% of runners, 85% of weight throwers, and 93% of swimmers performed better on amphetamines when compared with placebo. Even though 77% of the subjects did better with amphetamines, only 59% reported the drug to be subjectively helpful. The authors concluded that athletic performance in highly trained athletes can be significantly improved by administration of amphetamines.

A second study, by Karpovich [28], tested untrained subjects in running, swimming, and treadmill tests. Amphetamines were administered at dose of 10 to 20 mg given 30 to 60 minutes before testing. Nine to 12 athletes were tested in each event, and only 3 athletes improved with amphetamines. Karpovich's conclusion was that amphetamines at the tested doses neither augmented nor impaired performance.

Older reports suggested mixed effects of amphetamines on athletes. One report [29] suggested that amphetamines caused athletes to perceive that they are doing more work, while actual work load is unchanged. Another study [30] suggested that there was no improvement on a 100-yard swim by 12 untrained male subjects given amphetamines 1.5 hours before the test. A third pioneering study [31] observing the effect of amphetamines on soldiers challenged with an 18-mile hike and 24 hours without sleep suggested that the drug tended to decrease foot complaints and dropout rate on the hike by masking pain and fatigue. Although this study did note an amphetamine effect, one must extrapolate the findings to actual athletic performance.

During the 1960 Rome Olympics, Danish cyclist Kurt Jensen died after using amphetamine and a vasodilator. Two teammates also using the drug combination were hospitalized [24]. These events led many countries to consider bans on amphetamine use because of its danger. The International Olympic Committee investigated the use of amphetamines, and in 1968 drafted a list of banded substances, including amphetamines, due to concerns about unfair competitive advantage as well as health risk to athletes. Since the first list of banned substances there has been a continued effort to define banned substances and monitor compliance with drug testing. Subsequent to the stimulant drug ban, research investigating the specific benefits or consequences of stimulant use in athletes has slowed and been replaced with study of drug testing research. Williams and Thompson [32] tested athletes with a cycle ergotomy test 2 hours after a dose of amphetamine. On doses of 5 mg/70 kg, 10 mg/70 kg and, 15 mg/70 kg there were no differences in time to exhaustion. Chandler and Blair [33] studied untrained male former high school athletes using various physical tests in a placebo-controlled design. Using an amphetamine dose of 15 mg/70 kg, the study found performance enhancement from the drug on tests of knee extension strength, acceleration, time to exhaustion, peak lactate, and maximum heart rate. There was no advantage to amphetamine use in elbow flexion strength, peak speed on 30-yard dash, or aerobic power on treadmill test. The study authors concluded that amphetamines help maintain effort longer under anaerobic conditions, perhaps due to masking of fatigue or pain.

Concern about amphetamines in professional sports began in the 1980 with a review of amphetamine use in NFL players [34]. Skill players (ie, quarterbacks, wide receivers, and defensive backs) were found to be using low doses of amphetamines on game day (5–15 mg) to enhance concentration. Power players (ie, lineman) were found to be using very large doses of amphetamines (up to 150 mg on game day) to improve strength and aggressiveness and possibly to alter consciousness. This has led to the evolution and development of drug use policies by various professional sports leagues. Unlike the Olympic movements, which have commissioned an outside agency not associated with the promotion of sporting events to develop a drug policy monitoring program, the professional league policies are governed by collective bargaining agreements between the owners and players, with no outside agency to monitor compliance. Major league baseball, which has recently been rocked with scandal and subject to congressional hearings as players are accused of anabolic steroid use, has no current prohibition regarding stimulant use. The pressure to perform well and win is extreme in professional sport and difficult to avoid.

## SUMMARY

ADHD is a very common psychiatric disorder that affects children and can persist into adulthood. Impairment occurs in young developing athletes' ability to attend to coaching instruction and cooperate in team-related activities. These children may be seen as more coachable when treated with medication, and may be able to learn skills or strategies more quickly and more accurately. With treatment they may be able to focus better on a specific task, and may be more aware of position and time. These treatment benefits have not been empirically studied, but are inferred from other general studies of ADHD-affected children in school, home, and other group settings. Use of stimulants in treating ADHD symptoms in subelite and elite older athletes does not necessarily improve performance, and may lead to a decline in athletic functioning. Competitive athletes are a unique subpopulation, physically and mentally. They often have innate athletic talent that sets them apart from the recreational sport participant. Their competitive mind is seeking any physiological or psychological edge that will give them the performance advantage over their competition. Consequently, they may use or abuse stimulants or other substances if they believe that other athletes get their performance superiority from the substance, even if there is no clear scientific consensus of performance enhancement. Research on amphetamine effect on sport performance has been ongoing for over 60 years, yet the findings are equivocal. One consistent finding is that amphetamine use may mask pain and fatigue, allowing the athlete to ignore injury more readily. Although this may allow the athlete to finish one competition, the lack of somatic awareness may lead to more serious and permanent injury. Another important research finding demonstrated by the general psychiatric literature is that athletes affected by ADHD may benefit from stimulant medication in their nonathletic life responsibilities. To withhold effective medical treatment may adversely affect their social, educational, and vocational performance. Careful assessment of each athlete is important to develop a customized treatment plan that acknowledges the ADHD-affected athlete's impairing symptoms while complying with ethical and legislative rules of medicine and sport. More scientific study in the athletic population may help to debunk myths about the risks or benefits of stimulant and nonstimulant ADHD medication use in athletic function and performance, helping to define a more rational approach to the treatment of the ADHD-affected athlete involved in and outside the competitive arena.

References

[1] Committee on Quality Improvement Subcommittee on Attention-Deficit/Hyperactivity Disorder. Clinical practice guideline: treatment of the school aged child with attention-deficit/hyperactivity disorder. Pediatrics 2001;108:1158–70.

[2] Silver LB. Attention-deficit/hyperactivity disorder in adult life. Child Adolesc Psychiatr Clin N Am 2000;9(3):511–23.

[3] American Psychiatric Association. Diagnostic and statistical manual of mental disorders. 4th edition. Text revision. Washington (DC): American Psychiatric Association; 2000.

[4] Spencer T, Biederman J, Wilens T, et al. Pharmacotherapy of attention-deficit/hyperactivity disorder across the life cycle. J Am Acad Child Adolesc Psychiatry 1996;35(4):409–32.

[5] Conners CK. Forty years of methylphenidate treatment in attention-deficit/hyperactivity disorder. J Atten Disord 2002;6(Suppl 1):s17–30.

[6] Pliszka S. Patterns of psychiatric comorbidity with attention-deficit/hyperactivity disorder. Child Adolesc Psychiatr Clin N Am 2000;9(3):525–40.

[7] Conant-Norville D. ADHD and youth sports: a small opinion survey of child psychiatrists. Presented at the International Society for Sport Psychiatry Annual Scientific Meeting, Atlanta, May, 2005.

[8] Hupp SD, Reitman D, Northrup J, et al. The effects of delayed rewards, tokens and stimulant medication on sportsmanlike behavior with ADHD-diagnosed children. Behav Modif 2002;26(2):148–62.

[9] Stabeno M. The ADHD affected athlete. Victoria (Canada): Trafford Publ; 2004.

[10] August GJ, Stewart MA, Holmes CS. A four year follow-up of hyperactive boys with and without conduct disorder. Br J Psychiatry 1983;143:192–8.

[11] The MTA Cooperative Group. A 14 month randomized clinical trial of treatment strategies for attention deficit hyperactivity disorder. Arch Gen Psychiatry 1999;56:1073–87.

[12] Biederman J, Newcorn J, Sprich S. Comorbidity of attention deficit hyperactivity disorder with conduct, depressive, anxiety and other disorders. Am J Psychiatry 1991;148:564–77.

[13] The MTA Cooperative Group. Mediators and moderators of treatment response for children with ADHD. Arch Gen Psychiatry 2000;56:1088–96.

[14] Dunn AL, Trivendi MN, Kampert JB, et al. Exercise treatment for depression efficacy and dose response. Am J Prev Med 2005;28(1):1–8.

[15] Pelham Jr WE, McBurnett K, Harper GW, et al. Methylphenidate and baseball playing in ADHD children: who's on first? J Consult Clin Psychol 1990;58(1):130–3.

[16] NCAA. NCAA drug testing program pamphlet 2004–2005. NCAA Web site 2005. Available at: http://www.ncaa.org/library/sports_sciences/drug_testing_program/2004-05/2004-05_drug_testing_program.pdf. Accessed March 20, 2005.

[17] NCAA. NCAA drug testing. NCAA Web site 2005. Available at: http://www2.ncaa.org/legislation_and_governance/eligibility_and_conduct/drug_testing.html. Accessed March 20, 2005.

[18] US Anti-Doping Agency. Drug reference online. US Anti-Doping Agency Web site. Available at: http://www.usantidoping.org/dro/. Accessed March 20, 2005.

[19] United States Anti-Doping Agency. US Anti-Doping Agency Web site. Available at: http://www.usantidoping.org/. Accessed March 20, 2005.

[20] World Ant-Doping Agency. World Anti-Doping Agency Web site. Available at: http://www.wada-ama.org/en/dynamic.ch2?pageCategory_id=166. Accessed March 20, 2005.

[21] World Anti-Doping Agency. Prohibited drug list. World Anti-Doping Web site. Available at: http://www.wada-ama.org/en/dynamic.ch2?pageCategory_id=47. Accessed March 20, 2005.

[22] NCAA. Drug testing exception procedures. NCAA Web site. Available at: http://www1.ncaa.org/membership/ed_outreach/health-safety/drug_testing/exceptions. Accessed March 20, 2005.

[23] US Anti-Doping Agency. Wallet card of prohibited and permitted drugs. Available at: http://www.usantidoping.org/files/active/what/wallet_card.pdf. Accessed March 20, 2005.

[24] Jones A, Pichot J. Stimulant use in sports. Am J Addict 1998;7(4):243–55.

[25] Greydanus D, Patel D. Sports doping in the adolescent athlete. The hope, hype, and hyperbole. Pediatr Clin N Am 2002;49:829–55.

[26] Ryan AJ. Use of amphetamines in athletics [letter]. JAMA 1959;170:562.

[27] Smith GM, Beecher HK. Amphetamine sulfate and athletic performance. JAMA 1959;170:542–57.

[28] Karpovich PV. Effect of amphetamine sulfate on athletic performance. JAMA 1959;170:558–61.

[29] Folz EE, Ivy AC, Barborka CJ. The influence of amphetamine (Benzedrine) sulfate, d-desoxyephedrine hydrochloride (pervitin), and caffeine upon work output and recovery when rapidly exhausting work is done by trained subjects. J Lab Clin Med 1943;28:603–6.

[30] Haldi H, Wynn W. Action of drugs on efficiency of swimmers. Res Q Exerc Sport 1946;17:96–101.

[31] Cuthbertson DP, Knox JAC. The effects of analeptics on the fatigued subject. J Physiol 1947;150:253–62.

[32] Williams MH, Thompson J. Effects of various dosages of amphetamine upon endurance. Res Q Exerc Sport 1973;44:417–21.

[33] Chandler JV, Blair SN. The effects of amphetamines on selected physiological components related to athletic success. Med Sci Sports Exerc 1980;12:65–9.

[34] Mandell AJ, Stewart KD, Russo PV. The Sunday syndrome: from kinetics to altered consciousness. Fed Proc 1981;40:2693–8.

Clin Sports Med 24 (2005) 845–852

# CLINICS IN SPORTS MEDICINE

## Aggression and Sport

Robert W. Burton, MD*

*Department of Psychiatry and Behavioral Sciences, The Feinberg School of Medicine, Northwestern University, 446 East Ontario Street, Suite 200, Seventh Floor, Chicago, IL 60611, USA*

Without aggression there is no such thing as sport. The fast break in basketball, the breakout in hockey, and football's kickoff return all exemplify aggression in team sports. It is seen best in the coordinated push up the field toward the goal. In individual sports, aggression manifests itself more visibly as risk-taking behavior. Going over the bunker for the pin instead of laying up in golf, attempting the high degree-of-difficulty move in diving, skating, or gymnastics, or skiing all-out into a blind turn in the downhill are clearly aggressive maneuvers. In any sport, aggressive play is easily identifiable and valued. On the other hand, overly aggressive behavior is not allowed, and is penalized.

There is, in general, a consensus on what constitutes overly aggressive behavior. Whether set by explicit rules of play or by a more intuitive sense of appropriateness and fair play, boundaries exist. Differing sports and levels of competition allow for judgment calls in the gray areas, but a feature common to all sport is that aggression is desirable and confers a competitive advantage.

This situation mirrors nature. Aggressive behavior is inherent to life in the animal kingdom. It is understood as providing survival and evolutionary advantage to the individual or species that display it. Meanwhile, those who act in a way that crosses the line often put themselves at risk or pay a price. Although the competitive advantage of aggression in today's society may not be as readily apparent today as in prehistoric times, it still applies in principle. Human behavior is much more complex than that of other animals. To understand aggression in sport, it is helpful to use the three predominant perspectives of psychiatry.

The first perspective is what is observable. Descriptive diagnosis, exemplified by the Diagnostic and Statistical Manual of Mental Disorders, 4th Edition (DSM-IV) [1], which attempts to be atheoretical, provides a good starting point for discussion. From this perspective, we describe what we see and define what we mean by aggression, overly aggressive behavior, and violence. Historically, aggression has had many meanings and remains ambiguous. On balance, aggression has gotten a bad name. For the purpose of this discussion, the term aggression will refer to assertive, forceful, but constructive behavior synony-

* 636 Church Street, Suite 715, Evanston, IL 60201. *E-mail address:* rwbmd@comcast.net

0278-5919/05/$ – see front matter    © 2005 Elsevier Inc. All rights reserved.
doi:10.1016/j.csm.2005.03.001    sportsmed.theclinics.com

mous with self-directed attempts to achieve personal or group goals. While in pursuit of these goals, aggressive people do not intentionally injure or harm themselves or others. Rather, they attempt to control their environment—in sport, the playing field, and by so doing, the outcome.

Physical injury is an inherent risk of sport. Participants may behave quite aggressively, and as long as their primary goal is victory and not the infliction of injury, it is acceptable. Aggressive behavior that goes beyond the generally accepted standards of conduct or rules of the game, particularly that which appears to be intended to harm or endanger others or that shows recklessness, is considered overly aggressive. Violent behavior is most clearly defined as conscious, usually premeditated (but at times impulsive) acts designed to injure. Alternatively, the term violent behavior may be applied to that which is performed with blatant disregard for the welfare of others.

Most observers will easily discern overly aggressive and violent behavior from that which is aggressive but in accordance with the sporting context. An interesting example of an athletic moment that straddled this boundary was a player's headfirst tag of home plate during the 1970 Major League Baseball All-Star Game. His all-out and successful attempt to score disregarded the physical integrity of the opposing catcher, who stood in his way awaiting the throw home. The collision slightly up the line from the plate was stunning, to say the least. Given that it was during an exhibition game, it led to a debate over its appropriateness that transcended the usual inter-league allegiances of the fans and sportswriters. Several years later, a hard-throwing pitcher threw a fastball high and tight, inside and near the head of a batter in the same venue, resulting in an exchange of angry words and posturing. Again, the aggressiveness of the play was called into question. It will be helpful to keep these examples in mind while considering the discussion that follows.

Beyond observation and description, psychiatrists have developed the biopsychosocial model. This model takes into consideration biological, psychological, and social factors that contribute to behavior and relate to its cognitive and emotional underpinnings. A broad range of the factors can thus be considered. The objective is to develop a framework not only to assist in understanding aggressive behavior in sport in general, but also to aid in the assessment of problematic behavior, namely the inappropriate expressions of our inherent aggressive tendency in the context of sport.

Finally, in addition to the descriptive (or phenomenological) approach and a biopsychosocial formulation, it is imperative to keep a developmental perspective. Human behavior and its meaning evolve over the course of the life cycle. As a result, aggression in sport will look different at different ages, and the standards for appropriate behavior will vary as well. For the most part, more mature expressions of aggression will be expected in adults in sport, as elsewhere.

## BIOLOGICAL FACTORS

Aside from our basic aggressiveness as organisms attempting to survive in a sometimes hostile environment, a fundamental, biological differentiating factor between individuals is the presence of a Y-chromosome. Expression of the Y-chromosome determines male phenotype. Male members of most animal species are, in general, more aggressive than females. Masculinity is operationalized primarily by the male hormone, testosterone. The presence of this hormone circulating in the bloodstream has a large influence on the degree of aggressive behavior that an individual will exhibit. Related compounds, such as androgenic anabolic steroids and other substances that promote or mimic the relative abundance of testosterone in the brain and bloodstream, have the same effect. In fact, it might be argued that the increased aggressive behavior of athletes who use such substances is a greater contributor to performance than the increase in lean muscle mass that they promote.

Many of the other substances athletes take to gain competitive advantage also tend to increase aggressive behavior. Although athletes may think about taking these to increase their energy level, improve their endurance, or reduce their reaction time, an increase in aggression goes hand in hand. This group of chemicals includes caffeine, nicotine, the amphetamines, ephedrine, and other psychostimulants.

Alcohol is another substance with relevance to aggressive behavior and sport. Alcohol can promote aggressive behavior in susceptible individuals, and athletes do use alcohol [2]. The extensive association between alcohol and sport is disturbing, especially when one considers the nonelite athlete who may use it even during competition, and the acts of fan violence around sporting events that are so well known. In addition to the effects of intoxication, anxiety and irritability are common symptoms of withdrawal, and these can easily translate into overly aggressive behavior during the acute or postacute withdrawal state.

DSM-IV Axis I psychiatric disorders are generally considered to be behavioral syndromes caused primarily by the improper function of the brain. As such, they must also be considered biological factors of aggression. Athletes afflicted by illnesses such as bipolar affective disorder and attention deficit disorder are predisposed to exhibit overly aggressive behavior. Although athletes with bipolar disorder have reached elite levels in sport, they are at risk, especially during manic episodes of their illness. Athletes with attention deficit disorder, with their penchant for driven physical activity, may be drawn to sport, but may lack the interpersonal skills or the impulse control to limit their aggressiveness [3].

Another biological factor is the actual physical contact required by a given sport. The more physical contact that is considered to be acceptable in a given sport, the greater the likelihood that violence or overly aggressive behavior will be a part of that sport. Ice hockey may be the best example of this effect. There is clearly an aggressive response to physical discomfort inflicted by others. Hence, violence begets violence and players know "it is better to hit than be hit." It is probably the combination of the perception of pain and an accompanying sense of being threatened that produce this effect.

## PSYCHOLOGICAL ISSUES

Aggression is an inborn psychological feature of being human and alive. Rooted in the survival instinct and conferring an advantage to the individual and the procreation of the species, it is not strictly a learned behavior. It is an affective and behavioral capacity with which all of us are born, and a component of human temperament and, ultimately, of personality [4]. What differentiates individuals is the manner in which this capacity is expressed and used or, in contrast, contained and concealed.

As an inherent human characteristic, early experiences with aggression in childhood and infancy are extremely important. Youth sport participation is often one of the first times that children are allowed and encouraged to explore their aggressive capacity. It may be the first time a young athlete feels aggression and attaches this label to the subjective experience of making a constructive, assertive attempt to control his or her environment and master the situation at hand. Its opposite is more passive withdrawal and avoidance, which are not conducive to success in sport or in life.

The impact of the early sport and presport experiences of aggression is determined, in large part, by the response of adults involved, especially parents. Children's natural aggressive tendencies will be supported or inhibited by these significant others, whether parents, other family members, physical educators, instructors, or coaches. Ideally, young athletes will learn to control themselves in the presence of these acceptable aggressive feelings, and to express their feelings appropriately within the context of the game. Psychologically and socially, these are extremely important learning experiences: to feel the feelings, own them and the behaviors that manifest them, be responded to by a significant other, and to learn to contain or modify that behavior so that it fits the social context. Consider as well the somewhat different situation in which a young athlete is confronted by a teammate or coach with his or her lack of aggressive-ness. Without such experiences learning proper use of aggression, the world of opportunities shrinks considerably for that player. Never being able to use healthy forms of aggression means never being able to realize one's potential [5].

That aggression can be managed and controlled, contained, or amplified by self and others is an extremely important experiential lesson learned in the relative safety of the sporting context. Whether limited by the enforcement of rules by an official, or stimulated by an inspirational half-time speech from a coach or through the prompting of a teammate or taunting of an opponent, the vicissitudes of aggression are of tantamount importance for the individual, and ultimately for our society.

There are two intriguing concepts, one from child development and one from sport psychology, that connect this process of learning to manage one's aggres-sion with performance excellence in sport. Demos [6] described a "zone of optimal affective engagement" that refers to the parental influence that is avail-able to respond to the infant's earliest needs and expressions of emotion. He posits that there is a range of responsiveness from parents that best allows the infant to express him or herself. If the range is appropriate, it allows the infant to feel responded to, supported, and contained or held in the process that promotes a secure and developing sense of self. The experience of aggression is one of these early emotions to which parents must respond. If the response is neither too harsh nor too lenient, the infant learns to modulate it and his or her behavior. If the response is extreme in one way or another, the infant's aggression will be either inhibited or intensified.

In sport psychology, Hanin [7] developed the "zone of optimal functioning." It is a range of emotional states that allow an athlete to perform closest to his or her potential. The dimensions of these states are delineated using the athlete's own words to describe the subjective experience of his or her personal best performances. Techniques are then devised to achieve the optimal levels of the various dimensions during subsequent competitions. It is a given that the dimensions of the zone may be quite different for different athletes and those competing in differing sports. Power weight lifters, for example, will have a much different zone of optimal functioning than golfers.

The similarity of these concepts suggests further connections between playing sports and the development of self and personality. It may be, for example, that the foundation for an athlete's zone of optimal functioning is laid by the appropriateness of the zone of optimal affective engagement he or she experienced in childhood.

Returning to clinical considerations, certain personality disorders clearly present increased risk of overly aggressive behavior or violence. Borderline personality disordered individuals are, by definition, inclined to impulsive acts of physical aggression, not only toward themselves, but also toward others. Violent outbursts are common manifestations of their impaired interpersonal boundaries and fragile sense of self.

Narcissistic personality disorder has been considered to be an occupational risk to elite athletes [8]. The lifestyle of being pampered and catered to from a very young age limits development and promotes an entitled outlook. The special status, privileges, and constant adulation of fans and various supporters all contribute to the possibility of an athlete developing this disorder. The outward grandiosity attempts to conceal inner insecurity, feelings of incompetence, and doubts of worthiness, and the breakdown of the narcissistic defenses can result in raging outbursts both on and off the playing field.

## SOCIAL ISSUES

Sport is a strictly social phenomenon. The games do not exist in social isolation. At a minimum, an opponent is necessary, whether real or imagined. Most often a slew of others are involved, from parents and peers, to teammates, trainers, coaches and spectators. Any and all of these others can influence the level of aggression displayed through sport. Aggression, similarly, is largely social. Without others, the object of aggression can only be the self or an inanimate object, neither of which is as satisfying.

As mentioned, the role of parents is instrumental. In addition to their influence on children's development, as the primary role models, their own display of aggressive behavior or the lack thereof will have tremendous impact upon their children. Closely following the impact of parents are those of peers and coaches. Peer experiences will often be in opposition to parental ones, and thus provide contrast. They may, however, ultimately support, amplify, or diminish the parental influence, depending on their valence and the nature of the relationship. Confrontation from a peer, for example, may be better received than that coming from any adult authority figure.

Coaches' behavior, too, will either support or offset the initial influence of the parents. They can be supportive or corrective role models. When an unassertive parent has a child in a sport that requires aggression, coaches may be able to elicit the behavior without compromising the parents' position. Often consistent with and supportive of the parent, a coach, as an authority figure from outside the home environment, can wield considerable and potent reinforcement. On the other hand, a coach may be able to contain an athlete with overly aggressive tendencies. In essence, proper coaching can provide many developing athletes with a second chance to master their aggression.

There are two particular social manifestations of aggressive behavior that bear great relevance to sport. They are verbal abuse and mob behavior. Verbal abuse has become such a common scene in sport that observers may have become desensitized to it. It may seem naïve to point it out and discuss it, yet why is this type of violence so prevalent and tolerated? It has to do with aggression. When it occurs player-to-player, as in taunting, or "trash-talking" in today's vernacular, its message is clearly "I'm more aggressive than you!" Interestingly, a likely response is for the taunted to become more aggressive and fight back. The only possible strategic advantage of verbal aggression in sport, therefore, seems to occur when the increased anger and aggression elicited by it are unmanageable for the taunted opponent, and that emotion takes him or her out of the game. Otherwise, and possibly more often, it results in opponents raising their game to become more aggressive, and therefore more of a real threat to the taunter. On the surface, verbal aggression can be seen as simply distasteful posturing. Deeper down, it is clearly ill-advised, endangering not only players' physical well-being, but also their chances of winning.

When verbal abuse occurs between player and coach, the risks are greater. An athlete who is verbally abusive toward his or her coach risks losing playing time and career opportunities. When it happens coach-to-player, it can border on frank child abuse. A coach who yells from the bench and who berates players or officials publicly is modeling overly aggressive behavior. Attempts to motivate players in this manner are ill-advised and fraught with pitfalls. The abused player may feel humiliated, causing him or her to withdraw or shut down, the opposite of the desired effect. On the other hand, the player may feel understandably angry and act out in a way that is counterproductive to the athletic endeavor.

Granted, some athletes may respond as apparently is hoped by the abusive coach, and direct their anger into more aggressive play on the field, remaining within the confines of the game and their zone of optimal functioning. Even this apparently optimal response, however, will often co-occur with the development of a love-hate relationship with the coach, which leaves that working relationship in peril long-term. Every coach who has given the impassioned and inspired half-time speech knows the risk of going to the well once too often. Like the boy who cries wolf, the coach who incites to rage has a finite number of opportunities. Players become able to see through these manufactured scenes and start to feel used and abused, as they justifiably are.

When verbal abuse comes from fan or spectator toward participant, violence can erupt as well. For the athlete, it may require tremendous composure and self-control to restrain one's self in the face of angry or disappointed fans. Although this is assuredly a worthy life skill, is it really necessary in civilized sport or society?

Which brings us to a consideration of mob behavior and sport. The anonymity and sense of power that come with being a member of an unruly group, in this case at a sporting venue, promote behavior that would otherwise never be considered. The incidents of fan misbehavior, typically of large numbers of people either in eager anticipation of the beginning of an important contest or in celebration of victory, are well known. Breaking through restraining barriers and tearing down goalposts have resulted in significant injuries and even death. Aggressive fan misbehavior shows no signs of extinction, despite improve methods of crowd control. How else to explain these incidents other than that there is a powerful undercurrent of aggression that flows beneath the surface of sport? Liberated by the mob mentality, and often fueled by alcohol, overly aggressive behavior and violence spring forth. It appears that man's best attempts to contain this type of aggressive behavior in and around sport have been and will continue to be, at least at times, insufficient and unsuccessful.

## SUMMARY

Through sport, an individual athlete's psychological development can be promoted and perpetuated. As child, adolescent, and adult development continue, an optimal zone around sport and its attendant aggression should facilitate and further the capacity to be appropriately aggressive in life's many challenging situations. The experiences of sport should then lead people to be able to generalize their experience to other social contexts, in which it will be beneficial to either express or restrain their aggression. Guided and assisted by attentive parents, coaches, and significant others, involvement in sport offers promise for all kinds of athletes, in contrast to current impressions of arrested development and pathology among athletes.

Viewing aggression in its healthy form, in contrast to its extreme and inappropriate versions, and sport as a health-promoting exercise in psychological development and maturation may allow participants and spectators alike to retain an interest in it and derive further enjoyment from it. In addition, it will benefit all involved with sport to have a broader understanding of human aggression. Physicians, mental health professionals, and other health care providers can be influential in this process, and should be willing to get involved and speak out when issues and problems arise.

## References

[1] Diagnostic and statistical manual of mental disorders. 4th edition. Washington (DC): American Psychiatric Association; 1994.

[2] Giancola PR. Difficult temperament, acute alcohol intoxication, and aggressive behavior. Drug Alcohol Depend 2004;74(2):135–45.

[3] Burton RW. Mental illness in athletes. In: Begel D, Burton RW, editors. Sport psychiatry: theory and practice. New York: Norton; 2000. p. 73–4.

[4] Parens H. The development of aggression in early childhood. New York: Aronson; 1979.

[5] Summers FL. Transcending the self: an object relations model of psychoanalytic therapy. Hillsdale (NJ): The Analytic Press; 1999.

[6] Demos V. The early organization of the psyche. In: Barron J, Eagle M, Wolitzky D, editors. Interface of psychoanalysis and psychology. Washington (DC): American Psychological Association; 1992. p. 200–33.

[7] Hanin YL. Successful and poor performance and emotions. In: Hanin YL, editor. Emotions in sport. Champaign (IL): Human Kinetics; 2000. p. 157–87.

[8] Begel D. An overview of sport psychiatry. Am J Psychiatry 1992;149:606–14.

Clin Sports Med 24 (2005) 853–869

# CLINICS IN SPORTS MEDICINE

ELSEVIER
SAUNDERS

# Suicide in Athletes: A Review and Commentary

Antonia L. Baum, MD[a,b,*]

[a]The International Society for Sport Psychiatry, Chicago, IL, USA
[b]George Washington University Medical Center, 2300 Eye Street NW, Washington, DC 20037, USA

Not only are athletes at risk for psychiatric illness, but they are at risk for suicide. Although this act of self-annihilation may seem a stark contrast to the goals and ideals of the athlete, carefully honing his body to perfection, sadly, it is not. Freud [1] described the self-hatred seen in depression as originating from anger toward a love object, which was then turned on the self, with suicide therefore an expression of an earlier desire to kill someone else. It may seem less antithetical, then, to contemplate an athlete's suicide when considering the sometimes extreme aggression in an athlete being turned inward.

When reading accounts of athletes and sporting events, the word suicide frequently comes up, though in an unexpected context. There is the "suicide squeeze play" in baseball, in which, with a runner on third and usually not more than one out, the runner starts for home as soon as the pitcher makes a motion to pitch, and the batter bunts [2]. The "suicide squad" is the kickoff team in football. There are three blockers protecting the player returning the kick, and the mission of the suicide squad is to eliminate those blockers at all costs. In rodeo, a "suicide knot" is the way a bull rider ties his hands to his mount that makes it difficult to free them. Though these are not literal uses of the term suicide, the implication is that the stakes are high in sports, and that winning is do-or-die.

The notion of athletes as immune from the anguish of psychiatric illness—the concept that a sound body is somehow congruent with, or defines, a sound mind—has long been held It is not unusual to read, in the context of an athlete's suicide, that some of the bewilderment is expressed as, "But he was a gifted athlete!" The idea that athletes are not quitters is not mutually exclusive with suicidal behavior. Ron Rothstein, coach of the Miami Heat, had been coaching a New York high school team in back-to-back winless seasons 20 years earlier, and of that time he comments, "I contemplated suicide then, but never quitting [3]."

Suicide is the cause of 1.8% of all deaths. Between 1% and 4% of adults and between 2% and 10% of adolescents have attempted suicide [4]. Although

* 5522 Warwick Place, Chevy Chase, MD 20815. *E-mail address:* Doctorabaum@verizon.net

0278-5919/05/$ – see front matter
doi:10.1016/j.csm.2005.06.006

females more often attempt suicide, males more often complete suicide. Most who complete suicide meet *Diagnostic and Statistical Manual of Mental Disorders, 4th edition* (DSMIV) criteria for a major depressive episode, but just 15% of those who have a major depression commit suicide, whereas up to 25% of untreated bipolars commit suicide [5].

Studies evaluating whether athletes are at increased risk of suicide are inconclusive. In 1996, Kokotailo and colleagues [6] surveyed students at two large Midwestern universities (N = 1210). Evaluating factors including physical risk, mental health, alcohol and drug use, and sexual behavior. They concluded that male athletes demonstrated greater risk than nonathletes, whereas female athletes showed fewer risk behaviors than nonathletes. Paffenberger and coworkers [7], reporting on a 23- to 27-year follow-up period of Harvard alumni aged 35 to 74, found that depression rates appear to be lower among athletes, but that suicide rates were unrelated to physical activity.

Can one make predictions about the at-risk athlete? The professional sporting world would like to think so. Given their increasingly high financial stakes, professional sports organizations are routinely using extensive psychological screens on prospective players. The Wonderlic examination is a 12-minute intelligence test that has been used by scouts for the National Football League (NFL) for more than 30 years. Also used are the California Psychological Inventory, the 16 Personality Factor, a 105 question examination assessing aggressiveness and leadership, and Troutwine's Athletic Profile, which measures how individuals react to situations [8]. The goal is to go for "the right mix of on-field aggression and off-field character. No team wants to draft the next Dimitrius Underwood [a probable bipolar who attempted suicide under the stress of being a first-round draft pick]" [8].

## METHODS

In an effort to learn more about suicide in athletes and others connected to the sports arena, a review of the medical literature from 1966 to 2000 through Medline was conducted, and a review of the periodical literature from 1980 to 2000 through Infotrac was also done. These reviews found 71 athletes who had either contemplated, attempted, or completed suicide. These cases were analyzed by sport, gender, and age. Through inference, an attempt to establish the etiologic basis for these behaviors was undertaken.

## RESULTS

Of the 71 cases related to suicide in athletes, there were 66 completed suicides. The average age among the 71 cases was 22.3 years. There were 61 males and 10 females. The breakdown by sport revealed most to be in football, followed by basketball, swimming, track and field, baseball, and then other sports (Fig. 1).

Etiologic theories were developed and analyzed using the framework of George Engel's biopsychosocial approach [9]. Among the risk factors that appear to have a major influence on athlete suicide are injury, psychosocial stressors, the pressure to win, substance abuse, retirement, Axis I psychopathology, and

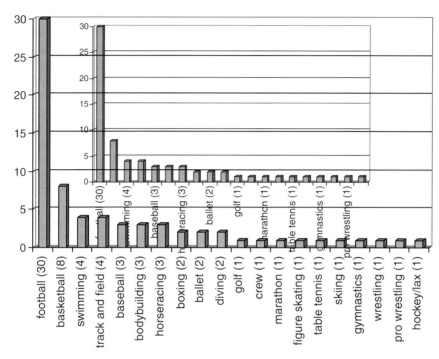

**Fig. 1.** Number of suicides by sport (N = 71).

anabolic steroid abuse. Other factors include a family history of suicide, eating disorder, homosexuality, cultural factors, and increased ownership of firearms by athletes (Fig. 2).

## ETIOLOGY OF SUICIDE IN ATHLETES: PROPOSED RISK FACTORS
### Injury

Physical injury is perhaps the most devastating event in an athlete's career. The body is the athlete's mode of expression, and when the body fails, there is a loss of mastery and control. Injury has been described as "the shattering of dreams, the blow sustained to invincibility" [10]. Through a series of five case reports of injured, suicidal athletes in a 1994 article in the *Journal of Athletic Training*, Smith and Milliner [10] identify risk factors for suicide in injured athletes. These include success in a sport before the injury, a serious injury requiring surgical intervention, a lengthy and difficult rehabilitation process restricting athletic participation for anywhere from 6 weeks to 1 year, the inability to recapture the success that had been attained before the injury, and replacement by teammates. The article authors emphasize the importance of the athletic trainer in identifying at-risk injured athletes (perhaps athletic trainers should have formal psychological training). From an epidemiologic standpoint, this is a population of people who are already at risk, because athletes seen by a trainer are often in

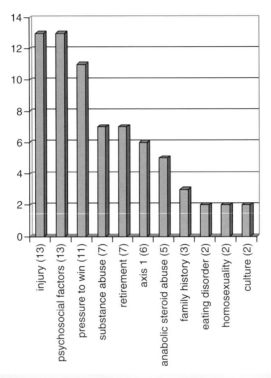

**Fig. 2.** Etiology of suicidal behavior (N = 71).

the 15- to 24-year-old age group, which is the high-risk age group for suicide–in the United States, suicide is the second leading cause of death in this age group. The potential for problems in this population is compounded by the fact that in this age range, there are 10 attempts for every completed suicide [10].

One injury that may have a more direct causal role in suicidal behavior is head injury followed by a postconcussive syndrome. "The core of the person can change from repeated blows to the head ... [better known as] the silent epidemic of football" [11]. Al Toon, a player for the Jets, described his history of concussion: "Each new concussion came from less of a blow, and recovery time increased" [11]. Afterward, Toon "retreated to a dark room for 6 weeks, turned into a recluse and even contemplated suicide. He never played again" [11]. Harry Carson of the New York Giants sustained 12 to 18 concussions in his 21-year career: "I thought I was going crazy ... . I entertained thoughts of suicide ... . I felt like I was in a state of suspended animation. I experienced headaches, anxiety, depression, blurred vision" [12]. Former Duke lineman Ted McNairy committed suicide years after brain deterioration felt to be secondary to repeated blows to the head [12].

The postconcussive syndrome as a potential etiologic factor in suicidal behavior is not an insignificant one. Of the 1.5 million high school football players in the United States, 250,000 have a concussion in a given season. A player who has a concussion is at a fourfold increased risk of sustaining another, in part because some athletes are more susceptible, and also because some players have a tendency to use their heads to block. Concussions on the ball field are probably underreported, both because they can be subtle, and because of football's "rub-dirt-on-it ethos" [11]. Ball players are becoming bigger and faster, and heads have a tendency to bounce off the relatively unforgiving artificial turf. Football's guidelines for returning to play can be more lenient than those of boxing, a sport associated with its own degenerative neurological disorders, notoriously dementia pugilistica. For example, the New Jersey Boxing Commission requires 60 days post-knockout and an electroencephalograph (EEG) before a boxer is allowed to return to the ring [11].

The Emotional Responses of Athletes to Injury Questionnaire (ERAIQ) can be used as an assessment tool to identify those injured athletes who might be at increased risk for suicidal behavior [10].

### Psychosocial Stressors

Anyone can encounter extreme circumstances that may make him vulnerable to suicide, and clearly athletes are not immune. In 1988, when heavyweight boxer Mike Tyson crashed his BMW into a tree, there was speculation that this had been a suicide attempt because of trouble with his wife at the time, actress Robin Givens [13].

Jeff Alm, of the Houston Oilers National Football League team, was speeding under the influence of alcohol, and lost control of his car on an exit ramp on a Texas freeway. His friend—and, some have speculated, his lover—Sean Lynch (a high school football buddy who had just come to town to boost Alm's morale as he prepared to return to the Oilers after a frustrating leg injury) was thrown from the car and died. After placing a frantic 911 call from his car phone, Jeff reached for the gun in his glove compartment and killed himself. "Alm wished that he could turn off the primal impulses that helped him flourish on the football field ... such aggressive behavior has been associated with a heightened risk of suicide" [14].

### Pressure to Win

It is the view of Richard Lapchik, who created the Center for the Study of Sport in Society at Northeastern University in Boston, that "... a disheartening trend among US sports fans is how they label everyone who fails to win a championship as a loser ... . The end of the 1986 baseball season provided ... the worst examples of calling winners 'losers.' In the American League playoffs, California ace Donnie Moore, his team on the verge of a World Series berth, yielded a game-tying home run to Dave Henderson of the Red Sox ... . The pressure was so intense that Moore had a breakdown and finally committed suicide. His wife said the pitch led to it all" [15].

The Canadian professional figure skater Rosalyn Sumner was at one point so depressed about her career that she "literally felt like committing suicide" [16].

Nadia Comaneci, the celebrated Romanian gymnast, attempted suicide at age 15 by drinking bleach. "She does not regret having tried to commit suicide; she does not regret having failed. She was tired. She rested in the hospital for 2 days and was therefore '… glad. Glad because I didn't have to go to the gym for 2 days, so I am happy'" [17]. She has since denied that this incident ever occurred.

Tito Lee was a 19-year-old Nashville football prodigy. He was financially disadvantaged and on a football scholarship at a tony private school. When applying to college, Lee's grades precluded any Division I offers. He went on to junior college, while 6 of his teammates went on to play Division I ball. Lee shot himself in the head [18].

Dartmouth College may never again see a female athlete as talented as Sarah Devens, who was captain of the field hockey, ice hockey, and lacrosse teams. She took a .22 caliber rifle and shot herself in the chest at age 21, not long after being named to the US B field hockey team, quite disappointed not to be on the A team—she also had had an earlier disappointment of failing to make the women's national ice hockey team: "… the stress of high expectations and her own competitive spirit may have contributed to her death by suicide … she seemed to go from game to game and practice to practice without coming up for air … . She told friends that she wanted to take a break, but she didn't dare … . How could she quit sports? Sports was probably the reason she was [at Dartmouth] … ." [19]. Interestingly, "Her blood could not have been bluer," and her family managed to keep a follow-up story about her death out of the Boston Globe [19].

When Greg Barnes, the basketball star of Columbine High School, hanged himself with an electrical cord in his garage at age 17, some blamed it on the fact that he had witnessed a coach bleed to death during the Columbine High School massacre of 1999, and "… assumed that the young man killed himself because of residual trauma from the shootings. Sadly, there are many reasons a young person might take his life, and the pressure of being labeled 'hands down the best schoolboy player coming back next year in Colorado' may have been one of them" [20].

The football coach at Holy Cross College in Massachusetts had had a very successful career; however, he committed suicide in the wake of an unlucky 4-6-1 season, when three of his victories escaped his grasp in the final 2.5 minutes of play [21].

## Substance Abuse

Substance abuse and dependence confer increased risk of suicidal behavior. Athletes are no exception, and may at times be more vulnerable because of the subculture existing in some sports. Walt Sweeny, a former National Football League (NFL) Charger, survived a suicide attempt and 23 hospitalizations for substance abuse. The judge's verdict was: "When the NFL creates such a tragedy … it may not turn its back." He mandated that the NFL's pension fund pay Sweeny $1.8 million. Although this might be viewed as a dangerous precedent, a survey of more than 1000 former players revealed that 1 in 10 felt they had had physical or emotional problems stemming from medications taken while playing professional ball, including steroids, amphetamines, and analgesics [22]. Unfortunately, this verdict was overturned on an appeal in 1997 by a federal district judge [23].

Darryl Strawberry of the Los Angeles Dodgers has had multiple hospitalizations for rehabilitation related to his difficulties with alcohol. He has struggled with back and shoulder injuries, has been arrested for assaulting his girlfriend, and has reported publicly that he has contemplated suicide [24]. Shannon Wright, an Arkansas middle linebacker who had had difficulties with alcohol, cut his wrists several years before completing suicide with a self-inflicted gunshot wound [25].

One of the American Ballet Theater's principle dancers, Patrick Bissell, had a long struggle with drug abuse before committing suicide. Each time he returned to the pressures of the dance world, he would resume his use of cocaine [26].

The pervasive but often hidden practice of hazing in university athletics involves alcohol at least 50% of the time, and often includes physically painful or humiliating demands; some "… have been ordered to exercise until they pass out or to inflict pain on themselves" [27]. It is conceivable that the consequences of such activities could include suicide, in addition to accidental death by overdose or injury.

### Retirement

Retirement for an athlete generally occurs at an earlier phase of development than it does for others. The Eriksonian stages of generativity and ego integrity [9] would ideally have been achieved before retirement. This is unlikely to be true for professional athletes, not only because physical limitations dictate their retirement at a chronologically younger age, but also because the training an athlete typically devotes himself to may preclude the development of emotional maturity.

The transition to retirement for an athlete may be more abrupt and dramatic than for one who does not rely on his body for his livelihood or his identity. Most are not prepared for the financial transition they face with retirement. Sixty-seven percent of retired professional football players suffer permanent injuries, and 20% have marital or emotional problems. "Some ex-players express bitterness over how fans who were so eager to buy them dinners and drinks while they were playing suddenly aren't so interested in them" [22].

Since 1980, seven ex-NFL players have committed suicide after retirement. Mike Wise, a pro lineman for the Los Angeles Raiders and the Cleveland Browns, killed himself just 3 weeks following his waiver by Cleveland. A few days earlier, he had told his fiancée "… that he equated having his name on the waiver wire with having it in an obituary" [28].

As A.E. Housman so eloquently describes in his 1944 poem, "To An Athlete Dying Young" [29]:

> … Smart lad, to slip betimes away
>    From fields where glory does not stay
>    And early though the laurel grows

It withers quicker than the rose.
Eyes the shady night has shut
Cannot see the record cut,
And silence sounds no worse than cheers
After earth has stopped the ears:
Now you will not swell the rout
Of lads that wore their honours out,
Runners whom renown outran
And the name died before the man.
So set, before its echoes fade,
The fleet foot on the sill of shade,
And hold to the low lintel up
The still-defended challenge-cup. ...

## Axis I Psychopathology

There are athletes who have attained a high level of success in spite of a co-existent primary psychiatric disorder (bipolar illness), some who have perhaps chosen the athletic arena as a means of coping with an Axis I disorder (attention deficit hyperactivity disorder [ADHD]), or others for whom psychiatric illness has been engendered through involvement in sport itself (eating disorder) [30].

Anthony Sherrod, a Georgia Tech basketball player reportedly suffering from bipolar illness, did not make it to the National Basketball Association (NBA) and shot himself [31]. Dimitrius Underwood of the Miami Dolphins, who also had bipolar illness, slashed his throat in a suicide attempt under the pressure of being a first-round draft pick [8].

Kenny Wright was a tight end on his high school football team. He shot himself at age 24. His history sounds consistent with ADHD. He did not go on to college: "... as much as the boy adored football, he knew that he couldn't take four more years of studying ... but to be in sports, to be active—that was always what motivated him, diverted him from the less active pleasures of life ... . He could not sit and read or even remain long before the TV ... . Sports put a lot of structure into Kenny's existence ... his grades were invariably better during the football season ... his temper was contained during football ... . And it's true that the only time Kenny really floundered in his life was after he finished school and there was no more football to point to in the fall" [32].

The Olympic diver Wendy Williams had such a severe major depressive episode that she became preoccupied with a finding a method for suicide, often contemplating driving her car off the cliffs of Maui. "I had clinical depression and I've probably had it all my life. It's just that, for most of my life, I couldn't admit to having something wrong. I was an athlete. I was supposed to be able to get over it. Mind over matter" [33]. Williams took the serotonin specific reuptake inhibitor sertraline to good effect (personal communication, 2002).

## Anabolic Steroid Abuse

In 1991 the Cleveland Clinic published a survey of 163 weight lifters, with the finding that of those using anabolic steroids (AS), 7% reported suicidal ideation within 1 month of discontinuing the drug [34]. A similar finding was reported in 1993 in a report on the use of AS [35].

When a 17-year-old body builder shot himself, his sister's view was that "The steroids pulled the trigger" [36]. A University of South Carolina senior defensive lineman, Tommy Chaikin, delivered an affecting first-person account of his experience with AS: "I was sitting in my room at the … dorm … with the barrel of a loaded .357 Magnum pressed under my chin. A .357 is a man's gun, and I knew what it would do to me. My finger twitched on the trigger. I was in bad shape, very bad shape. From the steroids. It had all come down from the steroids, the crap I'd taken to get big and strong and aggressive so I could play this game that I love" [37].

Terry Long, a guard for the Miami Dolphins, attempted suicide after testing positive for AS: "Your name's all over the paper. It's like a nightmare. You're afraid of what your friends and family might think" [38].

## Family History of Suicide

A family legacy of suicide can be a powerful influence on suicidal behavior, genetically as well as prophetically. There are some interesting examples of this among athletes.

Leon Hires III was a senior guard at Florida State. His father, grandfather, and great-grandfather had all shot themselves. Within a week of his father's funeral, he was back on the field but "… his passion for football was gone. Violent collisions brought tears to his eyes. He was an emotional wreck incapable of competing" [39]. He became suicidal, and is now on scraraline for his depression.

Willard Hershberger, a professional baseball player for the Cincinnati Reds, was the inspiration for Bernard Malamud's book *The Natural*. His father had shot himself in the bathroom. "Willard had found him and he was terribly shocked. Something snapped [and] ineluctably led him, 12 years later, to that bathroom in the Copley Plaza Hotel," where he in turn shot himself [40], ironically repeating his father's behavior.

## Eating Disorder

A number of sports have been associated with eating disorder, including aesthetic sports in which scoring is influenced by body shape, sports in which low body fat is advantageous, and sports in which there is a need to achieve a certain weight for competition [41]. The mortality rate associated with anorexia nervosa is 9% to 12%. One third of these deaths are from suicide. Self-annihilation through starvation is arguably a slow form of suicide. Christy Henrich, who had suffered from anorexia and bulimia nervosa, died in 1994 at age 22. She had just missed making the US Olympic gymnastics team in 1988. She weighed 60 pounds at the time of her death [42].

Chantal Bailey contemplated suicide at age 16. She was a figure skater who had anorexia nervosa, purging subtype. She eventually quit figure skating and her eating disorder resolved. "Bailey quickly found out that her 5′8″, 155-pound body was made for speed [43]," and she became an Olympic speed skater. She made an adaptive adjustment in her sport in the service of treating her eating disorder. Early identification of body types appropriate for particular sports is probably an important aspect of prevention.

Mary Wazeter, at Georgetown University on a track scholarship, dropped out after one semester. "The 'terrible thoughts' that drove Mary ... to attempt suicide revolved around food. Striving not just to be but 'to look like a serious runner,' she equated thinner with faster." She jumped from a railroad bridge and is now paralyzed from the waist down. The eating disorder was actually triggered by a hamstring injury; the inactivity created a fear of becoming fat [44].

## Homosexuality

In 1989, the US Department of Health and Human Services Task Force on Youth Suicide reported that homosexuals aged 15 to 24 had a two to three times increased risk of attempting suicide over age-matched heterosexuals [45]. A 1997 study of Massachusetts high school students cited that 46% of gays, lesbians, and bisexuals surveyed had attempted suicide within the last year [46].

There is a consensus that the world of professional sports is severely homophobic. "The most brutal sports, including football, have the tightest locks on their closet door ... . The vulnerability implied in men loving men is not part of the game plan" [47]. Even in the dance world there is a "don't ask, don't' tell" atmosphere. Many express the sentiment that "gay role models in sports would help eliminate stereotypes that they see as a major part of society's problems with homosexuality" [45].

Dave Kopay, a running back in the NFL, was the first professional football player to make his homosexuality known. This occurred 25 years ago, 2 years after he had retired from the sport. He comments: "I now think it may take another 25 years before an all-pro American ballplayer announces he's gay while in the sport ... . Most ballplayers could care less who you screw. It's the hierarchy—the management and marketing people—who get nervous" [47].

Though progress has been slow in the professional ranks, there are changes afoot at lower levels of athletic competition. These changes have been helped along by high school football players such as Greg Congdon, "... who survived two suicide attempts as he reconciled being a high school jock with being gay— [he]had never heard Kopay's story during his struggle" [47].

Ed Gallagher, of the New York Jets, attempted suicide by rolling off the Kensico Dam. He "... hated himself for being trapped in a 6'6", 275-pound offensive lineman's body. He hated the fact that he preferred sex with men, hated how the world liked him as the macho weight-lifting behemoth from Valhalla, NY ... . In the 5 years after his football career ended he grew more sexually repressed, paranoid, hypochondriacal and suicidal ... . Gallagher, 36, is a quadriplegic ... . 'When I went off the dam, I finally came to grips ... . What the hell am I hiding anymore ... . I was more emotionally paralyzed then, and I am physically paralyzed now'" [45].

Figure skater Rudy Galindo "... finds himself an icon to gay men and lesbians who admire his willingness to speak openly about being gay in a sport where homosexuality is often assumed but never discussed" [48]. He will receive letters: "I wanted to commit suicide, but [you] helped me get through it …" [48].

The decorated Olympic diver Greg Louganis was teased in childhood about being gay because of his attraction to dance, acrobatics, and theater. He attempted suicide three times before age 18 [49].

### Cultural Factors

Cultural attitudes toward suicide may influence suicidal behavior in the athletic arena. In Japan, the marathon is a more visible and respected athletic event than it is in many western cultures; "the perfect marathon" is seen as "draining one's body," a form of "ritual suicide" [50]. "Maybe it's the pain in a society that admires the bearing of pain … . The Japanese tend to be very moved by those who try to accomplish something that involves a lot of pain and suffering" [51]. Kokichi Tsuburaya was on medal pace in the 1964 Tokyo Olympic marathon when he was overtaken, thus losing the bronze medal. He felt he had let his country down, and committed suicide 4 years later [52]. Marathon coach Kiyoshi Nakamura, who died by drowning, was thought to have committed suicide in response to his protégé's defeat (he placed fourteenth) in the Los Angeles Olympics [53].

Suicide as a societal problem may have a negative impact on athletic achievement within a culture. Native Americans have a high suicide rate, which may prevent them from becoming serious contenders in the sports world; "Little Indian kids have the same Olympic dreams as white kids … but because of the high suicide rate, poverty and alcoholism, they haven't had the chance to open the door to that realm" [54].

### Firearms

One of the possible contributory factors to suicide in athletes is that increasingly, professional athletes, who are so much in the public eye, are carrying firearms for protection. In 1994, the NBA Player's Association developed a security division; one of their motivations was to educate their players about firearms [55]. Ownership of firearms is associated with a higher risk of suicide, particularly when combined with substance abuse.

### Sexual Abuse

The unique emphasis on the physical in the athletic arena can lead to sexual situations that may create the opportunity for abuse. Sexual abuse can lead to psychiatric sequelae that may put an athlete at risk for suicidal behavior.

Sexual abuse by coaches is not an uncommon occurrence. In particular, there can be "… problematic relationships between male coaches and female athletes … in the intensely physical and emotional world of sports" [56]. Ironically, since the passage and implementation of Title IX, the problem has been compounded; because salaries for coaching women became more lucrative, more males applied for these positions, and the number of female coaches has declined.

An elite tennis coach who had a history of inappropriate sexual advances committed suicide after unsuccessfully attempting to kidnap a 17 year-old former student athlete [56].

Four days after being accused of sexual assault, a Little League coach "sliced open his arms with a knife, called 911 to report his suicide attempt, and died before help could arrive, surrounded by photos of the boys he had coached" [57].

Aggression on the field may at times spill over into sexual aggression off the field. On one college campus, a football player raped the woman who was tutoring him. She contracted herpes, and subsequently committed suicide [58].

## DISCUSSION

That only 71 cases of suicidal behavior among athletes could be extracted from the medical and periodical literature over several decades suggests that there are data that are inaccessible. Given the stigmatization of psychiatric illness and suicide in general, magnified through the lens of the athlete and the world of sports, it is likely that secrecy and shame have prevented more cases from coming to light.

The male to female ratio of 5.5:1 in this sample is more exaggerated than in the general population, in which the rate of male suicide to female suicide is 3:1. This may represent a reporting bias, or the fact that athletics are still male dominated.

The preponderance of cases involving football players may in part be a function of factors unique to football that may enhance risk, including possession of firearms, emphasis on aggression, the culture of substance abuse and anabolic steroid abuse, and the frequency of serious injury. It may also be due to the immense popularity of football in the United States of America, however. The players garner a great deal of publicity and visibility, and therefore more press coverage. This phenomenon suggests that football players experience unique pressures that may put them at risk, and that the change in lifestyle with retirement may be more dramatic than with other athletes.

Self-injurious behavior, which can be regarded as being on a continuum with suicidal behavior, can be seen in athletes. Sports are a culturally sanctioned activity that may distract from pathology, though there is a danger in over-pathologizing as well. "Does the athlete who 'goes for the burn' harbor a secret pathology? ... the athlete who pushes herself to continue despite repeatedly torn ligaments, sprains, or the potential for cardiac arrest ... the differences are not merely a matter of quantity ... but also of motive ... . Often, the behavior develops to the point of being the person's primary method of regulating internal tension or distress" [59].

Extreme sports may also have a place along the continuum toward suicidal behavior. "Suicide can be conceptualized as a gamble, an act in which the individual acts in such away that the probability of death can range anywhere from 0% to 100% ... the parachute jumper has similar opportunities to vary the odds of death in his decision as to when to pull the ripcord ... . One jumper, who had experience in over 100 jumps, opened his reserve chute at 50 feet and was killed on impact" [60]. This is described in a letter published in 1971 reporting on 37 parachuting deaths in the year 1969, 10 of which were apparently due to failure to pull the ripcord [60].

"Suicide can often be performed in a manner that facilitates disguise of the suicidal intent" [60]. BASE (building/antenna/span [(bridge)/earth [cliffs]) jumping, a sport which involves propelling oneself off of the aforementioned structures and parachuting to the ground, has a fatality rate among the highest in sport. Though 46 BASE jumpers have been killed (the sport has a term for a BASE jumper's death: "He's gone in") over the sport's 18 years, it has surged in popularity in this country. It is known as "suicide with a kick" [61].

One extreme skier remarked: "I constantly have death in the back of my mind" [62]. Other extreme sports include mountaineering, gliding, bungee jumping, race car driving, and scuba and cave diving.

## ATHLETICS AS THERAPY

In contrast to these parasuicidal sports, to the stressors inherent in the sporting life, and to the coincidental occurrence of psychopathology in the athlete, athletics can also be seen as therapeutic, and therefore play a role in the prevention of suicide. Although a survey on occupational stress demonstrated an association between depression and substance abuse and sedentary television watching, it revealed an inverse correlation between depression and involvement in athletics [63].

Sports participation can contribute to self esteem. This may be particularly important in adolescent girls, who, in contrast to boys their age, tend to experience low self-esteem "… which can lead to such problems as negative body image, eating disorders and even suicide. Participation in athletics has been shown to promote positive feelings, positive body awareness and the courage to take risks" [64]. Although pregnancy in the adolescent is associated with an increase in the rate of suicide and attempted suicide [65], involvement in sports in the adolescent female has been correlated with the first sexual experience occurring at an older age, with less sexual activity, and with a lower pregnancy rate [41].

Athletic participation can play a preventive role in mental health through the restoration of self-esteem. Before his successful diving career, Greg Louganis had been a gymnast. A knee injury obviated his goal of becoming an Olympic gymnast, and "at 12 … he made a half-hearted attempt to kill himself. He recovered quickly from an overdose of aspirin and [laxatives] … . Conversations with a counselor did not help, but diving became a way of proving that he was someone special" [66]. "… Louganis kept diving competitively because he loved it more than anything else, perhaps because it provided a sanctuary from an abusive stepfather, dyslexia, the ugly taunts he endured because of his Samoan heritage, subsequent teen-age depression, and then three suicide attempts" [67].

For Karen Hartley, her success as a long-distance swimmer has been therapeutic. She survived a difficult childhood—one of ten children, a self described "street person," giving birth at age 14 to a baby she gave up for adoption–culminating in a suicide attempt, for which she was hospitalized for several months, before striking out on her own from age 15. "I'd just go really inside myself … I was a loner … . It helped in the end, because marathoners need to like to do that … . For these swims, you really have to know how to swim well, but I think a larger percentage of it is psychological … . After my breakdown, I had to be tough … . I had tried to kill myself, and I was very distraught that I didn't succeed … . And I felt, after I came out of it, that if I could do that, I could do anything. In a marathon, physical pain is secondary. And that's why I think that the tougher the conditions and the colder the water, the better I do … because I've been through so much before–this can't hurt!" [68].

Jack La Lanne, the California physical fitness pioneer, still going strong at age 90, who considered suicide at age 14 because of his small size and the frequent beatings he sustained as a result, became a legend in the world of fitness [69].

On occasion, there have been athletes inspired to Olympic competition through the suicide of a loved one, including the Canadian synchronized swimmer Sylvie Frechette, who followed through with her participation in the Barcelona Games after her fiancé committed suicide just 1 week before. A runner, he was to have been a track and field television analyst at the games [70]. One year after the suicide of her older brother, who was bipolar, Suzy Favor-Hamilton competed in the 1500 meters in Sydney with renewed motivation [71].

There are also examples of athletes who have served as role models to inspire others not to commit suicide, such as Rudy Galindo, described earlier, in the context of sexual orientation, or Muhammad Ali, who, when he happened upon a young man distraught over his unemployment and threatening to jump off a window ledge, coaxed him down, perhaps by virtue of his stature, and then made an effort to help him in his quest for a job [72]. Former Dallas Cowboy Troy Aikman financed a computer communication system among children in hospitals around the country, with one reported instance of a young basketball player, hospitalized herself, using the system to help another young patient at a distant location who had attempted suicide.

## PREVENTION

Education is perhaps the key to prevention of suicide in the athlete. An awareness of the existence of psychopathology in the athlete is an important first step, one that cannot be taken for granted in a sports culture characterized by denial of emotional frailty. Though efforts by professional teams to predict athletic performance have not necessarily been successful, there may be an ability to get a sense of how a player may respond to "… the varied pressures of professional football" [8].

The preparticipation sports physical may be the only time a young person has any contact with a physician. This is true for 80% of athletes [73]. It makes eminent sense to capitalize on this opportunity to perform a mental health screen on this vulnerable population. Unfortunately, these aspects are usually bypassed in favor of a cursory physical, in which the focus tends to be on the cardiovascular and musculoskeletal conditions that are most often associated with disqualification from athletic participation [74]. Additionally, the setting in which these screens are conducted often does not afford the privacy conducive to eliciting important psychosocial information. There is rarely an established relationship between the doctor and patient, further discouraging this type of discussion [73].

One helpful acronym to be used in the sports physical is STRESSED, or school, teenagers, relatives, economics, safety, sex, emotions, and drugs [75]. This examination is an excellent opportunity to screen for and educate about anabolic steroid abuse and eating disorders, as well as other areas of psychopathology, including depression and ADHD. When necessary, it is important to use the preparticipation examination as a forum to recommend against an athlete's participation in a particular sport. This might reflect a medical problem [73], or a mismatch between the body type of the individual and the sport in question. A physician in this role might be able to help advise a prospective athlete about what sports are logical for his physical makeup. Anticipation in this area could prevent the onset of eating disorders, or of anabolic steroid abuse. There might additionally be concerns about the psychiatric or psychological well-being of an individual with regard to the appropriateness of athletic participation.

Psychoeducational talks to athletes, their families, coaches, trainers, family physicians, and orthopedic surgeons are an important step in promoting the psychiatric health of athletes. A solid and cooperative consultation-liaison relationship among psychiatrists and orthopedic surgeons, coaches, and trainers is a vital part of this equation. With increased awareness comes the ability to anticipate, and then, ideally, to prevent tragic outcomes among those striving to be involved in the athletic arena.

References

[1] Freud S. Mourning and melancholia. The Freud reader. New York: WW Norton; 1995.
[2] Random House dictionary of the English language. 2nd edition, unabridged. New York: Random House; 1987.
[3] McCallum J. Turn up the heat, please. Sports Illustrated 1988;69:54–6.
[4] Jamison KR. Night falls fast—understanding suicide. New York: Alfred A. Knopf; 1999.
[5] Gallagher W. The dark affliction of mind and body. Discover 1986;7:66–74.
[6] Kokotailo PK, Henry BC, Koscik RE, et al. Substance use and other health risk behaviors in collegiate athletes. Clin J Sport Med 1996;6:183–9.
[7] Paffenberger Jr RS, Lee IM, Leung R. Physical activity and personal characteristics associated with depression and suicide in American college men. Acta Psychiatr Scand Suppl 1994;377:16–22.
[8] Hruby P. Tests of character. Insight on the News 2000;16:28.
[9] Sadock BJ, Sadock VA. Human development throughout the life cycle. In: Kaplan HI, Sadock BJ, editors. Synopsis of psychiatry. 5th edition. Baltimore (MD): Willimas & Wilkins; 1988. p. 22, 100.
[10] Smith AM, Milliner EK. Injured athletes and the risk of suicide. J Athl Train 1987;29: 337–41.
[11] Farber M. The worst case. Sports Illustrated 1994;81:38–42.

[12] Green Jr R. Former NFL linebacker Harry Carson says hits to head cause brain woes even years later. Knight-Ridder Tribune News Service June 6, 1997;606K6129.

[13] Anonymous. You did what? Sports Illustrated 1994;80:16.

[14] Tritsch S. I have a buddy dying. Chicago 1994;43:62–8.

[15] Lapchik R. Losing out on their time to shine. The Sporting News 1994;217:8.

[16] Sherman W. The sexy scandalous world of women sports stars. Cosmopolitan 1993;215: 202–6.

[17] Harrison BG. The fall from grace of an angel named Nadia. Life 1990;13:24–32.

[18] Montville L. Nobody saw it coming. Sports Illustrated 1998;89:36–9.

[19] Callahan G, Steptoe S. An end too soon. Time, Inc; 1995.

[20] Beggs J. Tragedy revisited. Sports Illustrated 1995;83:32–5.

[21] Reilly R. A wonderful throwback. Sports Illustrated 1986;65:34–8.

[22] Bayless S. When the cheering stops. Sport 1998;89:70–5.

[23] Finder C. Webster vs. NFL: a family's fight. Pittsburgh Post Gazette March 14, 2005.

[24] Anonymous. Scorecard. Strawberry's jam. Sports Illustrated 1994;80:14.

[25] Frei T. Why? The Sporting News 1993;216:42–4.

[26] Wadler J. Last dance for ballet's tragic prince; Patrick Bissell was a major star of his athletic art, but his hunger for drugs ruined his talent and destroyed him. People (Chicago) 1988;29:22–7.

[27] Rosellini L. The sordid side of college sports: many young athletes are subjected to hazing. US News World Rep 2000;102–3.

[28] Salguero A. NFL retirees cope with many difficulties after playing days are over. Knight-Ridder/Tribune News Service April 5, 1997;405K4688.

[29] Housman AE. "A Shropshire lad." In: The collected poems of AE Housman. New York: Henry Holt and Company; 1944. p. 90–6.

[30] Baum AL. Psychopharmacology in athletes. In: Begel D, Burton RW, editors. Sport psychiatry. New York: WW Norton & Company, Inc; 2000. p. 249–59.

[31] Newman B. The last loud roar; Anthony Sherrod of Georgia Tech dreamed of an NBA career; when reality set in, life became unbearable. Sports Illustrated 1990;72:54–8.

[32] Deford F. Kenny dying young. Sports Illustrated 1981;30–2.

[33] Pucin D. It's a depressing story with an uplifting ending. The Los Angeles Times February 2, 2001.

[34] Bower B. Pumped up and strung out: steroid addiction may haunt the quest for bigger muscles. Sci News 1991;140:30–1.

[35] Yesalis CE, Kennedy NJ, Kopsten AN, et al. Anabolic-androgenic steroid use in the United States. JAMA 1993;270:1217–21.

[36] Brower M. Steroids built Mike Keys up;then they tore him down. People (Chicago) 1989; 31:107–8.

[37] Chaikin T, Telander R. The nightmare of steroids; South Carolina lineman Tommy Chaikin used bodybuilding drugs for three years. They drove him to violence, and nearly to suicide. Sports Illustrated 1988;69:82–96.

[38] Mortensen C. Long struggles in "league of survival." The Sporting News 1991;212:16.

[39] Harry C. Leon Hires III is hoping to end a long history of male suicides in his family. The Orlando News, Knight-Ridder/Tribune News Service July 20, 2000;K2433.

[40] Nack W. The razor's edge; as the Cincinnati Reds chased a pennant in 1940, a dark family legacy tortured the mind of catcher Willard Hershberger. Sports Illustrated 1991; 74:52–61.

[41] Baum AL. Young females in the athletic arena. Child Adolesc Psychiatr Clin N Am 1998; 7(4):745–55.

[42] Huzinec M. Passages. People (Chicago) 1994;42:50.

[43] Robertson L. Speed skating was a way for American Chantal Bailey to get back control of her life. Knight-Ridder/Tribune News Service February 11, 1994;0211K7340.

[44] Levin E. A lethal quest for the winning edge; a runner's grim battle with anorexia nervosa underscores the peril of athletes on starvation diets. People (Chicago) 1983;20:18–22.

[45] Meisel B. Because of a lack of role models, some gay athletes see suicide as the only option. New York Daily News, Knight-Ridder/Tribune News Service July 30, 1993; 0730K4237.

[46] Special report. High school controversial; when two students in Baton Rouge, La. set out to form a Gay-Straight Alliance, they got a real education in the limits of tolerance. Newsweek 2000;135:54.

[47] Foster RD. Still short of the goal. Advocate 2000;60.

[48] Croft TS. Rudy Galindo. Advocate 1998;765:69.

[49] Dolen C. In his own words … Greg Louganis. Knight-Ridder/Tribune News Service November 1, 1999;K0485.

[50] Burfoot A. Home run. Runner's World 1991;26(12):90.

[51] Struck D. They're in it for the long run; Japanese see marathon as a symbol for life. Washington Post August 20, 2000.

[52] Beech H. Medalists with mettle. Time International 1998;150:48.

[53] Neff C. Money talked, nobody walked. Sports Illustrated 1987;66:34–5.

[54] Smith G. Birth of a nation. Sports Illustrated 1992;77:9.

[55] Shappell L. As world becomes more dangerous, increasing numbers of athletes say carrying a handgun has become a necessity. Arizona Republic, Knight-Ridder/Tribune News Service April 2,1994;0402K1935.

[56] Robertson L. Bond is delicate for female athlete, male coach. Knight-Ridder/Tribune News Service January 9,1994;0109K2873.

[57] Special report. Every parent's nightmare: the child molester has found a home in the world of youth sports, where as a coach he can gain the trust and loyalty of kids—and then prey on them. Sports Illustrated 1999;91:40.

[58] Eskenazai G, Quindlen A. Male athletes and sexual assault. Cosmopolitan 1991;210: 220–3.

[59] Conterio K, Lader W, Bloom JK, editors. Drawing the line: what is normal, what is not. In: Bodily harm: the breakthrough treatment program for self injuries. New York: Hyperion; 1998. p. 32–53.

[60] Lester D, Alexander M. Suicide and dangerous sports:parachuting. JAMA 1971; 215:485.

[61] Cover story. Life on the edge; is everyday life too dull: why else would Americans seek risk as never before? Time 1999;154:28.

[62] McCall C. To hell and back. People (Chicago) 1988;30:34–9.

[63] Johnsguard K, Buckley B, Miller B. Peace of mind. Runner's World 1990;25:73–81.

[64] Dooher D. A sporting chance; do girls benefit from sports as boys are said to do? Mpls St. Paul Magazine 1994;22:44–51.

[65] Jorgensen SR, Potts V, Camp B. Project taking charge: six-month follow-up of a pregnancy prevention program for early adolescents. Fam Relat 1993;42:373–80.

[66] Louganis G, Marcus E. Breaking the silence; in a moving memoir, an Olympic champion, facing AIDS, shares the secrets of a lifetime of private anguish. People (Chicago) 1995; 434:64–71.

[67] Wilbon M. A platform of grace and courage. The Sporting News 1995;219:9.

[68] Levin J. Endurance fever. Rolling Stone October 27,1983;61–8.

[69] 20 questions: Jack LaLanne. Playboy 1984;31:120–4.

[70] Farber M. Olympian strength. Sports Illustrated 1992;77:9.

[71] Shipley A. Back in favor after a family tragedy. The Washington Post July 18, 2000; section D:3.

[72] Jet. Muhammad Ali rescues a man. Jet February 5, 1981;52.

[73] Dyment PG. The triple-threat sports exam. Patient Care 1992;26:97–108.

[74] Kurowski K, Chandran S. The preparticipation athletic evaluation. Am Fam Physician 1990;61:2683.

[75] Donahue P. Preparticipation exams: how to detect a teenage crisis. Phys Sportsmed 1990; 18:53–8.

Clin Sports Med 24 (2005) 871–883

# CLINICS IN SPORTS MEDICINE

ELSEVIER
SAUNDERS

# Eating Disorders in Athletes: Managing the Risks

Alan Currie, MD, MPhil, MRCPsych[a,b,c,*], Eric D. Morse, MD[d,e]

[a]The Hadrian Clinic, Newcastle General Hospital, Westgate Road, Newcastle, England NE4 6BE
[b]University of Newcastle, School of Neurology, Neurobiology, and Psychiatry, The Royal Victoria Infirmary, Queen Victoria Road, Newcastle, England NE1 4LP
[c]UK Athletics Ltd, Athletics House, Central Boulevard, Blythe Valley Business Park, Solihull, Birmingham, England B90 8AJ
[d]University of Maryland Baltimore County, 1000 Hilltop Circle, Catonsville, MD 21250, USA
[e]Mental Health Services at University of Maryland College Park, 140 Campus Drive, College Park, MD 20742, USA

There are many potential pitfalls on the road to sporting achievement. In pursuit of excellence, athletes take risks. Many of these risks are calculated and well-managed, but they are risks nonetheless. Athletes risk traumatic and overuse injuries and make personal sacrifices in their education, career, and personal relationships. The well-prepared athlete and his or her support team take steps to minimize these risks in pursuit of a goal.

Since the 1980s it has been apparent that the possibility of developing an eating disorder is to be added to the list of risks to be addressed and managed. Having an eating disorder is associated with considerable morbidity and significant mortality. Athletes who have eating disorders tend to have shorter careers characterized by inconsistency and recurrent injury. How likely is it that an athlete will develop an eating disorder? Who is at risk? Can eating disorders be prevented? How can athletes who have eating disorders be identified? What are the consequences of developing an eating disorder? What action can be taken to help an athlete who has an eating disorder?

## PREVALENCE

Many attempts to quantify how many athletes have an eating disorder have been imprecise for a number of reasons [1]. Using screening instruments to measure prevalence is potentially inaccurate, because some standard rating scales have not been validated in athletic populations [2]. It has been noted that athletes may under-report eating problems and some symptoms more than others [3]. Eating

---

* Corresponding author. The Hadrian Clinic, Newcastle General Hospital, Westgate Road, Newcastle, England NE4 6BE. *E-mail address:* alan.currie@nmht.nhs.uk (A. Currie).

0278-5919/05/$ – see front matter
doi:10.1016/j.csm.2005.05.005
sportsmed.theclinics.com

disorders are not equally prevalent in all sports—sports in which low weight or leanness is related to the esthetic appeal of the sport, sports in which weight is related to performance (endurance sports and in particular running), and "weight-category" sports are associated with a higher prevalence of eating disorders [3–5]. Being an elite athlete may be associated with a lesser risk [5]. Competing successfully may either confer some degree of protection from developing an eating disorder, or may be incompatible with such a serious health problem. For these reasons, studies that use screening tools to examine heterogeneous groups of athletes across a range of sports and performance standards may provide unreliable estimates of prevalence.

Studies in which questionnaires are validated by clinical interviews, which involve large numbers of homogenous groups of athletes, and which contain a control or reference group are limited in number. Sundgot-Borgen and Torstveit's 2004 study [6] is the largest and most recent to meet all of these criteria. This study is also important because it is one of the very few to include male subjects. 1620 elite Norwegian male and female athletes and 1696 control subjects were surveyed by screening questionnaire. All subjects identified as being at risk of an eating disorder were subject to a clinical interview (as were a proportion of those identified as not at risk). Seventy-four percent of those surveyed completed the study. The study was similar in design to a previous study [3], although with approximately three times as many subjects. The latter study confirms the conclusions of the earlier work. The overall prevalence of eating disorders (anorexia nervosa [AN], bulimia nervosa [BN], and eating disorders not otherwise specified [EDNOS]) was 13.5% in the elite athlete group and 4.6% in the control group. Male eating disorder cases (32.4% in the elite group versus 5.4% in the control group) and anorexia nervosa cases (6.5% in the elite group versus 3.6% in the control group) form a more substantial proportion of the athlete group compared with the nonathlete control group. These data are summarized in Table 1.

**Table 1**
Prevalence of eating disorder by subtype

| Athletes | n | Anorexia nervosa | Bulimia nervosa | EDNOS and AA | Total (%) |
|---|---|---|---|---|---|
| male | 687 | 0 | 17 | 38 | 55 (7.7) |
| female | 572 | 11 | 36 | 68 | 115 (20.1) |
| % of cases who are male | 32.4 | | | | |
| % of cases who have anorexia | 6.5 | | | | |
| Controls | | | | | |
| male | 629 | 1 | 1 | 1 | 3 (0.5) |
| female | 574 | 1 | 17 | 34 | 52 (9) |
| % of cases who are male | 5.4 | | | | |
| % of cases who have anorexia | 3.6 | | | | |

Abbreviation: AA, anorexia athletica.
Data from Sundgot-Borgen J, Torstveit MK. Clin J Sport Med 2004;14(1):25–31.

There now seems little doubt that the association between sports participation and eating disorders exists. This represents a significant problem for the health and welfare of large numbers of athletes.

## DIAGNOSIS

According to the American Psychiatric Association's "Diagnostic and Statistical Manual of Mental Disorders, 4th edition" (DSM-IV) [7], AN is characterized by a refusal to maintain a minimally normal weight for age and height (less than 85% of that expected); intense fear of becoming fat despite being underweight; a body image distortion (denial of low body weight); and, in women, amenorrhea (the loss of three consecutive menstrual cycles). There are restricting and binge-eating/purging subtypes, although a mixture of the two is common. BN involves binge-eating with a sense of lack of control and inappropriate compensatory behaviors (purging or fasting) that occur, on average, at least twice a week for 3 months.

The criteria for EDNOS usually involve a similar picture to that of AN or BN. EDNOS may not meet the proper time frame or a part of a criterion for AN or BN, but still causes a general decrease in level of functioning. Binge-eating disorder is considered an EDNOS that involves recurrent episodes of binge eating in the absence of the regular use of inappropriate compensatory behaviors characteristic of BN [7]. Disordered eating is also part of the "female athlete triad," along with amenorrhea and osteoporosis [8]. This combination of pathological weight-control measures and associated hormonal disturbance (producing both the altered menstrual cycle and lower bone density) can have serious consequences, not just for sports participation but also for long-term health. It is especially important to note that although exercise may partially offset bone density changes, it does so only for load-bearing bones.

Many athletes who suffer from eating disorders have a greater lean body mass because of exercise, and may not be below the 85% expected cutoff. There is literature on "anorexia athletica" (AA) that removes the criterion of the 85% cutoff, and therefore it might be considered an EDNOS. Although AA may be a subclinical eating disorder, it can still lead to medical and mental health complications [9]. Sundgot-Borgen [3] set criteria for AA that must involve weight loss, gastrointestinal complaints, the absence of medical or affective disorder explaining the weight loss, excessive fear of becoming obese, and restriction of caloric intake. One of the following symptoms must also be present: delayed puberty, menstrual dysfunction, disturbance in body image, use of purging methods, binge eating, or compulsive exercising. Beals and Manore [9] presented similar criteria, except that distorted body image and limiting food choices or food groups were in the criteria absolutely necessary for diagnosis, and gastrointestinal complaints were in the relative criteria, only one of which is required for diagnosis. Beals and Manore suggested that further research was needed to determine what number of symptoms should be required to meet the criteria for AA. In this special population, the criteria should be validated for AA.

## BOX 1: CHARACTERISTIC FEATURES OF EATING PATTERNS AND CLINICAL SYNDROMES

### Athlete dietary concerns

*Meticulous attention to diet and weight*

*Goal-directed*

    Aim is performance enhancement

    Emphasizes adequate intake rather than restriction (what is needed rather than what is forbidden)

    Likely to "normalize" when sport ceases

### Disordered eating

*Use of pathogenic weight control measures*

    Laxatives, diuretics, enemas, diet pills, stimulants

    Self-induced vomiting

    Excessive exercise (eg, secret or extra training)

    Extreme, restrictive, or "faddy" diets

### Anorexia nervosa core symptoms

*Weight is 85% or less of expected*

*Intense fear of fatness/weight gain (even though underweight)*

*Body image disturbance*

*Amenorrhea*

### Anorexia athletica

*Fear of weight gain although lean*

    Weight is 5% or more below expected

    Muscular development maintains weight above anorexic threshold

    Distorted body image

*Restricted calorie intake*

    Often broken by planned binges

*Excessive or compulsive exercise*

    Often with other pathogenic weight control measures

*Menstrual dysfunction*

    May include delayed puberty

*Gastrointestinal complaints*

### Bulimia nervosa core symptoms

*Recurrent binge eating (excessive quantities with loss of control)*

*Compensatory purging, fasting, or overexercising*

    On average twice per week for 3 months

*Self-evaluation overinfluenced by weight/shape*

**EDNOS**

*Meets some/most clinical criteria*

*Does not meet full criteria for specific disorder*

**Female athlete triad**

*Disordered eating*

*Amenorrhea*

*Osteoporosis (or osteopenia)*

Making the diagnosis of an eating disorder can be a greater challenge in athletes. Denial, maintaining a sense of control, and secrecy are hallmarks of eating disorders. Because athletes are used to playing despite pain, and may have the "no pain, no gain" mentality, they may try to minimize their symptoms. Screening questionnaires may be helpful despite their limitations. A high suspicion for eating disorders is important. Screening for eating disorders should be part of the medical history-taking process for precompetitive physical evaluations. Eating disorders have one of the highest mortality rates of mental illnesses. Death may result from electrolyte abnormalities leading to seizures or arrhythmias.

Symptoms of eating disorders can include obsessions over food, weight, or body image; binging; and fasting. Purging can include self-induced vomiting; excessive exercise; and abuse of laxatives, enemas, diuretics, diet pills, or stimulants. The athlete may express feelings of guilt about eating or being "fat," despite normal weight or after a small meal. Some athletes fear eating with others, preferring to eat alone, or will visit the rest room within minutes of finishing a meal to vomit. Weighing oneself multiple times a day may be an indication. Most athletes will have previously attempted multiple restrictive diets and will have counted calories.

Physical symptoms of eating disorders include dry skin and hair, constipation, cold hands and feet, digestive problems, fatigue or weakness, parotitis, and insomnia [10]. Presentation may not occur until the athlete has a fainting spell due to dehydration, ketosis, or electrolyte imbalances caused by eating disorders. Diminished immune response may lead to complaints of recurrent infections and colds. On examination, the athlete may have a diminished or absent gag reflex and swollen submandibular glands. The diagnosis of an eating disorder may not be suspected until an athlete has a stress fracture with radiographic evidence of osteopenia. Dentists may make the diagnosis if the enamel of the backs of the teeth is worn away by gastric acids. The key features of normal elite athlete dietary attitudes and concerns, and the characteristic features of the principal eating disorder syndromes are listed in Box 1.

## ETIOLOGY

Why do athletes get eating disorders? In large part this is for the same reasons as anyone else does. In addition, there are general etiological factors that are more prevalent in a sporting environment, and factors that are genuinely specific to a particular athletic context; so called "sport-specific factors." In reality, many factors described as sport-specific apply to the general population as well.

In an early review, Wilmore [11] noted how those who have established eating disorders could become drawn to sports. Factors such as characteristics of "athletic" personalities (goal orientation, perfectionism [11], compulsiveness and an ability to block distractions [12]), unusual dieting or eating behavior [13], performance anxiety or negative performance appraisal [14], inappropriate weight loss to aid performance, and a rechanneling of the athlete's considerable drive from sport into eating [12] may combine with nonspecific vulnerability factors to promote the development of an eating disorder in sport. Conversely, in the absence of general vulnerability factors, unusual or apparently disordered eating may be relatively benign and resolve when sports participation ceases [13].

Burton [15] has also emphasized the interaction of athleticism and general vulnerability necessary to promote the development of an eating disorder. In particular, he has emphasized how an athlete's experience of him or herself can become more distanced and detached from reality by participation in sport. This might happen via high technology approaches and preoccupation with physiological parameters and their measurement. If this distancing occurs in an otherwise vulnerable individual, then an eating disorder may result.

It has been suggested that both bodily focus and bodily satisfaction are enhanced by exercise–which might therefore offer some protection against eating disorders. Weight preoccupation (which some sporting environments encourage), on the other hand, increases bodily focus while reducing bodily satisfaction, and therefore increases eating disorder vulnerability [16]. This is consistent with the findings of Smolak and colleagues [17] in their 2000 meta-analysis, which concluded that sports participation could be either a protective or a risk factor in the development of eating problems. Some recent and as yet unpublished data from the United Kingdom and Kenya may shed light on the interrelationship of general vulnerability and sports participation. Hulley and coworkers [18] surveyed four groups: elite UK athletes and nonathletic controls, and elite Kenyan athletes and nonathletic controls. Both UK groups had significantly higher prevalence rates than either Kenyan group, with the rate in UK athletes only marginally exceeding that in UK nonathletes. In the Kenyan groups, athletes had a lower prevalence of eating disorders than non-athletes. This might suggest that in the absence of significant sociocultural pressures, some protection is conferred by sports participation; however, when general vulnerability is at a higher level, the overall rate of eating disorders is significantly higher, with athletes at a marginally increased risk.

The risk and trigger factors operating in athletic populations include early dieting, prolonged dieting, weight fluctuations, early sport-specific training, traumatic events (including injuries), and participating in sports that emphasize leanness (either for esthetic or performance reasons or to "make weight" in weight-category sports) [12,19]. In sports in which aesthetic adjudication prevails, there is an identified need to reflect on setting standards that "compromise the health and well-being of all but the small minority who are constitutionally gaunt" [20]. Beginning early sports-specific training may be a particular vulner-ability factor, because participants may select a sport that is inappropriate to their body type [21]. Male gymnasts, in contrast to their female counterparts, are older, more experienced, and more aware of the need for adequate nutrition to fuel sporting performance. They also have a lower incidence of eating disorders [6]. A further factor may be that the hormonal changes of puberty have different impacts on male and female gymnasts. Increased muscle development in males may have a positive effect on performance. Conversely, pubertal changes in fat deposition in females may have a negative impact on performance for reasons that are at least partly esthetic and arbitrary. In weight-category sports, there is also often a culture of extreme weight loss measures from an early age that is likely to substantially increase subsequent risk [6]. Some athletes learn disordered eating behaviors from their peers. Weight loss may be encouraged or reinforced by teammates, coaches, weigh-ins, (especially group weigh-ins) and percentage body fat analysis.

Compared with their nonsporting counterparts, elite athletes are unusual individuals, subject to unusual pressures, who may therefore adopt unusual dietary practices. At times this will be goal-directed and associated with sporting excellence; however, in the presence of overwhelming pressures, general vulnerability factors, or both, weight-control measures can become pathogenic (disordered eating)—an especially high-risk situation for the subsequent development of an eating disorder.

A consideration of all etiological factors is useful for number of reasons. It illustrates how factors that promote sporting excellence can overlap with those that increase the risk of developing an eating disorder. The concept of a drive being rechanneled is a very useful one in this context. An understanding of which factors are operating in which sports will inform which preventive steps might be useful, the content of coach and athlete educational programs, and ultimately which issues are to be addressed in the therapeutic process for an individual athlete.

## TREATMENT

The ideal way of treating of eating disorders in athletes should involve a team approach that includes coordination and support among sports medicine physicians, athletic trainers, nutritionists, counselors, psychiatrists, coaches, family, and teammates. When the diagnosis of an eating disorder is made, a medical evaluation for safety to continue to play is necessary. Exclusion or deselection from the training group or from competition is only necessary if health or performance is compromised [20]. If participation is considered unsafe, the athlete should be evaluated by a mental health professional immediately, because this news could cause emotional decompensation. The athlete should be referred to a nutritionist to develop a dietary plan and to assist with nutritional assessments and education. Making the athlete's compliance with assessments compulsory for return to competition can assist in engaging the athlete into treatment.

Some basic principles of how an athlete who has an eating disorder should be approached have been described [12,20]. Addressing problems early and directly, but in a supportive and confidential environment, is central. By approaching the athlete as if he or she were injured, the athlete's performance expectations can be lowered in a manner that mitigates against the guilt and disappointment of apparent underperformance [20].

The key competencies of an athlete's therapist have been described as expertise in eating disorders combined with an understanding of sport (importantly, not vice versa) [12]. Sport psychiatrists match multiple types of therapies and sometimes medication to the athlete's symptomatology and personal preferences. For some athletes whose disordered eating habits are new and less frequent, education, hope instillation, encouragement, and continued follow-up might be all the treatment that is required. When symptoms are more severe or long-standing, individual, group, and family therapy are helpful in treating eating disorders [22]. The first step of therapy is establishing a good therapeutic alliance. This involves active listening, taking a good history, expressing empathy, and being supportive. The main goal of the first session is to get the athlete to continue treatment.

Cognitive behavioral therapy (CBT) is effective in treating eating disorders [23]. CBT can be used individually or in groups. The possibility of using athletes-only therapy groups has been suggested [12]. CBT is based on the idea that feelings and behaviors can be changed based on evaluating and challenging cognitive distortions and core beliefs [24]. By identifying what triggers disordered eating behaviors and learning new coping mechanisms and ways to work through difficult feelings, athletes are taught new skills that they can continue to use (sometimes in other aspects of their lives). Athletes have to keep mental logs and do homework with this type of therapy, so their level of motivation for treatment needs to be relatively high.

Ambivalence or resistance to change should be expected, and may be more pronounced if the athlete's disordered eating habits have coincided with weight loss and an initial improvement in performance. Motivational interviewing can be a helpful therapy in trying to move an athlete from precontemplation (when the athlete does not consider his/her disordered eating a problem), to contemplation (when the athlete is considering it to be a problem), to preparation (when the athlete is preparing to change the behavior), to action (trying to change the behavior) and eventually to maintenance (when the athlete is actively working on preventing relapse into disordered eating) [25]. This is the same approach that some sport psychiatrists use to treat addictions in athletes.

Psychodynamic psychotherapy may help the athlete deal with difficult feelings, including the loss of control that can stem from separating from parental figures. The parental figure may be the coach, and this role can eventually transfer to the therapist. This is why involving the family or coach in the therapy sessions can be fruitful.

Because the illness of an eating disorder is usually kept secret, encouraging the athlete to be open and to ask for support from family, friends, coaches, and teammates is an important step in the recovery process. When athletes share their experiences of disordered eating with their teammates, they get not only support but also advice from other athletes who are in recovery. Teammates and coaches can impact athletes getting into and staying in treatment. Intervening with teams by providing education can help to change the climate toward eating disorders.

Sport psychiatrists also prescribe medications to treat eating disorders. Selective serotonin reuptake inhibitors (SSRIs) and atypical antipsychotics (such as olanzapine, risperidone, or quetiapine) have been shown to be effective in the general population [26]. SSRIs may be particularly helpful in treating eating disorders in athletes when there is a large obsessional component. When the obsessional component is clearly limiting the athlete's level of functioning, asking the athlete for the percentage of waking hours spent worrying about weight, body image, diet, or exercise, and if the athlete would like to try to decrease that percentage with an SSRI can be an effective way to encourage a needed medication trial. Medication management should involve discussions about side effects, especially sexual side effects, because they are common reasons for discontinuation and relapse of symptoms.

Several areas of treatment need to be addressed to manage the female athlete triad effectively. Any underlying eating disorder must be identified and treated. If a full eating disorder syndrome is not present, pathogenic weight-control measures still need to be identified and modified. In milder or uncomplicated cases, a small reduction in training load accompanied by a small increase in nutritional intake with calcium and vitamin D supplementation may be sufficient. Occasionally it is necessary to provide estrogen replacement with an oral contraceptive pill [27].

## COMORBIDITIES

The evaluation and treatment of eating disorders requires screening and treatment of comorbid mental illnesses. Excessive exercise is an expected component of eating disorders. Exercise dependence or addiction goes beyond excessive exercise. Despite efforts and instruction not to exercise, athletes who suffer from exercise dependence cannot stop, even in the face of injury. Obsessions about food, body image, or weight are common symptoms of eating disorders, but when they extend to other aspects of life or if there are compulsions unrelated to disordered eating behaviors, then the athlete may be suffering from obsessive-compulsive disorder (OCD). The triad of eating disorders, exercise dependence, and OCD ("the over-doer triad") has been observed by Morse [28] to co-occur, and often requires an SSRI as part of the treatment plan.

Mood disorders are common comorbid mental illnesses of eating disorders. Hormonal and electrolyte abnormalities can contribute to mood fluctuations. Guilt, loss of self-esteem, and feeling out of control are common feelings when disordered eating behaviors worsen; however, when those feelings persist every day, all the time, the athlete may be suffering from depression. The DSM-IV criteria for a major depressive episode require that five of the nine symptoms are met for longer than 2 weeks. A history or current symptoms of mania (bipolar disorder) would change treatment significantly. A low-grade depression for more than 2 years in adults or 1 year in adolescents, called dysthymia (formerly named "minor depression"), can limit functioning and performance. Some athletes who suffer from dysthymia will also suffer from a major depressive episode, a so-called "double depression."

Although some body image distortion is expected with eating disorders, when an athlete complains that a body part is "ugly" or requires cosmetic surgery, the diagnosis of body dysmorphic disorder has to be considered.

Although misusing substances such as diet pills, stimulants, or laxatives is expected with eating disorders, when an athlete is unable to cut down on use, has withdrawal symptoms when not using, develops tolerance, continues to use despite knowledge of the dangers, spends more time focused on using or finding drugs, uses drugs to escape responsibilities, or increases the amounts used over time, then the diagnosis of substance dependence has to be considered. To meet DSM-IV criteria for substance dependence, three or more of these symptoms need to be present for more than 6 months. Other substance use disorders should be ruled out, because athletes may use "downers" such as alcohol or benzodiazepines to counteract the effects of stimulants.

## ORGANIZATION RESPONSE AND CULTURAL CHANGE

Although sports cannot truly be said to cause eating disorders, a sports environment may nonetheless be the context in which an eating disorder develops and becomes established. What then should be the response of those who work in sport?

Preventive steps in gymnastics that have been advocated include increasing the age minimum for competitive participation, training and education for athletes and coaches [29], and the abandonment of routine body composition assessments [30]. Educational programs have been promoted by several authors [6,12,13]. Sundgot-Borgen and Torstveit [6] have suggested that for some low-weight athletes, nutritional education may be all that is required, especially in view of the high prevalence of misinformation regarding diet in athlete populations—so-called "food myths" [21]. Others have stressed the need for screening programs for eating disorders [6,9,12,31] and importantly, the necessary diagnostic evaluation in response to a positive screen [12].

How have sports organizations responded to the increased awareness of eating disorders among their athletes and to these suggestions and recommendations? There are many examples of good practice, and what follows is an illustrative list only.

Sundgot-Borgen and Klungland [32] have described how a program of working with coaches and athletes over an 8-year period was able to reduce the prevalence of eating disorders in cross country skiers from 33% to 15%.

Largely in response to the work of Hulley and Hill [33], the Track and Field Authority in the United Kingdom has developed a comprehensive coach education program in collaboration with an eating disorder charity (The Eating Disorders Association). The program is designed for coaches of endurance runners, is delivered by experienced clinicians, and has been used in other high-risk sports.

The National Collegiate Athletic Association (NCAA) has a range of material available via their website (www.ncaa.org), including guidelines on good coaching practice, how to approach an athlete who has an eating problem, and nutritional guidelines and appropriate weight loss strategies. There is also a specific downloadable reference guide on disordered eating in the high-risk sport of Olympic wrestling, "Wrestling with Weight Loss" (www.ncaa.org/library/sports_sciences/wrestling_with_weight_loss.pdf). Most sports nutrition textbooks now include a section on eating disorders and help to dispel food myths. As an example of this, Jeukendrup [34] has written on weight loss strategies for athletes in a balanced way that minimizes risks, yet acknowledges the link between weight, nutrition, and elite performance, and therefore retains credibility with skeptical athletes and coaches.

Thompson and Sherman [35] have been powerful advocates for eating-disordered athletes to be considered as individuals, and for their eating disorders to be incorporated into a sporting context by therapists. This might even include helping an athlete to return to the sport in which the problem developed. Some treatment facilities have suggested ways to tackle this difficult problem [36]. It is likely to be important, for example, to consider whether an eating disorder is a secondary complication of sports participation or whether sports participation is a component of a primary eating disorder. A return to sport is much more likely to be recommended in the former scenario. A work-up that includes rating scales of eating attitudes (The Eating Disorders Inventory-2 [37]) and personality (the Minnesota Multiphasic Personality Inventory-2 [38]) and assessment of exercise attitudes, depressive symptoms, self-harm, and diagnostic comorbidity will help to indicate whether an athlete falls into a high- or low-risk group for return to exercise.

A return-to-exercise flowchart has been developed that can be incorporated into the treatment contract [35]. In order of priority, the chart covers medical stability, nutritional stability, abstinence from eating disorder behaviors, and finally whether sport is likely to exacerbate psychosocial stressors and therefore increase the probability of relapse.

There are now a range of recommendations and practical steps that can be taken by sports organizations, sports coaches, sports medical professionals, and eating disorder therapists to assist the individual athlete, and potentially to reduce the overall prevalence in high-risk sports.

## SUMMARY

Sport is not to blame for eating disorders. An underlying, general, and non-sports–related vulnerability is necessary for the development of such a multifaceted and multifactorial disorder in an athlete. To blame sports organizations and especially sports coaches may lead to marginalizing the illness, scapegoating, and missing an important preventive opportunity.

Nonetheless, the contribution of the sporting environment needs to be understood in order that organizations and individuals can appreciate their roles and responsibilities. These include adopting practices that reduce risk, identifying problems at an early stage, and facilitating appropriate therapy. In this way, there is a realistic prospect that risks that cannot be eliminated can at least be minimized, contained, and managed.

## References

[1] Byrne S, McLean N. Eating disorder in athletes: a review of the literature. J Sci Med Sport 2001;4(2):145–59.
[2] Sundgot-Borgen J. Eating disorders in female athletes. Sports Med 1994;17(3):176–88.
[3] Sundgot-Borgen J. Prevalence of eating disorders in elite female athletes. Int J Sport Nutr 1993;3(1):29–40.
[4] Byrne S, McLean N. Elite athletes: effects of the pressure to be thin. J Sci Med Sport 2002;5(2):80–94.
[5] Johnson C, Powers PS, Dick R. Athletes and eating disorders: the National Collegiate Athletic Association study. Int J Eat Disord 1999;26(2):179–88.
[6] Sundgot-Borgen J, Torstveit MK. Prevalence of eating disorders in elite athletes is higher than in the general population. Clin J Sport Med 2004;14(1):25–32.
[7] American Psychiatric Association. Diagnostic and statistical manual of mental disorders. 4th edition. Washington (DC): American Psychiatric Association; 2000.
[8] Otic CL, Drinkwater B, Johnson M, et al. ACSM position stand: the female athlete triad. Med Sci Sports Exerc 1997;29(5):1–9.
[9] Beals KA, Manore MM. The prevalence of eating disorders in elite female athletes [review]. Int J Sport Nutr 1994;4(2):175–95.
[10] Halmi K. Eating disorders. In: Sadock BJ, Sadock VA, editors. Kaplan & Sadock's comprehensive textbook of psychiatry. 7th edition. Philadelphia: Lippincott Williams & Wilkens; 2000. p. 1663–76.
[11] Wilmore JH. Eating and weight disorder in the female athlete. Int J Sport Nutr 1991;1: 104–17.
[12] Johnson MD. Disordered eating in active and athletic women. Clin Sports Med 1994; 13(2):255–69.
[13] Leon GR. Eating disorders in female athletes. Sports Med 1991;12(4):219–27.
[14] Williamson DA, Netemeyer RG, Jackson LP, et al. Structural equation modeling of risk factors for the development of eating disorder symptoms in female athletes. Int J Eat Disord 1995;17(4):387–93.
[15] Burton RW. Mental illness in athletes. In: Begel D, Burton RW, editors. Sport psychiatry: theory and practice. New York: WW Norton & Company; 2000. p. 61–81.
[16] Davis C, Fox J. Excessive exercise and weight preoccupation in women. Addict Behav 1993;18:201–11.
[17] Smolak L, Murnen SK, Ruble AE. Female athletes and eating problems; a meta-analysis. Int J Eat Disord 2000;27:37–80.
[18] Hulley A, Hill A, Njenja F, et al. Elite athlete status and culture: interactive influences on eating disorder development. Presented at the Conference of the North American Society for the Psychology of Sport and Physical Activity. St Pete's Beach, Florida, June 9–11, 2005.
[19] Sundgot-Borgen J. Risk and trigger factors for the development of eating disorders in female elite athletes. Med Sci Sports Exerc 1994;26(4):414–9.

[20] Garner DM, Rosen LW, Barry D. Eating disorders among athletes. Research and recommendations. Child Adolesc Psychiatr Clin N Am 1998;7(4):839–57.

[21] Sundgot-Borgen J. Eating disorders, energy intake, training volume and menstrual function in high level modern rhythmic gymnasts. Int J Sport Nutr 1996;6(2):100–9.

[22] Sim LA, Sadowski CM, Whiteside SP, et al. Family-based therapy for adolescents with anorexia nervosa. Mayo Clin Proc 2004;79(10):1305–8.

[23] Fassino S, Piero A, Levi M, et al. Psychological treatment of eating disorders. A review of the literature. Panminerva Med 2004;46(3):189–98.

[24] Williamson DA, White MA, York-Crowe E, et al. Cognitive-behavioral theories of eating disorders. Behav Modif 2004;28(6):711–38.

[25] Wilson GT, Schlam TR. The transtheoretical model of motivational interviewing in the treatment of eating and weight disorders [review]. Clin Psychol Rev 2004;24(3):361–78.

[26] Power PS, Santana C. Available pharmacological treatments for anorexia nervosa. Expert Opin Pharmacother 2004;5(11):2287–92.

[27] Birch K. Female athlete triad. BMJ 2005;330:244–6.

[28] Morse E.D. Eating disorders in athletes. Presentation given at the International Society for Sport Psychiatry's scientific session at the American Psychiatric Association annual meeting. New York, May 2, 2004.

[29] Powers PS, Johnson C. Small victories: prevention of eating disorders among athletes. Eating Disorders: The Journal of Treatment and Prevention 1996;4(4):364–76.

[30] Carson JD, Bridges E. Abandoning routine body composition assessment: a strategy to disordered eating among female athletes & dancers. Clin J Sport Med 2001;11(4):280.

[31] Rumball JS, Lebrun CM. Preparticipation physical examination: selected issues for the female athlete. Clin J Sport Med 2004;14(3):153–60.

[32] Sundgot-Burgen J, Klungland M. The female athlete triad and the effect of preventative work. Med Sci Sports Exerc 1998;30(Suppl 5):S181.

[33] Hulley AJ, Hill AJ. Eating disorder and health in elite women distance runners. Int J Eat Disord 2001;30(3):312–7.

[34] Jeukendrup A. Weight loss strategies for athletes. In: Sportscience. Available at: www.ukathletics.net. Accessed 2003.

[35] Thompson RA, Sherman RT. Helping athletes with eating disorders. Champaign (IL): Human Kinetics; 1993.

[36] Littlefield K, Zuercher RD. Recommendations for athletes returning to training/competition following an eating disorder. Presented at the 1st Academy for Eating Disorders Athlete Special Interest Group Conference. Indianapolis, Indiana, September 9, 2003.

[37] Garner DM. The Eating Disorders Inventory-2 professional manual. Odessa (FL): Psychological Assessment Resources; 1991.

[38] Butcher JM, Dahlstrom WG, Graham JR, et al. MMPI-2: manual for administration and scoring. Minneapolis (MN): University of Minnesota Press; 1989.

Clin Sports Med 24 (2005) 885–897

# CLINICS IN SPORTS MEDICINE

ELSEVIER
SAUNDERS

# Substance Use in Athletics: A Sports Psychiatry Perspective

David R. McDuff, MD[a],*, David Baron, DO[b]

[a]Division of Alcohol and Drug Abuse, Department of Psychiatry, University of Maryland School of Medicine, 701 West Pratt Street, Baltimore, MD 21201, USA
[b]Department of Psychiatry, Temple University School of Medicine, Philadelphia, PA 19140, USA

Professional and other elite athletes use some substances at higher rates than nonathletes in the general population [1–7]. This is especially true for substances that have actual or perceived positive impacts on athletic performance. Substances such as anabolic androgenic steroids, amphetamines, human growth hormone, or erythropoietin that combat fatigue, relieve pain, enhance injury recovery, alter intensity and aggression, sharpen focus, increase strength and endurance, or reduce or add weight are the most attractive (Fig. 1). Although these "performance-enhancing" substances may objectively or subjectively aid performance, they may also produce negative effects at higher dosages [8–15]. Other substances such as alcohol, marijuana, cocaine, or club drugs are used or abused for the same reasons by athletes as nonathletes. The reasons for starting these "drugs of abuse" (ie, fit in, boost self-confidence, produce pleasure, escape problems, have fun) are not always the same as for continued use (ie, stress relief, psychological dependence, negative emotions reduction, tolerance/withdrawal). Tobacco, especially if it contains high dosages of nicotine, can be viewed as either a drug of abuse or a performance enhancer (see Fig. 1).

This article focuses on the most common substances seen in professional, Olympic, and collegiate athletes; namely alcohol, tobacco, stimulants, and steroids. The prevalence and patterns of use, performance and health effects, and preventive and treatment interventions for each are discussed. For alcohol, its basic pharmacology and adverse effects on athletic performance through dehydration, hangover, insomnia, fights, and weight gain are emphasized [16–19]. The value of urine alcohol testing to reduce heavy drinking is discussed. For stimulants, the chemical structures of ephedrine, synephrine, phenylpropanolamine, and amphetamines are presented. The risks of "stimulant stacking" (ie, caffeine, nicotine, synephrine, amphetamine) and "upper-downer" pairings such as amphetamine and alcohol/marijuana are highlighted. Preventive efforts to

* Corresponding author. 4618 Brentwood Lane, Ellicott City, MD 21042. E-mail address: dmcduff52@yahoo.com (D.R. McDuff).

0278-5919/05/$ – see front matter
doi:10.1016/j.csm.2005.06.004

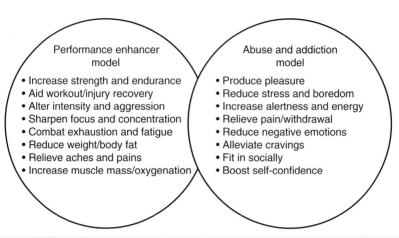

**Fig. 1.** Substances and athletics: reasons for use.

reduce stimulant use with several teams are described, and the problem of stimulant-induced insomnia and anxiety is discussed [20,21]. For tobacco, the patterns of use in baseball, football, and other sports are described. An organized prevention and early intervention program involving the team dentist is detailed. Successful substitutes for spit tobacco (moist snuff and chewing tobacco) are described [22–26]. For steroids, the complex issues of supplement contamination, adverse effects, designer drug detection, and prevention policy are reviewed [27–31]. The proper balance between sanctions and clinical interventions is discussed. For each of these substances, the different perspectives between addictive and performance-enhancing substances are used to highlight effective interventions.

## ALCOHOL

Beverage alcohol is a simple organic compound that easily crosses the blood-brain barrier quickly, affecting brain centers for balance and coordination, fluid retention, judgment and reasoning, emotional control, level of alertness, sexual interest, and socialization. Studies of the general population show that approximately 75% to 80% of young adults use alcohol, and that approximately 15% to 20% are heavy drinkers or binge drinkers [32]. Rates of alcohol use among college athletes are higher than the general public, with use rates for men of 75% to 93% and for women of 71% to 93% [32]. Use rates do differ by sport—swimming/diving, soccer, and baseball/softball rates are higher than basketball, volleyball, and track and field rates. Binge drinking is also more common among athletes compared with nonathletes, with recent episodic heavy drinking rates of 25% to 50% for athletes, compared with 16% to 43% for nonathletes [33].

Motivation to drink alcohol is usually divided into social, coping, hedonistic, or performance categories. Athletes cite all these reasons, and there is some evidence that these may differ by sport [33,34]. The National Collegiate Athletic

Association (NCAA) 2001 study [33] shows that college athletes drink mostly for social reasons (83.9%) compared with feeling good (12.9%), coping (3%), or performance (0.2%). Martens [34], however, demonstrates higher performance enhancement motives, especially among swimmers and divers. In addition, swimmers and divers and basketball players have higher levels of social motivation than track/cross-country athletes.

Alcohol use among athletes is associated with negative general health and athletic performance consequences. College athletes, for example, cite alcohol as the most negative substance on performance and health. Surprisingly, its harmful effects are cited two to three times more often than those of cigarettes, spit tobacco, or marijuana [33]. Injury rates among regular drinking athletes are also higher than among nondrinking athletes. One study [16] showed that athletes who drank at least weekly had injury rates that were twice those of nondrinkers (54.8% versus 23.5%). A recent study by Martens and colleagues [35] demonstrates that athletes who drink for coping reasons have more negative consequences than those who drink for other reasons.

Alcohol adversely impacts athletic performance in a number of different ways. Previous research has shown that alcohol consumption in the 24 hours before athletic activity significantly reduces aerobic performance, by about 11.4% [36]. This might not be significant, except that drinking the day before training and competition is extremely common, with rates by sport ranging from 18% to 84%. The lowest rates are seen for cycling, horse racing, and tennis, whereas the highest rates are seen in football, rugby, basketball, soccer, and golf [16]. Alcohol's negative effects on aerobic performance and psychomotor skills are thought to be due to its slow/fixed rate of metabolism (zero order kinetics) and its toxic interference with energy and carbohydrate metabolism. Additional negative effects come through dehydration, mood instability, and sensory motor system dysfunction. Interestingly, this "hangover effect" is seen even in low doses of just a few standard drinks, and may last from 24 to 36 hours, depending on its severity [16]. Alcohol is also poor nutritionally. Although it provides seven calories of energy per gram, it does not replace expended carbohydrates, and is often associated with significant weight gain caused by its "empty calories."

Alcohol can also adversely effect performance by interfering with sleep, disinhibiting aggression, and increasing high-risk behaviors such as drinking and driving, gambling, illicit drug use, or sexual promiscuity. Alcohol is notorious for its toxic effect on sleep. It is common for an intoxicated person to awaken 3 to 5 hours after falling asleep. This prevents adequate restoration, and can impair motor performance, concentration, and attentional shifting the following day. Some persons become aggressive or exercise poor judgment when intoxicated. Fights and injuries to the hands, wrists, and jaw are common. Negative behaviors such as those cited above can lead to arrest or suspension.

The authors discover heavy drinking in athletes in several ways. Any alcohol-related arrest or negative behavioral incident leads to automatic evaluation by a team assistance program professional. Referrals also come from concerned teammates, coaching staff, or the team's physicians and trainers. Heavy spit tobacco users often use alcohol heavily. Individuals who test positive for an illicit or performance enhancing drug are also more likely to be misusing alcohol. The University of Maryland's team assistance programs have found it especially useful to include alcohol in our urine testing program. When an athlete tests positive on a late morning or early afternoon test, it means that heavy drinking occurred the night before. Because alcohol's elimination is fixed at about one drink per hour, the quantitative results and the history can be used to determine the approximate peak blood alcohol concentration and number of standard drinks consumed.

## STIMULANTS

The use of amphetamines by athletes in the United States dates back to the 1940s for football and to the late 1950s for other sports [20]. Despite the lack of strong scientific evidence of a positive effect on athletic performance, amphetamines quickly became the most popular ergogenic aids, because of their demonstrated and perceived positive effects on self-confidence, mood, attention, aggression, and energy. Over-the-counter (OTC) stimulants such as phenylpropanolamine, ephedrine, and pseudoephedrine became regular substitutes for amphetamines after the passage of the Controlled Substances act of 1970. Although these sympathomimetic amines are not as potent as amphetamines, when used in combination with caffeine they became quite popular. The use of these OTC amphetamine "look-alikes" further expanded after the passage of the Dietary Supplement Health and Education Act of 1994 [9,20]. This act did not require manufacturers to prove the safety or effectiveness of their products. Consequently, the use of these OTC supplements for weight loss and athletic performance enhancement exploded, despite existing safety concerns. In 2000 and 2004 these safety concerns were fully recognized, when the Food and Drug Administration banned the sale of phenylpropanolamine and ephedra-containing supplements because of adverse events including sudden death, heat stroke, cerebrovascular accident, serious arrthymias, myocardial infarction, seizure, and serious psychiatric illness [11,21]. As soon as ephedra was removed from retail and internet suppliers, however, it was quickly replaced by bitter orange (*Citrus aurantium*), another sympathomimetic amine that contains synephrine. Because the chemical structures of amphetamine and these look-alikes are quite similar, it is no wonder that they are associated with similar risks and benefits (Fig. 2). In the last few years, the use of a new class of stimulants, the so-called "eugeroics" or "good arousal" drugs, has increased. The two drugs from this class, modafinal and adrafinil, were developed in France to treat narcolepsy and hypersomnia. Only modafinil is legally available in the United States, but both are easily obtained via internet pharmacies. Compared with amphetamine-like stimulants, they are marketed as having low abuse liability and fewer side effects such as insomnia, anxiety, and agitation. This is reportedly due to selective stimulation of noradrenergic neurons in the hypothalamus and brain stem [37,38]. Because these drugs are not chemically similar to amphetamine, they will not typically be picked up on stimulant urine drug testing.

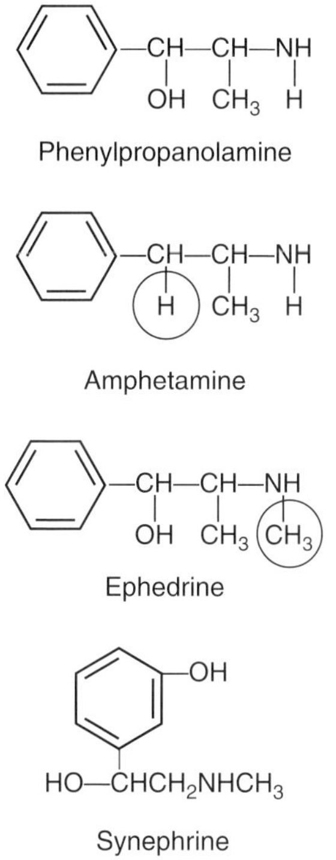

Phenylpropanolamine

Amphetamine

Ephedrine

Synephrine

**Fig. 1.** Chemical structures of amphetamine substitutes.

Much lower rates of about 5% or less have been seen over 10 years from the University of Maryland's team assistance urine drug testing program. Media and former player claims that 60% to 80% of baseball players use amphetamines are clearly exaggerations [39]. Much lower rates of about 5% or less have been seen from urine drug testing. This seems too low, however, because about 3.3% of college athletes in 2001 and 10% of 12th graders, 7% of college students, and 6% of young adults in 2003 self-reported amphetamine use [32,33,40]. Additionally, 3.9% of college athletes reported using ephedrine. For college athletes, social and personal reasons were the most common primary reason for use (27.4%), followed by performance improvement (23.8%), energy boost (21.5%), and weight loss (11.7%). Interestingly, for college athletes, use of amphetamines and ephedrine were more common in men for power sports (football, lacrosse, wrestling) and for those requiring enhanced concentration (rifle, fencing). For women, stimulant use was more common in ice hockey, gymnastics, and field sports (soccer, field hockey). Rates for women's sports were higher than for men for ephedrine but lower for amphetamines.

The adverse effects of regular amphetamine and other sympathomimetic stimulant use are quite relevant to athletic performance. The most common are anxiety, insomnia, tremulousness, irritability, and weight loss. Even though these effects are common and dose-related, when asked, athletes note more positive than negative effects. For college athletes, almost twice as many noted amphetamines to have a helpful rather than harmful effect on performance, whereas more than twice as many noted them to be harmful rather than helpful on health [33]. In the authors' practices with elite athletes, the most common problems that we have seen are insomnia and substance-induced panic attacks or generalized anxiety. In these cases, athletes were usually using high dosages of caffeine (>500 mg/day), nicotine, and either ephedrine or amphetamine [41]. In addition, many were also drinking alcohol regularly to counteract the side effects of the stimulant stacking. Some were also using short-acting soporifics such as zolpiderm or zaleplon. For insomnia, we are able to get athletes to reduce their stimulant use through informed discussion and improved sleep hygiene. For several cases of stimulant panic, we also used low-dose benzodiazepines short-term and then selective serotonin reuptake inhibitors later. To prevent these problems, we give regular preseason and in-season talks. After each, players will routinely bring us their stimulant-containing supplements and ask for advice about continued use.

## SPIT TOBACCO

Spit tobacco, primarily as moist snuff, is used extensively by male professional and collegiate athletes. In professional baseball, prevalence rates of 35% to 40% are seen, and even higher rates of 40% to 50% are reported for college baseball players [22,23,33,42,43]. Current rates of use in professional football players are estimated to be 20% to 30%, and rates in college were 35.6% in 1993 and 28.9% in 2001 [33]. Other male collegiate sports that had high rates of use in 2001 were wrestling (38.6%), ice hockey (35%), and lacrosse (32.2%) [33]. For professional athletes, the most common reasons cited for spit tobacco use are: (1) pregame and postgame relaxation, (2) improve concentration and focus, (3) relieve boredom, (4) boost energy/combat fatigue, (5) habit—need to have something in my mouth, (6) handling—dip and tin, (7) relieve withdrawal symptoms, and (8) improve performance. These are in contrast to those reported by college baseball players in a structured survey [33]. They cited recreational or social reasons (47.9%), pleasure (28%), stress relief (22.8%), and performance enhancement (1.4%). In sharp contrast with the positive reports on athletic performance that the authors receive from professional athletes, college athletes reported that spit tobacco use was nearly 20 times more likely to have no effect, and nearly twice as likely to have a harmful effect as a positive effect on performance.

Most athletes who use spit tobacco prefer brands that are more alkaline and therefore have more nicotine available for absorption. Remarkably, snuff's nicotine bioavailability can vary from 3% to 90%, depending on whether the additives make it more acid or alkaline [42,44]. This makes pH a much more potent variable for nicotine absorption than even the size of the dip or the fineness of the cut. Use can vary from a 30-gram tin every few days for those that use only when practicing or competing, to more than a tin a day for hard-core users. The best indication of nicotine dependence is use throughout the day, especially within 30 minutes of awakening and just before bedtime.

Spit tobacco users can develop many adverse health effects, including oral cancer, oral leukoplakia, caries, periodontal disease, hypertension, cardiovascular disease, sexual impotence, gastric ulcers, anxiety, insomnia, and nicotine addiction [42]. College athletes report that spit tobacco use is 20 times more likely to have a negative effect on general health than a positive one. These effects ,especially oral lesions, anxiety, and insomnia, are very helpful in getting athletes interested in cutting down or quitting [33,42]. One of the most effective approaches to tobacco cessation in high school, college, and professional athletes involves a dental examination and a brief motivational intervention by a dental hygienist [42,43,45]. One-year quit rates of 10% to 35% are seen after this type of intervention. The University of Maryland has supplemented this approach with a referral to our team assistance program (TAP). The TAP staff includes several addiction psychiatrists who are present during the preseason and throughout the season, and are able to prescribe nicotine replacement, buproprion, or antidepressant/anti-anxiety agents if needed. In addition, we provide ongoing relapse counseling targeting stress and craving control. We have discovered that many long-term users can stop during the season, but only if they find an effective oral substitute. Examples have included herbal snuff, nicotine gum, chewing gum, hard candy, plastic cigar tips, sunflower seeds, aromatic hardwood branches, and a low nitrosamine, spitless tobacco pellet.

## STEROIDS

The history of anabolic steroid abuse in American began in weight lifting [4,46]. Bob Hoffman, a World War I veteran, invented the barbell in 1923 and later established the famous York Barbell Company and Gym in York, Pennsylvania. His success as a trainer in York eventually led to him being named the head coach of the US Olympic weight lifting team. Mr. Hoffman became friends with John Ziegler, a physician from Maryland who trained at Hoffman's gym. As a result of this contact, Hoffman appointed Ziegler as the Olympic weight lifting team physician. At the 1954 World Championships in Vienna, Hoffman met a Soviet colleague who told him of a synthetic form of testosterone that produced dramatic improvements in strength and power. Ciba Pharmaceuticals provided Zeigler with this steroid and Nazi research records that had been confiscated by the United States after the War.

Ziegler decided to study its effect in weightlifting athletes. This resulted in the first mass-produced anabolic steroid, methandrostenalone, in 1958. Ziegler gave the steroid to the entire US Olympic weight lifting team in the 1960 Rome games, but still lost to the Soviets. They had already developed the next generation of anabolic performance enhancers. Although this was not in violation of existing Olympic rules, it was clearly inconsistent with the spirit of the Games or the Olympic Code. After the 1960 Games, York became the Mecca of US weightlifting. Former York lifters went on to become strength and conditioning coaches across the United States, taking what they had learned from Dr. Ziegler about anabolic steroids with them. By 1968, the use of anabolic steroids had become so common in Olympic competition that routine urine testing was instituted [4]. Dr. Ziegler died in 1984. Just before his death he was quoted as saying, "All those young kids, what a terrible price they'll pay. If only I'd known it would come to this. I wish to God I'd never done it" [46].

The use of anabolic steroids became widespread in Olympic and professional sports through the 1970s and 80s. Their use in football eventually led the National Football League to begin urine testing in 1987, and to impose sanctions in 1989. Nonusing players who wanted to "level the playing field" initiated this policy change. Finally, in 1990 the Anabolic Steroid Control Act was passed, placing anabolic steroids on Schedule III and requiring prescription by a physician. This act and the passage of the Dietary Supplement Health and Education Act in 1994 promoted a shift away from illegal anabolic steroids to legal nutritional supplements. Those supplements contained testosterone precursors or prohormones such as androstendione or dihydroepiandrosterone (DHEA). Studies of androstenedione have yielded conflicting results as to whether its use actually increases serum testosterone [4,47,48]. Other studies have shown that the dosages and contents of these supplements as reported on their labels may not be accurate, leading to the possibility of positive urines from contamination [5]. In the past few years with the Bay Area Laboratory Co-Operative (BALCO) steroid scandal in track and field and baseball, the important issue of designer steroids and other strategies to test negative has surfaced. Tetrahydogestrinone (THG), the active ingredient of the BALCO clear oral liquid was identified by the University of California at Los Angeles (UCLA) Olympic laboratory from syringe residue discovered at a US track and field meet. Although it took several months to identify this new anabolic steroid, it was eventually determined to be chemically similar to gestrinone and trembolone [49]. The BALCO body cream, on the other hand, was determined to contain both testosterone and epitestosterone. This combination presumably was designed to mask steroid use by keeping the ratio of testosterone to epitestosterone in the normal range (ie, under 6:1). The discovery of these compounds and their use in baseball led to the January 2005 changes in major league baseball's steroid testing and sanctions policy.

Anabolic androgenic steroids (AAS) are synthetic derivatives of testosterone. They induce protein synthesis in muscle cells and stimulate the release of growth hormone, which has robust anabolic effects. In addition to potent anticatabolic effects, these compounds allow athletes to overtrain and to achieve dramatic increases in muscle size and strength. Once training is stopped, size and strength gains rapidly disappear [50]. Steroid-abusing athletes report a dramatic increase in training and a faster recovery time. Ariel and Seville [51] demonstrated a significant placebo effect in competitive weight lifters who got stronger than matched controls when given placebos thought to be AAS. In addition to their strength effects, AAS have psychiatric side effects [14,15]. Interpreting the extant literature on psychiatric side effects is problematic. Doses used in clinical trials rarely reflect the supratherapeutic psychiatric doses by abusing athletes. Despite methodologic variations, the most consistent clinical psychiatric findings are increased hostility, aggression, irritability, and mood lability [52,53]. Pope and Katz [13], two of the leading steroid abuse researchers, evaluated 88 athletes using AAS. This nonblinded, retrospective, self-report survey study revealed that 23% of respondents reported major mood syndromes—12% with psychotic symptoms and 8% with drug dependence. No control group was used. Other self-reported effects are increased sex drive, acne vulagris, gynecomastia, and increased body hair [15]. Despite over half a century of steroid abuse by athletes, however, much remains to be learned about the long-term effects when taken in very high doses and combined with intensive physical training.

The current prevalence of AAS use in professional athletics has been greatly exaggerated in the media. In the 2003 major league baseball survey the urine positive rate was 5% to 7%, rather than the 40% to 50% suggested by former players. Admittedly the rate could be an underestimate, because survey testing was done only once during the playing season for each player on the 40-man roster; however, because testing was not tied to individuals as it was in 2004, it might not have had as strong a deterrent effect. The experience in minor league baseball, where steroid testing began in 2001, shows that urine drug testing and sanctions have a deterrent effect. Positive rates, 9% in the first year of testing [54], have dropped significantly.

Results from male college athletes in the 2001 NCAA report show that self-reported rates of use vary greatly by sport [33]. The lowest rates are seen in swimming (0.2%), soccer (0.9%), and gymnastics (1.1%), whereas the highest rates are in water polo (5.0%), football (3.0%), baseball (2.3%), and lacrosse (2.2%). Rates in football dropped dramatically from 9.7% in 1989, to 5.0% in 1993, to 2.2% in 1997, before rising to 3.0% in 2001. Women's use rates were much lower, ranging from 0.0% in several sports (field hockey, gymnastics, track and field, tennis) to 1.3% in swimming and 1.6% in lacrosse. Surprisingly, the average use rate for all sports of 1.4% is lower than self-reported community use rate of 2.4% in 12th graders for the same year [32]. The most common reasons for AAS use in this report were performance improvement (42.7%), appearance improvement (19.8%), and injury rehabilitation (16.7%).

The professional athletes that the authors see are referred for evaluation after a positive urine test. This provides an opportunity to discuss AAS initiation, recent patterns of use, and the impact on health and performance. A balanced discussion of the risks and benefits, with an emphasis on graduated sanctions, seems the best preventive approach. So far we have seen no cases of steroid dependence in baseball or football, and only one in another sport (competitive bodybuilding).

## DISCUSSION

Athletes use substances to produce pleasure, relieve pain and stress, improve socialization, recover from injury, and enhance performance. Given that the rates of use for many substances are substantially higher than in nonathletes, it is not clear whether this can be explained using abuse/addiction or performance enhancement models. Athletes may certainly develop substance-use disorders just as nonathletes do; however, the most common performance-enhancing substances (stimulants and steroids) have low addictive potential, despite moderate levels of neurobehavioral toxicity [55]. Because the most addictive substances (alcohol and tobacco) are often used episodically and the patterns of use can change dramatically from the playing season to the off-season, the rates of substance dependence may be kept low. An important clinical question is whether the treatment of athletes who have a substance-use disorder should in any way differ from the treatment of nonathletes? Also, should performance-enhancing drug abuse be viewed in the same way as alcohol, tobacco, marijuana, or cocaine abuse? In this article the authors have reviewed the existing literature on substance use in athletes, and we recommend future research into this highly emotionally charged topic.

Over the past 25 years, psychiatry has made great strides in understanding the complex interaction of biological and psychosocial factors that ultimately lead to drug abuse. Although there is much work to be done, clinical and basic research funded largely by the two National Institutes of Health (NIH) agencies responsible for studying this problem (National Institute on Drug Abuse [NIDA] and National Institute on Alcohol Abuse and Alcoholism [NIAAA]) have helped create the current interest in the science of addiction and abuse. This, in turn, has helped clinicians deal with the ever-present problem of stigma on drug abusers. Slowly but surely, the medical community and general population are realizing that drug abuse is not merely the result of a flaw in the moral fiber of the abuser, but a true medical/psychiatric disorder. This issue becomes even more problematic when an athlete is involved. World class and professional athletes are held to a higher standard by their adoring fans. When a prominent athlete is caught using drugs, it is a newsworthy event and almost always made very public. This is not the case for other professionals, such as doctors and lawyers, who strive to maintain confidentiality when one of their own has a drug problem. Why are athletes held to a higher standard? Conventional wisdom declares that athletes are role models who are looked up to by our youth, and who by setting this bad example may be encouraging drug use by others. Well-conducted survey research confirming this point is currently nonexistent. This is a very important point that needs to be addressed in future research.

Another prevalent conception is that drug use is cheating and sports are, or should be, all about fair competition. There is no doubt that some drugs do provide a competitive advantage to the user, but at what cost to the athlete? The psychiatric aspects of drug abuse include understanding the motivation to use, as well as determining effective treatment strategies. What role do pre-existing or emergent psychiatric symptoms and syndromes play in drug abuse in athletes [18]? This is a critical question that requires further study. None of the existing studies reporting on psychiatric effects of performance-enhancing drugs used by athletes match the dosing seen in the gym. No institutional review board in the country would approve giving high doses of black market compounds to study subjects. The extant literature on effective drug abuse treatment does not control for the unique aspects of athletes. The impact of intense training, along with other lifestyle differences between athletes and nonathletes, has not been addressed in the substance-use literature. Generalizing what has been learned from studies conducted in drug-abusing nonathletes to drug-abusing athletes may be problematic. Methodologically sound, large-scale clinical trials conducted on athletes are the only reliable way to study the issues surrounding athlete substance use. The unique role a coach plays in the life of an athlete is well known, yet little has been written about the coaches' contribution in identifying and intervening with substance use or abuse. A subtle but potentially important early warning sign of abuse may be a change in training habits or a drop-off in competition success. A coach is likely to observe this early on in the course of a developing problem, and may help initiate early treatment interventions. Training coaches on the early warning signs of sport-specific substance-abuse behaviors and providing confidential professional referrals may be an effective early warning system. This hypothesis needs to be studied.

Leshner published an excellent paper on science-based views of drug addiction and its treatment [56]. This work needs to be expanded to athletes. Validated and reliable screening instruments and effective treatment interventions for drug abusing athletes need to be studied using methodically sound research paradigms. For substance abuse researchers, this is an exciting area for future research.

Sports steroid-abuse scandals involving high-profile athletes continue to be front-page news across the country. The short- and long-term effects of headline articles, such as "The Bonds Bombshell" and "Tainted by Drugs" or Canseco's allegations [57] on drug use by athletes are yet to be determined, and are an important topic for sport psychiatrists to study.

## References

[1] Hoberman J. Sports physicians and the doping crisis in elite sports. Clin J Sport Med 2002; 12:203–8.
[2] Juhn M. Popular sports supplements and ergogenic aids. Sports Med 2003;33:921–39.
[3] Ambrose PJ. Drug use in sports: a veritable arena for pharmacists. J Am Pharm Assoc 2004;44:501–14.
[4] Millman RB, Ross EJ. Steroid and nutritional supplement use in professional athletes. Am J Addict 2003;12(Suppl):48–54.
[5] Lombardo JA. Supplements and athletes. South Med J 2004;97:877–9.
[6] Greene GA, Uryasz FD, Petr TA, et al. NCAA study of substance use and abuse habits of college student athletes. Clin J Sport Med 2001;1:51–6.
[7] Schwenk TL. Psychoactive drugs and athletic performance. Phys Sportsmed 1997;25:1–9.
[8] Samenuk D, Link MS, Homoud MK, et al. Adverse cardiovascular events temporally associated with ma huang, an herbal source of ephedrine. Mayo Clin Proc 2002;77:12–6.
[9] Lindsay BD. Are serious cardiovascular side events an unintended consequence of the dietary supplement health and education act of 1994? Mayo Clin Proc 2002;77:7–9.
[10] Landry GL. Ephedrine use is risky business. Curr Sports Med Rep 2003;2:21–2.
[11] Shekelle P, Morton S, Maglione M, et al. Ephedra and ephedrine for weight loss and athletic performance enhancement: clinical efficacy and side effects. Evidence report/technology assessment no. 76. AHRQ Publication no. 03-E022. Rockville, MD: Agency for Healthcare Research and Quality; February, 2003.
[12] Consumer Reports—Health and Fitness. Dangerous supplements: still at large and twelve supplements you should avoid. May 2004. Available at: www.consumerreports.org. Accessed June 21, 2005.
[13] Pope HG, Katz DL. Psychiatric and medical effects of anabolic-androgenic steroid use. A controlled study of 160 athletes. Arch Gen Psychiatry 1994;51:375–82.

[14] Harrison PG, Kouri EM, Hudson JI. Effects of supraphysiological doses of testosterone on mood and aggression in normal men: a randomized controlled trial. Arch Gen Psychiatry 2000;57:133–40.

[15] Hartgens F, Kuipers H. Effects of androgenic-anabolic steroids in athletes. Sports Med 2004;34:513–54.

[16] O'Brien CP, Lyons F. Alcohol and the athlete. Sports Med 2000;29:295–300.

[17] Kleiner SM. In high spirits? Alcohol and your health. Phys Sportsmed 1996;24:1–4.

[18] Miller BE, Miller MN, Verhegge R, et al. Alcohol misuse among college athletes: self-medication for psychiatric symptoms? J Drug Educ 2002;32:41–52.

[19] Nelson TF, Wechsler H. Alcohol and college athletes. Med Sci Sports Exerc 2001;33:43–7.

[20] Jones AR, Pinchot JT. Stimulant use in sports. Am J Addict 1998;7:243–55.

[21] Phenylpropanolamine and other OTC alpha-adrenergic agonists. The Medical Letter 2000;42(1094):113.

[22] Cummings KM, Michalek AM, Carl W, et al. Use of smokeless tobacco in a group of professional baseball players. J Behav Med 1989;12:559–67.

[23] Greene JC, Walsh MM, Letendre MA. Prevalence of spit tobacco use across studies of professional baseball players. J Calif Dent Assoc 1998;26:358–64.

[24] Severson HH. Enough snuff. 6th edition. Eugene (OR): Applied Behavior Science Press; 2001.

[25] Walsh MM, Hilton JF, Ellison JA, et al. Spit (smokeless) tobacco intervention of high school athletes results after 1 year. Addict Behav 2003;28:1095–113.

[26] Walsh MM, Greene JC, Ellison JA, et al. A dental-based, athletic- trainer mediated spit to-bacco cessation program for professional baseball players. J Calif Dent Assoc 1998;26:365–72.

[27] Catlin DH, Hatton CK. Use and abuse of anabolic and other drugs for athletic enhancement. Adv Intern Med 1991;36:399–424.

[28] Catlin DH, Leder BZ, Ahrens B, et al. Trace contamination of over-the-counter androstenedione and positive urine test results for nandrolone metabolite. JAMA 2000;284:2618–21.

[29] Kamber M, Baume N, Saugy M, et al. Nutritional supplements as a source for positive doping cases? Int J Sport Nutr Exerc Metab 2001;11:258–63.

[30] Major league baseball drug policy and prevention program. Available at: http://news.findlaw.com/legalnews/sports/drugs/policy/baseball/. Accessed June 21, 2005.

[31] National Football League. National Football League Player Development: player assistance services. Available at: www.nfl.com/player-development/story/6258756. Accessed July 8, 2005.

[32] Johnson LD, O'Malley PM, Bachman JG, et al. Monitoring the future national survey on drug use, 1975–2003, Volume II. College students and adults ages 19–25. NIH Publication No. 04–5508. Bethesda (MD): National Institute on Drug Abuse; 2004.

[33] NCAA study of substance abuse habits of college student-athletes. June 2001. Available at: www.ncaa.org/library/research/substance_use_habits/2001/substance_use_habits.pdf. Accessed June 21, 2005.

[34] Martens MP. Does alcohol consumption among intercollegiate athletes differ by sport type? Paper presented at the annual scientific meeting of the Association for the Advancement of Applied Sport Psychology. Minneapolis, Minnesota, September 30–October 3, 2004.

[35] Martens MP, Cox RH, Beck NC. Negative consequences of intercollegiate athlete drinking: the role of drinking motives. J Stud Alcohol 2003;64:825–8.

[36] O'Brien CP. Alcohol and sport: impact of social drinking on recreational and competitive sports performance. Sports Med 1993;15:71–7.

[37] Schwartz JR. Pharmacologic management of daytime sleepiness. J Clin Psychiatry 2004;65:46–9.

[38] What are modafinil and adrafinil? Available at: www.modafinil-adrafinil.com. Accessed June 21, 2005.

[39] Barker J. Low priority of "Greenies" questioned. Baltimore Sun Sports Section January 15, 2005.

[40] Johnson LD, O'Malley PM, Bachman JG, et al. Monitoring the future national survey on drug use, 1975–2003. Volume I: Secondary schools students. NIH Publication No. 04–5507. Bethesda (MD): National Institute on Drug Abuse; 2004.

[41] Sinclair CJ, Geiger JD. Caffeine use in sports. A pharmacological review. J Sports Med Phys Fitness 2000;40:71–9.

[42] Cooper J, Ellison JA, Walsh MM. Spit (smokeless)-tobacco use by baseball players entering the professional ranks. J Athl Train 2003;38:126–32.

[43] Severson HH. What have we learned from 20 years of research on smokeless tobacco cessation? Am J Med Sci 2003;326:206–11.

[44] Henningfield JE, Radzius A, Cone EJ. Estimation of available nicotine content of six smokeless tobacco products. Tob Control 1995;4:57–61.

[45] Gansky SA, Ellison JA, Kavanaugh JF, et al. Oral screening and spit tobacco cessation counseling: a review and findings. J Dent Educ 2002;66:1088–98.

[46] Fitzpatrick F. Where steroids were all the rage. Philadelphia Inquirer. October 20, 2002.

[47] King DS, Sharp RL, Vukovich MD, et al. Effect of oral androstendione on serum testosterone and adaptations to resistance training in young men. JAMA 1999;281:2020–8.

[48] Leder BZ, Longcope C, Catlin DH, et al. Oral androstenedione and serum testosterone concentrations in young men. JAMA 2000;283:779–82.

[49] Green G. Update on issues in drug testing. Presentation given at the winter meetings of Major League Baseball. San Francisco, December 12–13, 2003.

[50] Elashoff J, Jacknow A, Shain S. Effects of anabolic-androgenic steroids on muscular strength. Ann Intern Med 1991;115:387–93.

[51] Ariel G, Seville W. Anabolic steroids: the physiological effects of placebos. Med Sci Sports 1972;4:124–6.

[52] Su TP, Pagliarilo RN, Schmidt PJ, et al. Neuropsychiatric effects of anabolic steroids in male normal volunteers. JAMA 1993;269:2760–4.

[53] Moss HB, Panzak GL. Steroids use and aggression. Am J Psychiatry 1992;149:1616.

[54] Robertson L. Baseball's new drug policy still way off base. Miami Herald Caution D; p. 1. January 17, 2005.

[55] Siri F, Roques BP. Doping: health risks and relation to addictive behaviors. Ann Med Interne (Paris) 2003;154:S43–57.

[56] Leshner A. Science-based views of addiction and its treatment. JAMA 1999;14:1314–6.

[57] Canseco J. Juiced: wild times, rampant roids, smash hits, and how baseball got big. New York: Regan Books; 2005.

Clin Sports Med 24 (2005) 899–928

# CLINICS IN SPORTS MEDICINE

ELSEVIER
SAUNDERS

# Invisible Players: A Family Systems Model

Jon Hellstedt, PhD

*Department of Psychology, University of Massachusetts, One University Avenue, Lowell, MA 01854, USA*

The family is the most important influence in any athlete's life. The family unit is where the young athlete develops the skills and coping mechanisms needed in the demanding life of competitive sport. The family is the primary social milieu in which the athlete develops identity, self-esteem, and the motivation for athletic success. Successful athletes often credit their families for encouragement, instilling discipline (both self- and externally driven) and the value of achievement, and above all, the experience of feeling love and support not primarily contingent on success or performance.

Unfortunately, however, a family can also have deleterious effects on an athlete's development. Parental demands and expectations can foster an atmosphere of rigid rules and unrealistic expectations. A poorly functioning or underorganized family system and genetically mediated underlying psychopathology can result in a lack of internal modulation (controls) and self-discipline, substance abuse, inadequate interpersonal relationships, poor stress management skills, and difficulty accepting authority and limits from coaches. An athlete's performance can be negatively impacted from either excessive or ineffectual family influence.

The demands on athletes and their families have intensified in recent years. The wealth and glamour of professional sport and the proliferation of youth sport programs have greatly impacted the American family. In a historical review of the rise of youth sports for children, Berryman [1] states, "Children's sport organizations led to changes in the American family structure and, in many instances, added a new aspect to the socialization of children."

This historical development provides a context for the scene described in the case example of the Stanley family detailed below. This scenario is often repeated in other families after ski races, gymnastics events, hockey and baseball games, or any other athletic event. The drama involves a talented youngster competing in an athletic event and not meeting high parental expectations. The disappointed parents who have put time, money, and emotional energy into

Ian R. Tofler, MB, BS, made editorial contributions to this article. Correspondence can be sent to him at: robertoff@aol.com.

their child's athletic development are frustrated by their son's or daughter's performance. The parents appreciate but may exaggerate the talent their child has, and are frustrated by what they perceive as lack of effort. This family drama results in a young athlete's internal conflict ("I can't please them, so I must be a failure") or tension between parent and child ("If they don't lay off, I am going to scream").

## THE CASE OF THE STANLEY FAMILY

Amy Stanley was ahead in the semifinal match for 14-year-olds at the regional tennis championships. She was leading well into the match when she seemed to get overconfident and stopped playing aggressively. She lost in a second-set tie breaker—a match it seemed she could have won.

Her parents Fred and Betty were watching. Betty was quiet and withdrawn. Fred was visibly upset at Amy's performance and mentioned to Betty, "Why does she always do this to herself. She's so good, yet she doesn't seem to want to win."

In the car on the way home from the match, Fred turned to Amy and said, "You didn't seem to really want to win today." Amy was quiet, looked out the car window and said to herself, "Maybe you're right."

Fred was concerned about Amy's erratic play, and after the most recent match he discussed the situation with Amy's coach. The coach indicated to Fred that over the past year, he has observed Amy questioning her commitment to tennis. He has noticed that she doesn't practice with much intensity, and often needs to be talked into workouts and competitions. The coach acknowledged her considerable talents and told Fred that of all the juniors he has worked with, Amy has the most natural ability. The coach then suggested that Amy talk to Dr. Jane Hawthorne, a sports psychologist who had worked with many tennis players in the area. "She's very good, and knows a lot about the sport," the coach said. Fred, though somewhat uncomfortable about the idea, talked it over with Betty and Amy, and Fred called Dr. Hawthorne for an appointment.

Dr. Hawthorne has an interesting perspective as a clinical sport psychologist. In addition to her skills in helping athletes improve their performances using relaxation, visualization, and goal setting, she also has a background in family systems theory and intervention. During her graduate training she took courses in systems theory, and during her clinical internship she received supervision in family therapy. At many workshops and sport psychology conferences, she has learned skills in working with individual athletes, but she is also interested in working with their families. She remembers attending a sport psychology conference where a psychologist who works with elite athletes said that over-involved parents were often a problem. His policy was to "bar parents from his office" and to work only with the athlete. Dr. Hawthorne felt uncomfortable with that model of intervention. It overlooked an important reality. Parents can't be kept in the waiting room. Family influences are ever present, either overtly or unconsciously, in the athlete's mind and performance.

The Stanley family (a composite of several families worked with in clinical practice) and the interactions that form their family system became invisible players and had a direct impact on Amy's performance on the court. As sports at all levels become more professional, and as elite athletes compete at increasingly younger ages, the assessment of family-based problems and interventions in the family system become essential skills for the sport psychologist.

## REVIEWING THE LITERATURE

Rainer Martens [2] was the first to alert parents, coaches, and psychologists about the potential emotional risk factors in youth sports. Accounts of problems in athletic families have been common in the media ever since. The image of the "little league parent" who inflicts emotional (and sometimes physical) abuse on children, referees, and even other parents is commonly portrayed. Sport magazines, newspapers, and television documentaries have featured stories about young athletes who have been apparent victims of overbearing parents. This media attention raises an interesting question that needs to be addressed with empirical research: What are the positive and negative factors in families of young athletes? Unfortunately, there are still few studies that address this issue.

### Family Interactions

The research on athlete families underscores the major influence of the family on the developing athlete. For example, studies by both Greendorfer and Lewko [3] and Sage [4] found that parents are the major influences on introducing a youngster to youth sport. The role of the father is notable in both studies, in that he appears to be the major influence on the sport participation of both male and female children.

Other studies document the major influence of parents. For example, McElroy and Kirkendall [5] concluded that parents are the primary "significant other" in the formation of children's (especially males') attitudes toward winning and skill development. In a study of Israeli athletes, Melnick and colleagues [6] found that parents of sport-gifted children held very high expectations for their children's performance, and offered more encouragement for sport participation than did parents of a control group of nonathletic children.

The influence of the parents is strongest in the early years of development. There is a shift in influence toward peers and other adults when the child reaches adolescence. Higgenson [7] found that in preadolescent years, the parents are the primary influences, but as the child reaches adolescence, the influence shifts from parents to the coach and peers. During adolescence, the influence of the parents is still profoundly present, but more subtle. For example, Berlage [8], in a study of father's career aspirations for their hockey playing sons, found that fathers of 11- and 12-year-old hockey players have pronounced aspirations for their children continuing in sport. Most of the fathers surveyed hoped their sons would play hockey in high school and college, and almost all fathers believed that continued participation would benefit their sons in their adult lives. It is an easy assumption to make that this type of family environment has a major impact on the attitude of the developing athlete.

The issue of stress and pressure from parents is a complex problem, and is difficult to research. Attempts have been made, however, to determine what are the factors within the family that create a stressful environment for the child. Gould and coworkers [9] described many sources of stress in the youth sport environment, and indicated that a major stressor is the young athlete's fear of failure. Although this fear of failure can emanate from different sources (self, peer, or coach), a major source appears to be the young athlete's parents. In his research on the development of competitive trait anxiety, Passer [10] has concluded that negative performance evaluation from parents has a major role in the development of high trait anxiety. Conversely, in a study that looked at the other side of this issue, namely, the factors which support positive sport participation, Scanlan and Lewthwaite [11] found that male wrestlers who experienced positive parental performance reactions and a high level of positive parental involvement in the sport experienced greater enjoyment than those who did not.

Research on family influences is complex and difficult. Quantitative methodology is often unable to explore the intricacies of the family processes that exist in athletic families. The subtle interactive factors that exist in family life lend themselves more to qualitative methods using interviews and content analysis. In recent years, some studies have used this methodology to highlight some of the issues and processes that provide helpful insight into clinical assessment with these families. Among this research are the studies of Bloom [12], Scanlon and coworkers [13], and Kesend [14].

## Developmental Events

The work of a research team headed by Bloom studied the developmental events in the lives of exceptionally talented young people. Included in this study were samples of artists, musicians, mathematicians and scientists, as well as athletes. Bloom's report included studies of Olympic level swimmers [15], professional tennis players [16], and an integrative analysis of their home environments by Sloane [17]. The results of this team of researchers is important to the model developed in this article, because they provide both a developmental perspective and the system qualities of the home environment.

The developmental process is similar for the swimmers and tennis players. Three distinct phases of development occur that involve early parental influence, followed by the gradual emotional separation of the parents from the athlete:

1. In the early years (ages 4–12) the child is introduced to a variety of sports, mainly by the parents, mostly the father. The emphasis is on playfulness, fun, and family involvement in athletic activity. The parents provide early instruction, but soon locate a coaching/instructional program that will expose the child to a higher skill level. Toward the end of this phase, the parents enjoy taking the child to entry-level competitions in which the emphasis is ostensibly on fun rather than winning.

2. In the middle years (ages 13–18) there is a shift from fun and playfulness to the development of sport specialization, and a commitment to higher levels of training and competition. Both the athlete and the family center their leisure-time activities around the sport. The parents now provide transportation, structure practice time, arrange competitions, and secure the best coaching available. Some problems are reported in the parents' negotiating the transition to the coach having primary influence on skill development. Conflicts between parents and coaches often develop, and coaching changes become rather frequent [15].

3. In the later years (ages 19–late 20s) the athlete usually separates from the family and moves on to college or independent living. The family is mainly a support system and an emotional refuge from the stress of competition. Monsaas [16] reports that this stage was negotiated well by most of the parents. Some, however, "missed traveling to tournaments and felt a bit left out in these later years." It is also interesting to note that a few of the fathers continued in the role of coach and traveled with the athletes until they were in their late 20s. Examples from elite women's tennis come to mind.

There were similarities in the systemic composition of these families. Sloane [17] noted three main qualities of the home environment.

1. First, the families shared a strong value system that emphasized success through hard work. This value system was clearly communicated by the parents to the children through verbal teaching and role modeling.

2. Second, the families, most notably the fathers, valued athletic activity as a way to learn important character traits such as the motivation to achieve and the dedication to hard work.

3. A third characteristic was the willingness of the family system to organize itself around the athletic activities of the child-athlete. Parents sacrificed by forfeiting other activities to take the child to the pool or the tennis court. Family vacations were organized around training or competitions. Large sums of time and money were devoted to sports to the exclusion of other possible family activities.

## Family as Source of Support or Pressure?

In a retrospective study of sources of stress in the lives of elite figure skaters, Scanlon and colleagues [13] illustrated the multidimensional nature of stress in an elite athlete's life, and also the paradox of the family system as both a source of, and a refuge from, those pressures. Family influences were found to be both a source of valuable support and also a source of stress.

The positive nature of family influences is indicated by the fact that most of the athletes in the Scanlon study [13] report that the support they received from their families was essential in helping them to achieve the high level, and to cope with the pressures of being a competitive athlete. Some athletes, however, reported stressful family interactions, such as performance criticism and pre-competition lectures from parents. "Psychological warfare" (backstabbing) from other competitors' parents and guilt over the large sums of money spent on the athlete's training were major factors vis-à-vis siblings and other family members.

Financial pressures came overtly from parents constantly reminding them of the costs involved, and covertly from the athletes observing parental sacrifices such as how hard they were working to support them.

Another study using a similar methodology was done by Kesend [14]. Using interview material obtained from 20 Olympic level athletes (15 males and 5 females), Kesend examined sources of encouragement and discouragement in the athletes' development. The data showed that the family is the athlete's main source of encouragement. Parents and siblings were more widely cited for providing support than coaches, peers, and members of various sport organizations.

Specific mechanisms for family support were introduction to sport in the early years, support for sport participation, positive role modeling by parents, verbal and nonverbal approval of competitive accomplishments, and emotional acceptance of decisions and ideas regarding elite level sport participation.

Parents and family, however, were also sources of discouragement. Parental behaviors interpreted by the athletes as discouraging were suggestions of pursuing alternative careers and parental anxiety or lack of anxiety over physical injury. Unrealistic parental expectations also were discouraging (one athlete had scored 67 points in a basketball game and was criticized by a parent for not playing more aggressively!) to some of the athletes. Overt parental "pushing," however, was not a frequently mentioned factor, and probably often went under the child's radar as normal parenting. Hellstedt [18,19] investigated the parent-athlete interactions in a group of athletic families as they made the transition from the early to the middle stage of athletic development. In a longitudinal study of ski racers and their families [18], he found that the 12- and 13-year-old elite ski racers perceived their parents as having a strong influence on their development as athletes. The specific mechanisms by which parents were influential were parental "coaching" (teaching and advice giving), off-season monitoring of conditioning and dry-land training, emotional and financial support, and expectations to continue participation in the sport.

In addition, the changes in perceptions of parental pressure that developed between ages 13 and 15 were examined by Hellstedt [19]. Parental pressure was measured along three dimensions: (1) general participation in the sport, (2) performance appraisal, and (3) pressure to continue competing. At age 13 there was a substantial group of young athletes who indicated they were "unhappy" with the amount of parental pressure, especially the pressure to continue participation in the sport. Two years later, however, the athletes perceived less parental pressure, and were beginning to shift the source of this pressure away from parents (particularly father) to their coaches. Fig. 1 indicates the changes in pressure ratings over the 2-year interval.

The data generally showed that these athletes felt quite positively about the contributions of their parents to their development as athletes; however, at least two problem areas were apparent. One was a higher perception of parental pressure in the younger age group, indicating that this may be a time of higher sensitivity to this type of influence. Secondly, affective reactions of dissatisfaction were positively correlated with the amount of parental pressure in both age

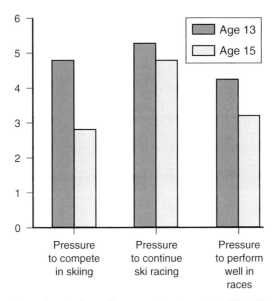

**Fig. 1.** Changes in perceptions of parental pressure in a group (N = 67) of developing ski racers. Mean scores on scale of 1.

groups [19]. This finding suggests the possibility that anger toward parents can be a motivating factor in sport withdrawal, athlete burn out, or simply transition to another life phase.

### The Paradox of the Athlete Family

In summary, the research on athletes and their families suggests that though the family may be a source of stress to some athletes, in general the family is an indispensable source of support to the athlete. Contrary to the negative images of the athletic family in the media, studies on athletic families seem to indicate that for the majority of young athletes, the family is a vital social support system that nourishes and encourages the athlete's development. The families of successful athletes appear to be tightly organized systems with very concerned, albeit competitive, parents who have high expectations for their children. A common denominator in these families is strong parental role models who provide the energy and motivation for the young athlete. These families also have very clear rules concerning hard work and achievement.

Here is where a paradox emerges. The strengths of these families may also be their weakness. What is perceived as a positive attribute by some young athletes may be a negative, disabling, and damaging experience for others. There is a fine line between positive achievement motivation and excessive pressure. What for some young athletes may be seen as parental encouragement may feel like a lack of freedom and breathing space to others.

In addition, the research shows another problem area for families. Perhaps because of the tight organization that develops, and the close parent-child relationship, some of these families had difficulty negotiating the transition from one stage of family development to the next. For example, the transition from the parents to the teacher/coach as the dominant influence on the athlete's training was sometimes difficult. Parents and coaches often disagreed over what was necessary in the athletes' skill development.

There is also an athletic family developmental process that unfolds along a somewhat predictable course. During the early years of sport involvement, the emphasis is on fun and skill development. There is a shift, however, in the commitment stage of development, in which both the athlete and the family system invest major levels of energy and financial resources into sport involvement.

In the later stages of the athlete's development, the athlete separates from the parents and family, and is influenced primarily by other adults such as coaches, agents, and members of athletic organizations. For some families, these transitions seem to be difficult, and can result in conflict between extrafamilial adult influences and parents. This issue of transitions in the developmental process of the families is looked at more closely in the next part of this article.

Finally, the balance between healthy encouragement and excessive parental involvement is a precarious one. When the parents cross over the line they are in danger of becoming too "child-focused" [20]. This is a process in which the spousal subsystem in the family loses its vitality, and the child's success in sport becomes the emotional epicenter of the family. The result can be marital conflict or family dysfunction, during or subsequent to the period of active athletic involvement of the child.

## A DEVELOPMENTAL MODEL FOR THE ATHLETIC FAMILY

To fully understand the difficulties facing a young athlete such as Amy Stanley, psychologically oriented sports medicine professionals need a model for assessing the structural health and developmental maturity of the athletic family. In this section, a model based on the research on athletic families and on concepts from family systems theory is presented. This construct is applied to the Stanley family.

Family systems theory developed from the work of therapists and researchers who observed that symptom formation in an individual is connected to developmental or structural problems within the individual's family. Although there are many different perspectives (and emphases) among family theorists, there is basic agreement that the family is an interacting social system in which the component parts affect one another. A useful framework for understanding the structural properties of a family is found in the work of Minuchin [21]. According to his model, the main structural components of the family are the power hierarchy, rules, interactional patterns, subsystems, and types of boundaries between the subsystems.

A family is more than structural components, however. A family system undergoes a constantly changing developmental process. A useful perspective on this process of change and the connections between generations as the family develops is provided by Bowen [22,23]. Bowen's insights have recently been enhanced by the developmental framework provided by Carter and McGoldrick [24]. This framework underlies the model developed in this article. Following the stage theories of individual developmental paradigms such as Erikson's [25], Carter and McGoldrick [24] state that the family is a social organism that passes through a life cycle in much the same way as the individual does. This life cycle is a series of stages with certain tasks that need to be accomplished before the next stage of development can be successfully mastered. If these tasks are not completed during early stages, there will be problems in later stages of development. The transitions from one stage to the next are particularly stressful for families, and are often the intervals of time when symptoms appear in individual members or in the family system as a whole.

The demands of athletic competition and training often present to families unique circumstances that are deviations from the "normal" family life cycle. For example, a young gymnast and her family may have premature separation brought on by her leaving home to receive specialized coaching. A swimmer or figure skater must train many hours a day and absorbs family resources with great impact on the entire family. A career-threatening injury after years of training creates a grief experience for an athlete and a family to resolve. Such developmental delays, barriers, or impasses can negatively affect the young athlete.

Carter and McGoldrick [24] have pioneered approaches to the stages and tasks families need to master as they develop. A caveat regarding this model is that it addresses the issues of intact, middle to upper class families, which are no longer the demographic norm in our society. Many athletes emerge from less organized families or from families that experience major disruptions, such as abandonment, separation, and divorce, that are not specifically addressed in this article because of space limitations. The general developmental tasks required of these families can be found in Peck and Manocherian [26] and Fulmer [27], and can be adapted to the athletic family system as it is presented in this article.

Although the following analysis will demonstrate how the Stanley family is having difficulty negotiating certain developmental transitions and tasks, it is not the authors' intent to "pathologize" this family or athletic families in general. Although this family is having some difficulty, it must be emphasized that it is a healthy family that has many strengths. It is important to restate what was stated earlier in the article—that in most cases (including this one), the family is still the main source of support and encouragement for the developing athlete.

## THE STANLEY FAMILY: A DEVELOPMENTAL ANALYSIS

To an outside observer, the Stanleys are a model family. They are a successful, financially comfortable, professional family with two attractive children who are both gifted athletes.

Fred Stanley, aged 43, is a lawyer and an avid recreational tennis player. His wife Betty, 41, is a former school teacher who is currently enjoying her role as a full-time parent to their two daughters, Caroline, 17, and Amy, 14. Caroline and Amy are both competitive tennis players, and since Caroline was 11 the Stanley family has organized itself around the tennis court. Both girls used to play other sports, but because of their potential and his own love of the game, Fred (with Betty's support) has encouraged them in tennis. At around age 12, both girls chose to specialize in tennis, and are year-round competitors. Coaches, summer camps, indoor winter training, tournaments, travel, a racket stringer in the garage, and a station wagon full of tennis gear are visible symbols of the family's avocation. The family used to go on family vacations, but now all their travel is for the girls' tennis tournaments. Fred goes to as many of the tournaments as he can, and both he and Betty attend the local matches.

A close look at the course of this family's development reveals some unresolved developmental tasks that are affecting Amy's performance in tennis. Developmental analysis of this family begins at the time when Fred and Betty met, dated, and decided to marry.

## Stage One: The Unattached Young Adult

A developmental analysis of the Stanley family begins with the life experience of Fred and Betty Stanley when they met in college as single, young adults. A genogram [28] of this period of the family's development appears in Fig. 2.

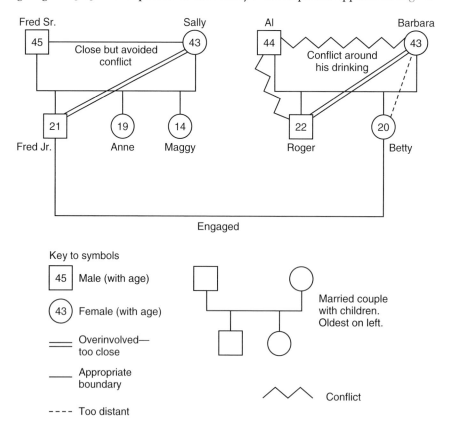

**Fig. 2.** Genogram of Fred and Betty Stanley at the time of marriage.

Fred and Betty met during college. Fred was a senior prelaw student. Betty was a junior. Fred's stable, middle class family encouraged his college education and law school. Fred had, however, struggled throughout his life for his father's acceptance. Fred Senior was an emotionally closed person who had a difficult time expressing his positive feelings for his son. He was a workaholic, and he owned his own manufacturing company. He struggled financially at various times when the children were young. He was set in his ways and demanded a great deal from his children. His pattern was to encourage Fred Junior to excel in sports and academics, but give him little positive feedback. Fred's mother, on the other hand, was very nurturing to her three children. She was a submissive figure, however; she let Fred Senior dominate most aspects of the family decision-making. She avoided conflict in her own marriage by letting her husband dominate, and encouraged her children not to challenge their father's role in the family.

Among the Stanley children, Fred was clearly the star. Throughout school he was a capable athlete and good student. Athletically, Fred played baseball, swam, and played tennis at their local club. In high school he played basketball, though he lacked height and often played in a backup role. He also played on the tennis team and was elected captain his senior year. When he tried out for the college tennis team, he was cut because there were many talented players at his school. Although frustrated by this setback, he continued to play recreationally.

In contrast with the Stanley family, which was tightly organized and devoid of overt conflict, Betty's family was marked by high "expressed emotion"(EE). Open conflict in Betty's family centered around her father Al's drinking and her mother's anger at Al's irresponsibility. Betty's older brother Roger was the hero in this family, and was often put in the role of surrogate father by taking over many of Al's duties and becoming Barbara's helper. Betty took on the role of the peacemaker in the family. The conflict between her parents bothered her and she would mediate their disputes. Betty became emotionally controlled, and internalized pain and sadness that she never expressed to others.

Betty was active in high school sports. She ran cross country and track, and participated in gymnastics. She was also a solid, hard-working student. Because of her unhappy home life, she enjoyed getting away from home, and when she met Fred she was immediately attracted to him.

To the casual observer, Fred and Betty were able to accomplish most of the developmental tasks of this stage of family development, which are:

- Establish a sense of self in work and gain financial independence
- Develop intimate peer relationships
- Differentiate themselves from their families of origin

To the casual observer, Fred and Betty appeared happy and self confident. Some unresolved developmental tasks, however, were present that became problematic in the development of their own family. Both have failed to fully differentiate from their families of origin. Fred was, and still is, working to please his father. He is self-centered and fixated on being financially and professionally successful. Betty is a capable person, but has low self-esteem and rigid emotional control. Her inability to differentiate from her family of origin manifested in a desire to avoid conflict, and a need to recreate a marital relationship in which Fred was the dominant player.

Athletically, the main task for the young couple was the development of an active and competitive lifestyle. This was relatively easy for both of them because they were both active in sports. Fred taught Betty to play tennis, and she influenced him to enjoy running for exercise. During their courtship and early marriage they remained active in sport.

## Stage Two: The Newly Married Couple

The major tasks for this stage of family development is to build a strong spousal relationship with equal power sharing. In addition, the couple must develop workable communication patterns, the ability to nurture and express affection for one another, and the mechanisms to resolve conflict [29]. Finally, the newly married couple needs to establish itself as separate and autonomous from their respective families of origin.

Fred and Betty married. Both families were present, though Fred's father and Betty's mother seemed to be the major players in the arrangements and events surrounding the wedding. Fred had finished his first year of law school and Betty had graduated from college. They moved to an apartment at Fred's university and Betty began teaching in an elementary school in a nearby town.

Betty taught school for the first 2 years of their marriage, which helped pay the bills while Fred went to law school. He graduated from school, passed the bar examination, and got an excellent job with a large law firm in the city.

Their marital contract was based on complementary needs. The result was a marital system with an unequal balance of power. In choosing a partner, Betty sought stability, and a strong male figure that she lacked in her own father. She also chose to avoid conflict as a way of making a marital relationship work. Fred was comfortable with Betty, who was similar to his own mother. He was pleasing his father by being successful and having visibly successful children. He also followed his father's model by becoming a dominant and demanding father figure. Fred's fantasy when he met Betty was that they would create a close family of high achievers. Betty's fantasy was that they would be stable and free of conflict. Their marital roles were also influenced by their complementary sibling positions in their own families. Fred was the oldest and dominant male child, and Betty was the younger subordinate female child.

Fred remained on a successful career trajectory. They were very busy during these years. Tennis became a favorite pastime for Fred. He played at the club level and entered local tournaments. Their social life centered around tennis. Mixed doubles events and parties were their social life. They also fell into a pattern of becoming active in activities outside their relationship, and began to find little time for each other. The major task that was not met at this stage was to establish mechanisms for resolving conflict. Betty's desire to avoid conflict and her collusion in the establishment of Fred's dominant role in the power hierarchy became problematic as the family developed.

### Stage Three: The Athletic Family with Young Children

In athletic families the main task of this period is to introduce the children to a variety of sports. In the families studied by the Bloom research team [12,15–17], this was a time of great excitement and playfulness. The excitement of seeing a child learn a sport skill is intense for parents. The child often loves the first encounter with sport because of the playful, noncompetitive nature of the environment.

Soon after Fred began his career as a lawyer they had their first child. Betty left her teaching position and became a full-time mother. Three years later their second child was born. The children developed without having any major physical problems or illness. Fred and Betty stayed active in sports and gradually introduced the children to gymnastics, then soccer, swimming, and skiing. At 6 years of age, Caroline began tennis lessons.

The Stanleys were rather typical of athletic families at this stage of development. The parents introduce the children to sport and spend time teaching the children these skills. The family clearly values the sport, the play, and the nonverbal connection and attachment it engenders. The parents are willing to spend large amounts of family time with lessons and practice. For families who negotiate this stage well, the playful and fun quality of sport activity is never lost. The child enjoys the activity and the development of athletic skill is the dividend.

There are potential problems at this stage of development for athlete families, and they were beginning to appear with the Stanleys. The main task of the family with young children is to make space in the family for the children. The Stanley's had no problem with this; in fact, they went too far in the other direction. The children became an enormous presence in the family. Fred and Betty had grand expectations for their children, and engaged in what is called "the family projection process" [22], in which one or both parents project their own "unfinished business" from their own history onto their children.

Most parents have grandiose fantasies about their children, but in the Stanley family these fantasies developed considerable intensity. While their daughters were very young (probably even before they were born) both Fred and Betty ambitiously imagined that they would be exceptional children and top athletes. Fred's images were the strongest, and derived from his relationship with his own father and his inability to be "good enough" to please him. This pattern of enmeshment with both Caroline and Amy stemmed from his own family experience. His two daughters became involved in this multigenerational need to achieve to please Fred's father.

Another task of this developmental period is for parents to share in the nurturing and care of the young children. In the Stanley family, however, these roles became restrictive. Fred handled the important sport role. Betty took care of most other things.

As the children grew, Betty did most of the parenting in the home and in relationship to school activities. Fred's parenting role was largely centered around the sport involvement of the girls. Evenings and weekends, Fred threw a ball to the girls and took them to the tennis court to practice. As Caroline became more involved in tennis, Fred met her at the club after work and hit balls with her. He became disenchanted with the club professional and soon found another to work with her.

Another unresolved issue at this stage was that Fred and Betty were not able or willing to make adequate space in the family for their own spousal relationship. When too much space is made for the children, the family becomes child-focused, and the boundaries in and around the family become rigid, because most of the family involvement is in youth sport. They can become a tennis family (or hockey, skiing, football, equestrian, or any other sport). The children develop friendships with other children in the same sport, and tend not to meet other children. The parents neglect their own relationship by focusing too much of their time and energy on the children. This was evident in Fred and Betty's relationship; they were unable to draw a boundary around their own relationship and the initial level of intimacy diminished.

### Stage Four: The Family with Adolescent Children

For many families, adolescence can be the most difficult period of development. It is often a time of great turmoil. The child begins to change from being dependent and compliant to being independent (or counterdependent) and more dedicated to peer group than family. The authoritative structure of the parental subsystem is challenged, and the ability of the parents to adapt to this change is severely tested. If the parents are not able to adapt and retain the respect of the child, the ability of the family to function smoothly is diminished. The main tasks involve a realignment of the boundaries and power hierarchy of the family. The child must gradually be given more power in the family and more involvement in the decision-making processes: Mom and Dad saying "no" to a request to stay at a friend's house for the night changes to their asking the adolescent what is a reasonable hour to come home from a party, and all agreeing to a mutually acceptable time.

It is also a difficult time for athletic families, in that there is an evolution from sports as fun to sports as serious business. Whereas adolescents in many families are dropping out of youth sport programs to pursue other interests [30], the pattern is reversed in athletic families. The major task for them is to develop or maintain a commitment to sport and the role demands of the serious athlete.

Adolescence is also a period of time where the primary influence on the child-athlete should shift from the parents to the coach and peers. The parents' role change. They become the support structure of the athlete. The coach becomes the primary influence for skill development and competitive motivation and development. Some parents have major difficulty with this. Diffuse boundaries in the parent/athlete relationship result in conflicts in the coach/parent/athlete relationship [31].

At the same time that the shift in influence is away from them, the parents must continue to be influential in the child-athlete's development by emphasizing a goal orientation and a strong work ethic. A critical need is for parents to strike a workable balance between teaching discipline and determined effort while also fostering a sense of independence in the child-athlete.

The first major "derailment" from the normal family life cycle occurs at this stage in the athlete family. This is a prolonged "adolescent moratorium," adolescence for the adolescent athlete, often markedly different from the adolescence of most of his or her peer group. The demands of athletic training and competition often result in a social deprivation of free time, "hanging out," and dating. Also, non-sport related career issues are put on hold as the youngster focuses on the role of the athlete. This prolonged adolescence is reinforced by the child continuing to be dependent on the family for financial and functional support during the early stage of elite competition. During this derailment the athlete and the athlete's family do not experience summer jobs, peer relationships, or decision-making around college choice or career options. Instead the family continues to concentrate on the young athlete's sport involvement. The result is a calculated sacrifice that creates a developmental impasse.

The family can help the athlete through this period in several ways. One is to support, wherever possible, the athlete's sense of independence. A practical way of accomplishing this is for the parents to let the athlete travel and compete without their presence. Another is to let the athlete have major input into decisions about coaching, training programs, and competition schedules. Because they are often sheltered by coaches and sport organizations, some elite athletes need to find within their families the psychological permission and the necessary skills to establish independent thinking and decision-making patterns.

A major task of the parents is to allow the influence shift from parents to coach by establishing a clear boundary between their roles as parents and their roles as coaches to their own child. This boundary will help the developing athlete view family as a safe and supportive refuge from the pressures of competition and training. Also, the family can encourage the adolescent's social maturity by supporting efforts to have meaningful relationships with peers. Attending concerts, going to friend's homes for the weekend, and dating are all important formative experiences, and should be encouraged by parents. A life beyond sports is a healthy present and future resource, and a psychological buffer for the athlete. It helps establish a protective but permeable boundary for both the athlete and the family to the extrafamilial social environment (Fig. 3).

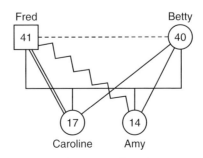

**Fig. 3.** The Stanley family with adolescent children.

The Stanley family hit some snags at this stage of athletic family development (see Fig. 3). Fred was overinvolved with the two girls. Betty was underinvolved and conflict-averse with Fred. Caroline accepted the compliment of overinvolvement with her father. She became so absorbed in competitive tennis that she had limited peer relationships outside of tennis. She had done little dating or partying, but had devoted herself to competition and training. Her parents colluded in this delayed adolescence by continuing to monitor and supervise her decisions. Career decisions were not important for Caroline or her parents. She had a chance to be a professional tennis player, and that became a family ambition. She was granted a college scholarship for her tennis, but the choice of school was made primarily on the basis of the quality of the tennis program and not on academic factors.

Although this parenting approach seemed to have worked with Caroline, it was not appropriate for her younger sister. Amy was uncomfortable with the prewritten family script. She wanted more independence, and was not eager for the life of a competitive athlete. Her individual desires were in direct conflict with the family rules. The crisis that was about to explode had its roots in previous developmental tasks not being met by the parents within their marital relationship.

Amy was about to challenge the family's "child-as-athlete" focus. She wanted more nonsport social involvement and generally more independence in decision making. In addition, Fred and Betty had not developed interests outside of tennis, and would have difficulty if Amy pursued other directions. Finally, Fred had problems with accepting other nonfamily adults as influences on Amy. This led to conflicts with her coaches.

## Stage Five: The Launching of Children

The major tasks at the launching phase of family development involve the parents letting go of their children, developing adult-to-young-adult relationships with them, and refocusing energy on their own marital relationship. These tasks produce a second major problem area or potential derailment of athlete families from the normal family life cycle. In athlete families, the prolonged adolescence of the previous stage results in a launching delay. The delay can result from the parents maintaining an overinvolved position by managing an abundance of the athlete's life decisions. The emotional separation and letting go of the young adult athlete is complicated by the overinvolvement that may have developed during the previous stages.

The normal process, at least for the middle and upper classes in the United States, is for the young adult (aged 18–22) to attend college, move away from home, and begin career or graduate training. Marriage and the formation of the adult child's own family may follow. Although some young adult offspring will return home for brief periods of time, the goal is to establish independent living apart from the family. In athletic families there can be a delay in this launching process. These families may find they are "out of synch" with other families because their child has put off important life decisions in order to train and compete. There is a trend in many sports for athletes to delay or interrupt college to train more intensively. Career preparation is also delayed.

If the young adult athlete has committed to sport, the family needs to be aware of and to tolerate this delay. Otherwise there will be additional stress or pressure on the young athlete. Athletic families may not have the "empty nest" that other families experience, so they must tolerate numerous entries and exits from the family caused by the young athlete leaving home for periods of time to compete and then returning.

The launching delay and frequent practice launches may present problems in families in which the parents tend toward overinvolvement. The parents may gain emotional gratification from the young adult delaying independent living, and this may work to the detriment of the emerging professional athlete. For example, in the tennis families studied by Monsaas [16], two fathers were still actively coaching the young adult athletes well into their late 20s, a process which would likely inhibit the critical self-differentiation of the adult athlete.

The major task for the athlete family during the launching phase is to perform a delicate balancing act between encouraging financial and emotional independence on the one hand, and providing a source of emotional support and refuge from the stress of competition on the other. Finding and trusting a coach outside the family is an essential component in this process.

The Stanleys were in transition toward the launching phase. Fred and Betty continued to overmanage Caroline's life and make decisions that were inhibiting her growth to young adulthood. Fred and Betty had difficulty adjusting their own marital relationship without Caroline's (and Amy's) tennis as a focus. The process of separation was a difficult one for this family.

## Stage Six: The Family and Adult Children in Later Life

The athlete has completed the highest competitive phase and has retired from sport, and is now making the transition to career and the establishment of the athlete's own kinship family. The major issues for the parents are the completion of any unresolved issues around the athletic accomplishments of the adult offspring. It is a time for the parents to enjoy their own spousal relationship and retirement, and feel a sense of dignity about their accomplishments as a family. The major issue for them relative to their offspring is to assist and support the athlete around retirement issues and the establishment of a new career and a separate family. A healthy permeable boundary is appropriate here, so that the parents are perceived as supportive of but not fused with the adult offspring.

This phase was difficult to predict for the Stanley family. If Fred and Betty were not able to separate from their two daughters and establish their own marital relationship as a distinct and valued subsystem, this stage would also be a difficult time for them.

This completes the developmental model. Now it is time to return to the Stanleys as a family with adolescent children and examine the assessment and treatment issues that emerge when a sport psychiatrist or psychologist becomes involved with the family.

## CLINICAL FAMILY ASSESSMENT AND TREATMENT

The assessment of the family system of the athlete is an important component to any sports-related assessment procedure. Family processes are often important factors in problems such as eating disorders [31], rehabilitation from injury [32], burn-out and overtraining [33], substance abuse [34,35] parental overinvolvement [36,37], and problems in the coach/parent/athlete relationship [38]. Even problems that present as individual concerns, such as performance blocks or retirement from sport, may involve family issues, and a family analysis should be included in the assessment, and possibly in the treatment.

## ASSESSMENT OF THE ATHLETIC FAMILY

Based on the model presented in this article, two basic questions need to be answered in the process of doing a family system based assessment. The first question is "What are the developmental impasses?" The second is "What are the structural/interactional strengths and weaknesses of the family?"

The best procedure for collecting information is a cluster of interviews with key family members. All family members do not need to be present for all assessment interviews. It is important, however, to have the principal players in the family together for at least one session in order to observe the patterns of communication and interaction. A suggested format is to see the athlete alone for a session, the parents together for another session, and the entire family together for one or two sessions. The order in which these sessions take place is interchangeable, depending on the circumstances, motivation, and time schedules of the family members.

To provide a framework for assessment of the family's developmental and structural characteristics, some assessment categories are helpful. Doherty and Baird [34] present a succinct assessment formula based on four themes: (1) the level and the source of stress in the family, (2) the ability of the family to adapt to change, (3) the degree of cohesiveness in the family, and (4) the interaction patterns in the family. Brief examples from the Stanley family will illustrate these themes.

### Levels of Stress

The first task of the clinician in family assessment is to determine the intensity and source of stress in the family.

Fred Stanley called Dr. Hawthorne and asked for an appointment for Amy. "She's a promising young tennis player, but she is easily distracted. And since her last match, which she lost because she lacked the effort, she is talking about quitting tennis and giving up the opportunity to be a top level player. Her coach suggested I give you a call, and hopefully you can sit down and talk with her."

Dr. Hawthorne explained to Fred that she likes to do a three- or four-session evaluation, at the end of which she will make some treatment recommendations. She explained that the purpose of the evaluation was to get to know both Amy and the family, so that a treatment contract can be designed to meet everyone's particular needs. Because Caroline would be leaving soon for college, it was agreed that the family would come together for the first session.

Based on the tone of the phone conversation, Dr. Hawthorne sensed that Fred Stanley saw the problem as Amy's alone. He did not define the issue in a broader context. She speculated that the Stanleys appeared in a moderate state of stress. There was no major life crisis facing any of the family members, but it was likely that feelings of anger, disappointment, and frustration were being felt but not expressed. Their intensity was not as elevated, however, as other athlete families Dr. Hawthorne was seeing, such as the family of an elite diver whose mother was dying from cancer during the peak of the diver's career, or the family of a gymnast whose father was in the acute stage of alcoholism. Nevertheless, there seemed to be more stress in the Stanley family than Fred acknowledged.

In addition to the degree of stress in the family, it is important to identify the source of stress. Is it coming from within the family or from outside the family system? Internal stressors such as parental pressure on a vulnerable adolescent athlete, financial strain due to a child's training and coaching costs, alcoholism or other substance abuse, death of a family member, or marital conflict and divorce are examples of stressors within the family. Examples of external stress are job loss, discrimination and racism, or conflict between the family and a coach or sport organization.

Based on the brief phone conversation with Fred, Dr. Hawthorne formed her initial impression of the source of stress in the family. It seemed to be emanating from a developmental impasse in the transition for the Stanleys from a family with young children to a family with adolescent children. She also got the impression that Fred's domineering nature may have been a problem in the family, and that he may have been an overinvolved parent. She would wait and see how they interacted in her office before she formed any more impressions.

## Levels of Cohesion

A second dimension for assessing a family is cohesiveness. The main structural element in determining the level of cohesiveness is boundary formation. The rigidity or flexibility of boundaries within and around the family determines the degree of cohesiveness in the family. A family that is too cohesive will have diffuse boundaries and will be overinvolved with one another. This will be apparent in a diagnostic interview in which family members think and speak for one another, sit close together, or try to mute the expression of affect. A family lacking in cohesion will have rigid boundaries, evidenced by an unwillingness to look or speak to one another. This type of family will sit far apart, look distracted or recalcitrant, and not listen when a family member is talking about thoughts or feelings.

In the waiting room Dr. Hawthorne observed that Fred spoke first and introduced the family members to her. Betty seemed quiet and soft spoken, and Amy seemed sullen and moody. Caroline appeared pleasant and smiled frequently. When they came into the consulting room (with two love seats in an L shape and the therapist's chair forming a triangle) Fred sat next to Caroline and Amy sat next to her mother. After some pleasantries, Dr. Hawthorne's first question was "I'd like to hear what each of you likes about your family." Fred was the first to respond by saying "We have two really outstanding daughters."

Dr. Hawthorne's initial impressions were that Fred was overinvolved and controlling. He spoke for the other family members and controlled the flow of the communication. The cohesion in this family seemed centered around Fred's efforts and agenda. Dr. Hawthorne thoughts to herself, "How do the others respond to him?"

## Adapting to Change

All families need to be able to adapt to changes that are required as the family passes through the stages of the family life cycle. Adaptability implies flexibility in communication, problem solving, and conflict resolution, particularly when a family member asserts a need for change. The impetus for change can come from within the family, such as a developmental change in a member, or from outside the family, such as the death of a friend or relative. For example, the developmental task of the family with adolescent children is to begin to share the authority in the family. The children need to be given more power to make their own decisions. Many families find this difficult to negotiate, and the Stanleys were no exception. They were having difficulty changing the boundary and power arrangements in the family as the children became adolescents and young adults. A key indicator of the family's adaptability is how flexible the parents are when Amy asserts some independence. A hint of the Stanley parents' rigidity emerged early in the interview.

Dr. Hawthorne asked Amy to describe what, if anything, she would like to see changed in her family. Her answer was, "I wish they would let me do more things with my friends and not always want me to be practicing tennis. My wishes don't seem to count." She went on to describe a situation in which she wanted to go to a party at her friend's house and her parents wouldn't let her, because she had what she described as a "minor" tournament that same week-end. "I don't see why I can't do both," she said in a sullen voice.

## Interaction Patterns

Recurring patterns of interaction form the fourth assessment dimension. Here the clinician looks for communication patterns, ability to tolerate closeness, decision-making processes, time structuring, conflict resolution patterns, and the mechanisms by which the family accomplishes its daily tasks. Does the family have fun together? Do they spend time apart as well as together? Are they able to negotiate when they disagree on an important issue? Are they able to express intimacy to one another? How do they deal with conflicts between family members?

Betty had been attentive but quiet for the first 15 minutes of the session. When asked what she liked about the family, she said "I think we get along pretty well compared with a lot of families." Dr. Hawthorne agreed with her, but then went on to ask, "What does happen in the family when you don't agree on something." Betty indicated that she usually went along with the wishes of others, especially Fred. Amy said, "We don't negotiate; they tell me what to do and I'm expected to do it." Caroline said, "The only two that fight in the family are Dad and Amy. I think they are too much alike. Mom and I get along with everyone just fine."

Dr. Hawthorne then asked Fred and Betty what things they did for themselves without the children. They both indicated that right then they had very little time to do things as a couple because they were always going to the girls' tennis matches. The travel and time involved made it difficult to do anything else.

A week after the interview with the entire family, Dr. Hawthorne met with Amy. In that session she talked about her ambivalence about tennis—her love for the game and the people she has met through the sport, and her occasional desire to quit and do some other things. She expressed her frustrations about being pressured by her parents to stay with the sport. "They want me to get a college scholarship just like Caroline did."

She shared with Dr. Hawthorne the fact that there were times when she didn't want to train any more, but was afraid to say that because her father would get upset. She felt her mother was more understanding, but was weak and would not stand up to her father.

At the end of the session, Dr. Hawthorne asked Amy if she was willing to be involved in family therapy sessions to help improve the communication within the family and establish herself in a more effective way than she had in the past. Dr. Hawthorne explained to her that she would also like to see Amy in some individual sessions to talk about her feelings regarding tennis, and that by working together the family could explore ways they could live together more productively. Amy agreed to participate.

As a final step in the assessment process, Dr. Hawthorne met with Fred and Betty alone. She asked them questions about their own parents and families, how they met, what their courtship was like, and for a brief picture of the development stages of their own family. She focused on their involvement with tennis, their stance around training, going to matches, and what they said to the girls before and after a competition.

Fred did a lot of the talking, but Dr. Hawthorne skillfully drew Betty into the conversation at key times. For example, when Fred was describing the scene in the car after Amy's last tennis match, Dr. Hawthorne turned to Betty and asked "Betty, how did you feel at the time?" Betty said she felt Fred was being a bit hard on Amy but she hadn't said anything. "Do you often feel this way and not say anything"? Dr. Hawthorne asked. "Yes, I guess so," Betty replied. "I don't like to have disagreements in front of the kids." "Did your parents fight in front of you"? Dr. Hawthorne then asked Betty. "All the time," said Betty. "I couldn't stand it, and vowed I would never do that in front of my own children."

## TREATING ATHLETE FAMILIES

Though some therapeutic insight develops during the assessment phase, most of the change in perspective within the family takes place during and after a treatment contract is negotiated. It is important to involve the family in the treatment whenever possible, depending of course on the extent of family involvement in the level and source of stress, and the definition of the problem from the athlete's perspective.

## The Treatment Contract

The treatment contract often helps the family reframe a problem from an individual perspective to a broader family perspective. When Fred initially called for an appointment, he defined the problem as Amy's. Dr. Hawthorne's skillful assessment helped the family see Amy's difficulties on the tennis court in a broader perspective.

At the end of the final evaluation session, Dr. Hawthorne explained to Fred and Betty that her experience with athletes had led her to see that the problems they face in the competitive situation have a direct impact on the family and vice versa. She explained that she believed that families of elite athletes experience unique pressures and stress that many other families do not. She also explained that her belief was that Amy was facing a personal crisis on two levels. One is her own self doubt about her ability and desire to be an elite athlete. The other level is how her decisions about tennis impact the family.

Dr. Hawthorne suggested that treatment must take into account both these levels, and asked Fred and Betty if they would be willing to be involved in some family sessions to explore how the family communication and decision-making patterns were related to Amy's feelings about her sport in general, and her performance on the court.

Dr. Hawthorne recommended a series of 12 sessions, with a mixture of individual, couple, and family meetings. She explained that in the individual work with Amy she would help Amy with competition-related problems of stress, and would teach her relaxation and mental imagery skills that would help her performance. In addition she would give Amy a chance to talk about some of the feelings she had about her self-image, her identity as an athlete, and her goals in the sport. The couple sessions would focus on their ways of dealing with the pressures and stresses of being athletic parents. The goal of the family sessions would be to help all members of the family communicate with one another and feel that their own needs were being addressed. Fred and Betty agreed that the format made sense and would be helpful. They began treatment together.

## Goals of Treatment

Therapeutic intervention with athletic families has the following goals:

1. To assist the family in resolving developmental impasses
2. To improve the structural functioning of the family by strengthening boundaries, power hierarchies, communication patterns, and conflict resolution mechanisms
3. To develop the necessary support network both inside and outside the family that the young athlete needs to achieve her goals

To help her set her treatment goals, Dr. Hawthorne drew a "treatment genogram" (Fig. 4). This drawing helped her develop strategies for her interventions with the family. She then began to work with them using the following types of interventions: education/prevention, support, facilitation, and challenge [34].

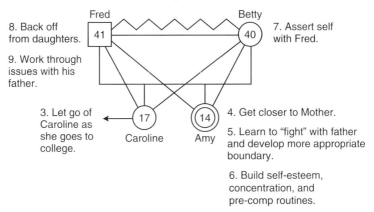

**Fig. 4.** Treatment goals genogram of Stanley family.

## Education/Prevention

The interventions that are aimed at helping the family resolve developmental impasses are often educational in nature. The family needs help in understanding and adapting to the changes that are required as it negotiates the stages of the life cycle. Educational interventions are geared toward helping the family resolve past and present impasses so that they can better meet the challenges which lie ahead of them. With the Stanleys, a major impasse was the inability of Fred to untangle himself from the drama that he had played out as a young man with his own father. In one of the family sessions, Dr. Hawthorne helped Fred to see the relationship between his inability to please his own father and his desire for his daughter's prowess in tennis.

Dr. Hawthorne asked both Fred and Betty to talk with their daughters about their own athletic experiences when they were in high school. Betty talked about how little encouragement she received from her parents, because they were always involved with her father's drinking. Fred recounted how he felt hurt when his father seldom watched him play. One year he won the high school district singles tournament, and his father didn't come to see the match. His eyes teared as he talked of how his father later told him that "I couldn't get away from the office."

Dr. Hawthorne then asked Fred," What did you decide at that time about how you would act when you became a parent"? Fred clenched his fist and replied, "I vowed that I would never miss one of my kid's matches. Never."

Dr. Hawthorne was able to use this therapeutic breakthrough to help the family see the need for a change in the boundary between the parents and the adolescent children. She showed her appreciation for Fred's wanting to be at all of Amy's matches, but she was able to help him see the reciprocal developmental need for Amy to learn to deal with competition pressures without her parents' sometimes suffocating presence. She shared with them an article by a former champion tennis player [39] on how to be an effective tennis parent. One of the author's suggestions was to attend no more than 75% of the child's matches. Dr. Hawthorne explained the reasons for this suggestion, then she worked with them in setting up a behavioral change contract to practice during the coming week.

The family agreed that her parents would not attend Amy's next match. When she returned home, they would ask her how she felt about her performance. Fred and Betty were helped to see that a question such as this shifts the focus from a concern about outcome to a concern for Amy's feelings about her performance. "I believe that the important thing for parents," Dr. Hawthorne said, "is that they not be so concerned about winning and losing, but about how their child feels about the experience."

This intervention was educational and preventive in that it helped the family resolve their present impasse and prepared them for the tasks of the next stage of family development. They were about to enter the launching phase, and having more flexible boundaries is essential for the successful resolution of that phase.

## Support

An athletic family faces a unique set of stressful events and conditions. The win/lose pressures of competitive sport as well as the demands on time and financial resources often contribute to the tension in these families; however, these families also have a great deal of strength, and their positive qualities need reinforcement. For example, their emphasis on goal attainment and the work ethic is certainly a positive quality. They need to feel understood and supported in what they are seeking to accomplish. In meetings with subsystems of the family, the sport psychiatrist or clinical sport psychologist affirms their struggle to develop the talent in the family.

In one session, Fred and Betty shared with Dr. Hawthorne the personal and financial sacrifices the two of them had made to further their daughters' tennis careers. They spoke of the pain that they sometimes felt when Amy didn't appreciate these sacrifices. They also shared that many of their friends had pulled away, both because of the time commitments to tennis and because they didn't think their friends could relate to the kind of intensity the family put into tennis. "I think many of our friends think we are crazy," Betty said at one point. Dr. Hawthorne listened empathically to these feelings and reinforced them. "You both have to understand that what you are working on is producing excellence in your daughter's tennis, and with that comes a lot of pain and sacrifice and isolation. I am sure few people, other than other tennis families, understand the difficulties you face. Perhaps you need to share more of these feelings both with one another, and with some of your tennis friends."

### Facilitation

One of the main tasks of the clinician in working with athletic families is to open the communication channels process within the family. This can be done by encouraging the family members to communicate directly with one another. This openness produces meaningful changes in the boundaries and interactional patterns within the family.

In the second session at which all family members were present, the incident that took place in the car after the regional championships was discussed. Dr. Hawthorne asked Fred to share with Amy what he was really feeling after the match. After some hedging he finally said, "I was angry and disappointed. I thought you could have won if you had played harder." Amy responded, "I knew you were angry. I was angry too. I felt like I tried hard [the tears began to flow]. When I felt the match slipping away, I knew you were over there watching and getting upset. I thought of how you would be disappointed in me during the whole third set!"

Facilitation is more than simply allowing a catharsis to take place. It leads to positive behavioral change. Dr. Hawthorne was able to do this by first commenting on how feelings are often communicated without words, and that Amy sensed how Fred was feeling. Then she pointed out that it is better to be direct so the issue can be talked about and resolved.

At the end of the session, Dr. Hawthorne helped the Stanleys establish a behavioral contract that involved Fred, Betty, and Amy. They agreed that the next time one of them felt anger, they would acknowledge it, and then state what they saw as the problem and how they would like it resolved.

### Challenge

The family structures that are not working well need to be challenged. A firm nudge is often what helps a family respond more creatively to the needs of its members. In designing challenging interventions, the clinician hopes to rock the boat, shake up the system, and guide it toward reorganizing at a more adaptive level. Two of the major areas in which the Stanleys needed to be challenged were in the area of the power imbalance in the spousal system, and the inability of Betty and Fred to deal openly with conflict in their own relationship. Betty needed to empower herself to the point where she was willing to challenge Fred's role in the family. Betty's softer and more understanding approach to problems was an undervalued source of energy in the family.

In a session with just Fred and Betty present, Dr. Hawthorne asked them about their fighting style. "We don't fight," said Betty. "What are some issues that you don't fight about?" asked Dr. Hawthorne. "And, could you look at Fred and tell him some of the things you have been avoiding." Betty went on to say that she was really upset with him during and after the regional championships, but she didn't say anything. "I didn't want to start a fight."

Dr. Hawthorne suggested they engage in a role play in which the car scene got re-enacted and the problem got discussed between them. She asked Betty to begin with a clear description of Fred's behavior that she was upset about, and her attendant feelings. Fred was asked to listen, and respond with his own feelings about what Betty had said. The role play went well. A contract was established that the next time Betty felt a strong disagreement with Fred about something, she would tell him what the problem was. He would then respond with one of two statements Dr. Hawthorne taught him: either "I understand," or, "I don't understand your feelings, please help me."

### Termination

At the end of the 12 sessions, the family terminated their family sessions with Dr. Hawthorne. Already Amy was feeling better about her tennis, and was experiencing less pressure from Fred and Betty. Betty believed that they were getting their own issues out on the table more openly with one another. Caroline had left for college, and they had been able to let go of her. They missed Caroline, but were planning to visit her at the fall parents' weekend. Fred agreed with Dr. Hawthorne that he would let Caroline make her own decisions now about tennis, and that he would support her choice of direction. Amy agreed to come in for a session once a month to discuss her feelings about her tennis and her decisions about whether to continue or not. They would also continue working on imagery and concentration to enhance her tennis skills. The family also agreed to a follow-up session with all members present in 3 months to assess the changes in the family.

## ETHICAL ISSUES IN WORKING WITH FAMILIES

There are certain ethical and value issues that are more complex than other interventions with athletes. For example, the issue of confidentiality is more complicated when working with multiple members of a family. If and when to share information obtained in a separate interview is often a dilemma for the clinician. Corey and coworkers [40] present an excellent discussion of these general ethical issues. This article concludes with a brief discussion of a few major guidelines that are important to follow when intervening in a family system.

### Training and Competence

Working with the family system of the athlete is more complex and challenging than working with the individual athlete. It is therefore important that a clinician who takes a family-centered approach with athletes have specialized training and supervision in conducting family therapy. The clinician also has to have a background in sports psychology and a familiarity with the unique pressures that face a competitive athlete.

### The Family as Client

There is a difference in value orientation when taking a family-centered approach to assessment and treatment. The goal of family treatment is to facilitate change in the whole family, not simply in an individual family member. A basic principle of family system theory is that anything that affects any one family member has an impact on all other parts of the system. It is conceivable, for example, that an individually oriented clinician working with Amy on issues of self differentiation might have provoked a marital crisis between Fred and Betty. Amy might have gotten stronger, but others might have gotten worse in the process. The "family as client" approach allows all family members to negotiate the salient developmental task at the same time.

## Avoiding Subsystem Alliances

Thirdly, the clinician must stay out of the triangles, alliances, and entanglements that develop in families, and between families and coaches and sport organizations. In working with families, it is important not to become an advocate of any one member of the family, but to remain neutral and be seen as an ally of all members of the family. A basic rule when working with couples or families is that there are no villains and victims, and that everyone shares some responsibility for what goes on in the family. Had Dr. Hawthorne become only Amy's advocate (or Fred and Betty's), the family would not have been able to make the changes that it did. On the other hand, when reportable abuse has occurred and is presented in family therapy, the therapist is a mandated reporter and must take steps to protect the abused athlete child or adolescent.

## Countertransference

In avoiding the entanglements and unhealthy alliances in families, it is essential that the clinical sports psychologist be aware of his or her own family of origin role so that these countertransference issues will not interfere in the work with the client family. Just as we expect overinvolved parents to see their own unresolved issues that they may be projecting onto their children, clinicians needs to see that they too engage in the family projection process. If a clinician empowers the adolescent athlete at the parents' expense, or encourages parents to set limits on a rebellious adolescent because of residues of the clinician's own experience, the family will not be helped.

## A MODEL FOR THE HEALTHY FAMILY

Finally, the clinical sports psychologist who takes a family-centered approach should base interventions on a model for healthy family functioning that serves as a guide to the complexities of family life. This article has attempted to present a developmental model, and it is hoped that it is a beginning for dialogue and refinement that will lead to an improvement in the quality of life for our young athletes.

An issue that did not come up with the Stanley family but that frequently presents itself in athletic families is whether a young athlete (under 15 years old) should leave the family home to train in a favorable geographical environment (eg, warm climate for tennis or mountains for skiers) or with specialized coaching (eg, tennis, gymnastics, and figure skating). This can be a dilemma for a family oriented clinician, because it presents a conflict between the value of family cohesion against the training, coaching, or competition needs of the young athlete.

In keeping with the ethical guidelines of our profession, it is important for the clinical sports psychologist to help the family explore the issues involved in this decision and not impose a predetermined solution or answer. The developmental model can help both the clinician and the family assess the developmental readiness of both the family and the young athlete. For example, in one family, a relocation for the young athlete may be appropriate; in another, it may be premature. The important questions for the clinician to help the family answer are: "What are the major developmental issues in the family now?"; "How have they handled previous stages of family development?"; "Is the young athlete developmentally ready for this kind of move?"; and "How would it affect the various subsystems in the family, such as the parents, the siblings, and the extended family?" Once a decision is made, the family oriented clinician can also help the family negotiate the separation so that the negative aspects of the separation are managed as well as possible. Also, during the period of separation, the clinician can be of value to the family solving various problems that develop, such as conflicts between the family and the coach or training academy. Finally, the clinician can be helpful by consulting with sport organizations and academies for whom this issue is a frequent problem. The consultant can help the organization both in managing these transitions, and in rethinking training and competition philosophies so that families can stay together and the athlete's needs can be met at the same time.

## THE FINAL SESSION

Three months later, Dr. Hawthorne met with the Stanley family and discovered that the family had been able to maintain the changes they had made earlier in treatment. They were communicating their feelings to one another, and Fred and Betty were discussing their differences and even fighting occasionally! Amy was happier; she was still playing tennis, but was taking more time away from the game to have fun with her friends. She was playing in fewer tournaments, but with good results. Dr. Hawthorne gave them positive reinforcement for the changes they had made.

Dr. Hawthorne ended the session by asking Betty, Fred, Amy, and Caroline to create a "sculpture" of how they saw the family now and the changes that had been made.

Betty started by placing Fred and herself together so they couldn't reach out and touch one another. She put Caroline near the door to the office, indicating her psychological departure for college. Amy was in front them, but standing sideways so that she half faced them and half faced the door. When family members were asked if anyone wanted to change this at all, Amy says she did. She walked over to her parents, who had been facing toward her in the sculpture and moved their heads so they looked more at each other.

"This is a good place to end," Dr. Hawthorne said. After a family hug, Dr. Hawthorne said goodbye to the Stanley family. She was confident that Amy would be a better tennis player and a happier person as she continued her journey.

## SUMMARY

The authors hope that this article has demonstrated that the family is a key player, in the athlete's development and performance, sometimes invisible, but often all too visible. The practice of clinical sport psychology is enriched by a family-based orientation to the assessment and treatment of athletes. Creating a workable family system is a challenge for parents. They have many difficult decisions to make, and are often without support and direction in making those choices. Sport psychiatrists and psychologists can be helpful to parents as well as athletes by using family-based assessments and treatment interventions that provide education, challenge, and support as they negotiate the tasks and transitions in the family life cycle.

References

[1] Berryman JW. The rise of highly organized sports for preadolescent boys. In: Smoll FL, Magill RA, Ash MJ, editors. Children in sport. Champaign (IL): Human Kinetics; 1988. p. 3–16.

[2] Martens R. Joy and sadness in children's sports. Champaign (IL): Human Kinetics; 1978.

[3] Greendorfer S, Lewko J. Role of family members in sport socialization of children. Res Q 1978;49:146–52.

[4] Sage G. Does sport affect character development in athletes? The Journal of Physical Education, Recreation & Dance 1998;69(1):15–8.

[5] McElroy M, Kirkendall D. Significant others and professionalized sport attitudes. Res Q Exerc Sport 1980;51:645–53.

[6] Melnick M, Dunkelman N, Mashiach A. Familial factors of sports giftedness among young Israeli athletes. Journal of Sport Behavior 1981;4:82–94.

[7] Higginson D. The influence of socializing agents in the female sport-participation process. Adolescence 1985;20:73–82.

[8] Berlage G. Fathers' career aspirations for sons in competitive hockey programs. Paper presented at the Regional Symposium of the International Committee for the Sociology of Sport. Vancouver, British Columbia, May 1981.

[9] Gould D, Horn T, Spreemann J. Sources of stress in junior elite wrestlers. Journal of Sport Psychology 1983;5:159–71.

[10] Passer M. Competitive trait anxiety in children and adolescents. In: Silva J, Weinberg R, editors. Psychological foundations of sport. Champaign (IL): Human Kinetics; 1984. p. 130–44.

[11] Scanlan T, Lewthwaite R. Social psychological aspects of competition for male youth sport participants: IV. Predictors of enjoyment. Journal of Sport Psychology 1986;8: 25–35.

[12] Bloom B, editor. Developing talent in young people. New York: Ballantine Books; 1985.

[13] Scanlon T, Stein G, Ravizza K. An in-depth study of former elite figure skaters: III. Sources of stress. Journal of Sport and Exercise Psychology 1991;13:103–19.

[14] Kesend O. The elite athlete's sources of encouragement and discouragement affecting their motivation to particpate in sport: a qualitative study from a development perspective [unpublished dissertation]. Cincinnati (OH): The Union Institute; 1991.

[15] Kalinowski A. The development of olympic swimmers. In: Bloom B, editor. Developing talent in young people. New York: Ballantine Books; 1985. p. 139–92.

[16] Monsaas J. Learning to be a world-class tennis player. In: Bloom B, editor. Developing talent in young people. New York: Ballantine Books; 1985. p. 211–69.

[17] Sloane K. Home influences on talent development. In: Bloom B, editor. Developing talent in young people. New York: Ballantine Books; 1985. p. 439–76.

[18] Hellstedt J. Early adolescent perceptions of parental pressure in the sport environment. Journal of Sport Behavior 1990;13:135–44.

[19] Hellstedt J. The family pressure cooker: reflections on parents, coaches and young athletes.

Paper presented at the 98th annual convention of the American Psychological Association. Boston, August, 1990.

[20] Bradt J, Moynihan C. Opening the safe—the child-focused family. In: Bradt J, Moynihan C, editors. Systems therapy. Washington (DC): Groome Child Guidance Center; 1971.

[21] Minuchin S. Families and family therapy. Cambridge (MA): Harvard University Press; 1974.

[22] Bowen M. Family psychotherapy with schizophrenia in the hospital and in private practice. In: Boszormenyi-Nagy I, Framo J, editors. Intensive family therapy. New York: Harper and Row; 1965. p. 213–43.

[23] Bowen M. Family therapy in clinical practice. New York: Jason Aronson; 1978.

[24] Carter B, McGoldrick M, editors. The changing family life cycle: a framework for family therapy. Boston: Allyn and Bacon; 1989.

[25] Erikson E. Childhood and society. New York: Norton; 1950.

[26] Peck J, Manocherian J. Divorce and the changing family life cycle. In: Carter B, McGoldrick M, editors. The changing family life cycle: a framework for family therapy. Boston: Allyn and Bacon; 1989. p. 335–71.

[27] Fulmer R. Lower-income and professional families: a comparison of structure and life cycle process. In: Carter B, McGoldrick M, editors. The changing family life cycle: a framework for family therapy. Boston: Allyn and Bacon; 1989. p. 545–79.

[28] McGoldrick M, Gerson R. Genograms in family assessment. New York: Norton; 1985.

[29] Nichols W. Marital therapy. New York: The Guilford Press; 1988.

[30] Gould D, Horn T. Participation motivation in young athletes. In: Silva J, Weinberg R, editors. Psychological foundations of sport. Champaign (IL): Human Kinetics; 1984. p. 359–70.

[31] Minuchin S, Rosman B, Baker L. Psychosomatic families: anorexia nervosa in context. Cambridge (MA): Harvard University Press; 1978.

[32] Rotella R. The psychological care of the injured athlete. In: Bunker L, Rotella R, Reilly A, editors. Sport psychology. Ithaca (NY): Movement Publications; 1985. p. 273–87.

[33] Odom S, Perrin T. Coach and athlete burnout. In: Bunker L, Rotella R, Reilly A, editors. Sport psychology. Ithaca (NY): Movement Publications; 1985. p. 213–22.

[34] Doherty W, Baird M. Family therapy and family medicine. New York: Guilford Press; 1983.

[35] Krestan J, Bepko C. Alcoholic problems and the family life cycle. In: Carter B, McGoldrick M, editors. The changing family life cycle: a framework for family therapy. Boston: Allyn and Bacon; 1989. p. 483–513.

[36] Ogilvie B. Psychology and the elite athlete. Phys Sportsmed 1983;11(4):195–202.

[37] Tofler IR, Knapp P, Drell M. The Achievement by proxy spectrum: recognition and clinical responses to pressured, high-achieving children and adolescent. Child Adolesc Psychiatr Clin N Am 1998;7:803–20.

[38] Hellstedt J. The coach/parent/athlete relationship. The Sport Psychologist 1987;1:151–60.

[39] Smith S. Are you a good tennis parent? Tennis 1990;26(3):42–4.

[40] Corey G, Corey M, Callanan P. Issues and ethics in the helping professions. Pacific Grove (CA): Brooks Cole; 1988.

Clin Sports Med 24 (2005) 929–942

# CLINICS IN SPORTS MEDICINE

# Systemic Issues Involved in Working with Professional Sports Teams

Joshua W. Calhoun, MD[a,b,]*, Kennise M. Herring, PhD[c],
Teresa L. Iadevito, BS[a]

[a]United Behavioral Health, 13655 Riverport Drive, Marylan Heights, MO 63043-8560, USA
[b]Department of Psychiatry, St. Louis University Medical School, 239 Westgate Avenue, St. Louis,
MO 63130, USA
[c]Department of Psychology, Roosevelt University, 440 South Michigan Avenue, Chicago, IL 60605, USA

I n recent years the consultation-liaison service (CLS) psychiatrist has moved beyond serving the traditional medical surgical unit to working in various nontraditional settings. Bourgeois and colleagues [1] note several incentives for this expansion, including pressures from managed care policies, and the realization that applied psychiatric consultation has value outside of the traditional hospital unit. Consequently, contemporary CLS psychiatrists have new and exciting opportunities to offer psychiatric (illness intervention) and psychological (prevention/wellness/organizational intervention) services in familiar settings such as the corporate workplace, and more enigmatic settings such as professional sports organizations. For some time, sports organizations have employed the services of behavioral health care specialists; however, the consultant was typically used to help the athlete enhance performance. Currently, there seems to be broad recognition that the mental health needs of athletes must receive attention comparable to the attention given to the athlete's physical health needs. At the collegiate sports level, there is a clear campaign to destigmatize psychiatric care and increase the use of psychiatric services. In a November 8, 2004 edition of NCAA News online [2], Hosick reported that the NCAA education service staff would actively address the mental health needs of the student-athlete at the January 2005 NCAA Convention and again during a panel discussion of clinical sport psychologists in February 2005.

Despite the likely long-term involvement of a small number of psychiatrists and other mental health professionals in sports at the collegiate, Olympic, and professional sports levels, we still do not have a systematic body of literature. This is needed to deepen our understanding of the precise role of the behavioral health care specialist in the sports organization; to address the needs of the athletes at

* Corresponding author. Department of Psychiatry, St. Louis University Medical School,
239 Westgate Avenue, St. Louis, MO 63130. *E-mail address:* Joshua_w_calhoun@uhc.com
(J.W. Calhoun).

0278-5919/05/$ – see front matter
doi:10.1016/j.csm.2005.06.005

various levels, and the efficacy of our intervention efforts; and to address issues of salient importance for both the health care professional and the athlete [3,4].

We have minimal data about performance psychology and the collegiate athlete. There are interesting and indeed helpful anecdotal and case study data about Olympic and occasionally professional athletes. Notwithstanding the authors' preference for empirically supported findings, we have none to offer in this article. Instead, we must follow in the steps of our colleagues and provide what we hope will be useful anecdotal data and theoretical considerations about the athlete. It will remain for others to examine our ideas and contribute empirical research.

In the first section of the article, the authors provide a review of the existing literature on the role of the mental health professional in sports clubs. Next, we examine the usefulness of systems theory as a framework to understand the sports clubs' milieu. In the third section of the article, we examine two systems variables that impact the work we attempt with professional athletes—organizational systems and intra-psychic systems. The authors maintain that there is too little understanding of the impact of the therapist's internal psychological processes on the athlete. We also examine the reciprocal relationship between the therapist (as a system) and the sports club system, and the impact of these variables on the athlete. We highlight inter-systemic conflicts that may arise between the therapist and the professional athlete by discussing seven intrapsychic processes that manifest as countertransference matters that we have observed working in this area. It is the authors' contention that psychiatrists working with professional athletes must thoroughly understand the unique, internal, emotional, and cognitive processes activated while working with the athlete, as well as the fluid, complex system in which the athlete works and lives.

During the 1990s, Begel [5] and Tofler [6] noted the striking dearth of scholarly work to guide mental health professionals trying to work in sports medicine. Both strove to use their case experiences to help create discussion and research interests. In these early works, the authors examined the primary role of the sport psychiatrist as a mental health professional working with illnesses, performance problems, psychological correlates to injury, interpersonal difficulties both on the team and in the athlete's personal life, life skills, and psychological factors impacting training [7].

In reference to the authors' work with the National Football League (NFL), it has been our experience that most professional sports organizations remain ambivalent regarding the use of psychiatric consultants, and most athletes have minimal interest in understanding the relationship between their psychological well-being and their physical performance. Psychiatrists, working with sports organizations, must conceptualize work with the athlete in a systems framework, and should therefore consider all matters related to the sports organization. These matters include hierarchical and political as well as personnel issues [8].

Since the publication of Begel and Tofler's work, there have been several other contributions to the field, largely in the sport psychology publications, in the

*Australian and New Zealand Journal of Psychiatry* [3,9–11], and in an edited text about sport psychiatry [12]. Although these articles are welcome additions to the literature, the total extant work does not comprise a systematic body of knowledge. Even though the professional sports system in the United States is expansive, there is no published scholarly work about the organizational structure of the professional sports club or about the psychological characteristics of professional athletes. For a host of complex and not well understood reasons, psychiatrists who are working with professional athletes are not publishing their experiences or insights.

The authors submit that one of the professional sports clubs' implicit, and perhaps explicit, requirements is that the psychiatrists retained to provide services must maintain utmost discretion about their work with the clubs' employees and their sensitive areas of operation. Although we appreciate the clubs' presumed need to protect their employees, the absence of useful clinical insights and empirically derived understandings impedes progress.

Macleod [3] noted the high prevalence of substance abuse and eating disorders in elite athletes, as well as the possibility of other psychiatric illnesses involving impulse control, affective disorders, anxiety disorders, and brain injuries. He argued that the role of a sport psychiatrist should primarily be that of a clinician treating illnesses. He delineated separate functions for sport psychologists, whom he saw as providing performance enhancement, stress management, life skills coaching, and development. Mcleod also suggested that many elite and presumably professional athletes might deliberately seek to avoid the mental health practitioner retained by the team and select a "neutral" doctor to ensure autonomous and anonymous mental health care.

Despite the efforts to destigmatize mental illnesses, the stigma associated with using psychiatric services remains strong among today's young adults, as noted by Glick and coworkers [4]. Such taboos, along with an ideology of strength and machismo, may preclude athletes seeking or using psychiatric services. Glick notes the intense media scrutiny that the average professional athlete receives, and implies that media vigilance may contribute to the professional athlete's reluctance to seek mental health care. Hosick [2] also talks about the stigma "attached to mental-health issues in the sports environment" and notes that the culture of sports, which tends to characterize athletes who use psychiatric services as weak or cowardly, is an impediment to a troubled athlete seeking help.

Implicit in the existing work is the caution that mental health practitioners who work with the professional athlete must develop a unique kind of cultural competence in order to both understand and to navigate the complex organizational system in which the athlete works. The practitioner-consultant who takes a job with a sports organization is often put in an unfamiliar and compromising situation professionally. For example, Anderson and colleagues [10] note that sport mental health professionals are often required to work in nontraditional settings and in nontraditional ways. The work often includes home visits, telephone and e-mail consultations, therapy sessions in locker rooms, playing fields, courts, or airplanes, and other porous boundary patient-doctor inter-actions that the typical psychiatrist does not encounter.

It is easy for the uninitiated practitioner to become simultaneously over-stimulated and overwhelmed by the frame deviations that working with profes-sional athletes sometimes require. Consequently, the inexperienced sport psychiatrist may develop erroneous and ultimately counterproductive treatment formulations. A dyadic model of treatment that focuses primarily on the thera-pist and patient does not allow the sport mental health consultant to effectively intervene with the professional athlete.

## APPLIED SYSTEMS THEORY AND THE PROFESSIONAL SPORTS ORGANIZATION

In organizational psychiatry and psychology, mental health consultants increas-ingly rely on systems theory in their work with executives and corporate employees [13–16]. Psychiatric and psychological work within organizations has facilitated the consensus that one must understand the integral relationship among all of the variables in any setting before trying to effect change in any key part of the organization. Within systems theory, one variable in a system necessarily influences and is influenced by all other variables in the system. Because systems are comprised of interconnected parts, change in one part impacts change in another part of the system. Thus any actions taken with an athlete might impact the entire organization!

In light of these thoughts, if we are to further develop the systemic model of a sports organization [7], not only must we understand the complex relationships between sports club owners, coaches, and players, but we must also consider the impact of what Fuqua and Kurpius [17] term "near and remote external systemic variables." Examples of these variables include fans and the media. Professional sport clubs are for-profit companies that wish to entertain the public while generating a substantial profit. The perceptions of the fans, influenced by the media, greatly impact the organization's bottom line.

Fuqua and Kurpius remind us that all organizations are fluid systems with natural and predictable life cycles. They offer a model of the developmental stages of organizations comprised of four predictable cycles/stages of organiza-tional change: (1) development, (2) maintenance, (3) decline, and (4) crisis. This model lends itself nicely to the professional sports organization.

Following the player draft, the acquisition of new players requires that the sports organization repeatedly review its developmental processes. During this time, rookies, and other players new to the team meet and participate in the team's training camp, where the plan for the season is developed. Simulta-neously, relationships between the players, the coaching staff and players, and among the coaching staff are developing. Athletes who do not demonstrate the ability to fit in with the team's charted developmental course are dealt with differently than athletes who are a good match for the team. In some instances, athletes are traded to another team; in other instances, depending on the kind of sport's organization, the athlete may be waived and left unemployed. At the end of the development phase, the organization enters the maintenance phase.

During this phase, the plan for the season has been hatched and the goal of the club's employees is to implement the plan and win as many games as possible. Whether the athletes have a smooth or a very tumultuous course is dependent upon many systemic variables. If the athlete is injured or takes ill, the course is particularly hard, because at a minimum he is momentarily unavailable to help promote his organization. An athlete's injury or illness has a potentially devastating impact on the sports system. A winning season may be halted if a key player is on injured reserve or is away for treatment of an illness. Injury and illness are often the precipitants of the inevitable third stage in the model, the decline stage.

Sooner or later all organizations will experience a cyclical decline in their productivity. Star players age and retire, and teams are often left without a key component of their winning strategy. Because of the athletes' vulnerability to injury, the sports organization may be more vulnerable to unanticipated decline than most organizations. The decline stage of an organization often produces systemic crises, particularly if the club was a highly competitive, winning organization, and is now a losing team. This repetitive cycle is an inherently stressful one for any organizational employee, but more so for the athletes, given the kind of work they perform. It is imperative that the behavioral health care consultant grasp and tolerate the fact that a sports club is an open system, and that much that happens to the player is truly out of both the player's and the consultant's control.

In systems theory, human organizations are thought of as open systems in which there is a continuous, reciprocal relationship between the organization and the environment in which it operates. This interaction between the organization and its environment is critical. This quality of the sports club is particularly challenging for the sport psychiatrist, because it is often difficult to discern whether aspects of the athlete's behavior are attributable to variables associated with the organization and its open-system characteristics, or to variables associated with the athlete's internal-psychological makeup. Some interaction of both processes is always at play. It is relatively easy for the mental health specialist to erroneously attribute psychopathology to an athlete if the unique broader system in which he or she lives is insufficiently understood.

## THE ATHLETE AND THE INTRA-PSYCHIC SYSTEM

Professional athletes are celebrities. Their off-field/off-court actions often make the front page—not the sports page—of major newspapers. A portion of the daily television news broadcast is devoted to professional sports. Some television programs are solely devoted to the activities of professional athletes, and they are frequently the subjects of "rich and famous" type television shows. Professional athletes are associated with charitable events, causes, car accessories, clothing, palatial houses, and glamour. The psychiatrist consulting to a sports team has, in some ways, more data about his athletic patient than any other person seen in the practice, save perhaps for the patient who has committed a highly publicized crime. The media afford the most senior corporate executives more privacy than the highest paid athlete. The athlete's salary, marital status, job performance, injury history, and a wealth of other personal data are available to any who are willing to comb the Internet or read sports publications.

Working with professional athletes puts the consultant in an unusual position. Because athletes are treated like public figures, the psychiatrist does not have the routine work condition of simply learning what patients are able or willing to share about themselves during talk therapy on their timelines. Access to a myriad of wanted and unwanted data about the patient requires that the therapist diligently filter personal psychological systems in order to minimize negatively impacting the athlete-patient.

The minimal data that exist suggest that most of the mental health professionals who work with professional athletes employ a cognitive behavioral framework in their interventions. There is vast empirical support for the efficacy of cognitive behavioral techniques for a variety of psychological disturbances. Social cognitive theory also addresses the complex cognitive processing that occurs between the therapist and patient [16]. Another particularly applicable concept that must be considered when working with professional athletes is countertransference.

For at least 50 years, the concept of countertransference has held a prominent place in the psychodynamic literature [18–24]. Originally discussed by Freud in the context of the patient's transference to the analyst, the conceptualization of countertransference has evolved from a narrow definition of a destructive process related to transference and analysis, to a broader meaning of the thoughts and feelings that the therapist has about a patient. Included in these thoughts and feelings are love and fondness as well as hatred and contempt. The expanded definition allows that the therapist's thoughts and feelings need not necessarily adversely compromise the therapeutic efforts with the patient if the processes are well understood by the therapist. There is evidence in the literature that mental health practitioners who are currently working with athletes are aware of the countertransference vulnerability unique to the sports mental health consultant. Anderson and colleagues [10] urge therapists to be aware of the "slippery slope" when treating athletes. They caution against multiple role relationships, while acknowledging that such relationships are inevitable in treating the athlete because of the systemic variables that impact the athlete's life.

## COUNTERTRANSFERENCE ISSUES

The authors' experience with professional athletes suggests several potentially damaging countertransference areas that all sport psychiatrists, working with professional athletes, will confront (Fig. 1).

### Identification

Begel [5] cautioned that "A psychiatrist who is a sports fan may derive vicarious gratification from the exploits of the patient." Implicit in this comment is the realization that the clinician may lose therapeutic posture and inadvertently

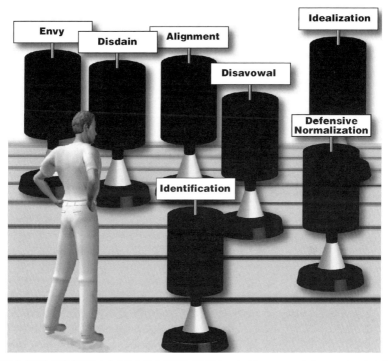

**Fig. 1.** The team psychiatrist and countertransference issues. (Courtesy of George I. Viamontes, MD, PhD, St. Louis, Missouri.)

overidentify with the athlete. The authors find that mental health professionals who are not fans are also vulnerable to identifying with the athlete. At some point, all of us have longed to have seemingly unconditional acceptance and near-universal appeal. Despite the fact that we do not have celebrity status, we can fantasize about what it is like to be the achiever of great athletic feats. It is easy to identify with the athlete's greatness, and in so doing, neglect the parts of the athlete that are overwhelmed by a life that offers few public opportunities for normalcy. Anderson and coworkers [10] note the problems with "overidentification" and boundary blurring, and caution the behavioral health care consultant to be aware of internal processes that suggests he is living "vicariously through the athlete." They remind us that we are not immune to "hero worship," and caution that even psychiatrists may be awed by the athlete's celebrity status, athleticism, fame, and wealth.

Alignment

Related to identification, Moore [22] notes that alignment is our tendency to collude with the athlete patient against the misunderstanding system. "We may be a bit reluctant to force him to change his ways knowing how we would feel if we were forced to do this."

Ordinarily, our athlete patients are at least a generation younger than the consultant. Many of the athletes have not yet grappled with the developmentally expectable life demands as they transition from adolescence to young adulthood. As such, their behaviors are often more similar to the adolescent's struggles with identity development than to the adult's efforts at synthesis and cohesion. Many of us struggle with unresolved adolescent issues involving authority, autonomy, and identity. We are not always aware of the degree to which the matters are active in our lives because of the structure and order in our professional and personal lives. Regarding alcohol dependent persons, Moore [22] states, "we may find ourselves aligning with him against those people in the environment who would seek to deprive him, such as a spouse, a judge, an employer, or other persons seen as the depriving and punitive parent that is part of our background by necessity"; background that is quite applicable to our work with the athlete. The inability of the therapist to recognize this process within himself can compromise the athlete's mental health care.

### Disavowal

Correlated to the aforementioned processes, the behavioral health consultant may unwittingly find himself minimizing behaviors that should arouse concern. Often these behaviors are not blatant indicators of clear psychopathology, but warnings that some problem is lurking. Behaviors associated with aggressive and violent acts, substance misuse problems, problematic eating behaviors, compulsions, and excessive exhibitionism are too often dismissed as "stuff athletes do."

### Disdain

Rarely do we discuss the concept of disdain in our work with patients. Therapists treating athletes must carefully monitor the strong negative reactions our athlete patients provoke, particularly those feelings in response to variables associated with the athlete's decorum and class. Many of our athletes spent their childhoods in settings that were economically deprived and marginalized by society. Although the authors are not aware of a body of statistical data that lists the demographic characteristics of all professional athletes, anecdotal data suggest that perhaps as many as 40% of professional athletes grow up with insufficient parental supervision, domestic violence, open displays of aggression, drug activity, sanctioned bigotry, criminal behavior, and other social-psychological conditions that mental health professionals consider risk factors. There is no clear, positive correlation between athletic giftedness and social adjustment. An athlete can have remarkable athletic talent and equally remarkable difficulty functioning in society.

Many professional athletes are of African-American descent, and many behave in ways that are sanctioned within the African-American community, but frowned upon by other parts of society. Behavior that has created spirited discussion in most strata of society includes speaking glibly to reporters, publicly using dialect/slang, wearing "doo-rags" and other clothing characteristic of young black men (dubbed "urban gear"), driving large sport utility vehicles and other luxury cars, dancing in end-zones, passionately dunking, and other behaviors typically associated with contemporary African-American athletes. Television and radio programs have countless "grist for the mill" discussions of athletes' antics and the disdainful responses these behaviors provoke. As members of society, psychiatrists are as vulnerable to feeling revulsion and contempt for the athlete's antics as other members of society. Our cognitive processes are often a reflection of the environment in which we live. The sport psychiatry consultant must vigilantly monitor interactions with the athlete for any evidence of disdain. Such feelings may be manifest in harsh sentiments about the athlete's need to "assume responsibility," "grow up," "stop behaving like a thug," or in verbal references to the athletes as "these guys." Although these sentiments may be understandable in context, they are potential land mines in the consultancy.

### Envy

It is easy to understand how the sport mental health consultant might feel envious of the athlete, but there is no recent professional literature that discusses countertransference, fame, and wealth. The authors also could not find any literature that discussed the treatment of celebrities or of countertransference and celebrity envy. We are struck by how little is understood about the views of psychiatrists and psychologists that treat the wealthy. Working with athletes can easily stimulate feelings of envy within the consultant. It is easy to imagine what it must be like to have all of the accoutrements associated with youth, wealth, and fame. At some point, one likely covets and envies all of the perquisites that accompany the professional athlete's lifestyle. At this writing, there is a published report of an athlete who is currently paid an annual salary of over well 14 million dollars. He is displeased with the proposed salary extension of 27 million dollars over 3 years—calling the offer an insult [25]. The entire readership of this article is not likely to make 27 million dollars over the next 3 years. The money, fame and celebrity, as well as the seeming omnipresent feelings of entitlement, are all enviable irrespective of our contentment and happiness with our lives and our intellectual understanding that being rich, famous, and entitled does not make for a happy, healthy existence.

In a 1974 paper, Wahl and coworkers [26] offered thoughtful discussion about psychoanalysis with the rich and famous. As far as the authors can determine, their work has not been further developed. They noted that rich patients provoke complex feelings within the therapist, stressing the need for therapists to screen for evidence of envy when treating the rich. They note the possibility of covertly hating parts of the patient, reifying the patient, and unconsciously derogating and idealizing the patient. The paper's authors state, "There is no doubt that social structures and social tensions have influenced and shaped psychical structures and psychical tensions" [26]. They remind us that as members of a societal system, familial system, and class system, we inevitably have attitudes about how much money certain people should be paid, how people should manage their money, and how those who have money should behave. Because many of the athletes acquire large amounts of money with little to no socialization about managing the psychological and social demands created by money, they manifest seeming adjustment difficulties related to wealth. The therapist may overlook the athlete's struggles if the athlete's behavior provokes countertransference processes.

## Defensive Normalization

One often hears the consultant working with professional athletes comment on the importance of "treating these guys just like everyone else." Although there is some appeal in offering a level playing field to all in the interest of offering nondiscriminatory care, the reality is that the athlete is simply not like everyone else.

Few people can afford to effortlessly pay psychiatric fees. Rarely will clinicians see patients actively working at their jobs. During baseball, basketball, football, soccer, hockey, or racing season, the CLS psychiatrist can turn on the sports channel and conceivably find his patients working. Most patients reside in one place and are typically available at scheduled times. This is not the case with the athlete patient, who may live in one locale during the season and another while in the off-season. The athlete's lifestyle is different, and he has been socialized differently than most working people. Throughout his career, the professional athlete has been deemed special and has had to manage both the advantages and disadvantages that accompany special treatment. To insist that he is just like everyone else and therefore "not entitled to special treatment" puts the consultant in a position of missing an opportunity to respond with genuine empathy to the professional athlete-patient's efforts to manage his world.

## Idealization

Begel [5] cautions, "A tendency to idealize athletics leads observers to deny the existence of psychiatric symptoms." Occasionally, holding athletic prowess in awe may be an inevitable outcome of treating professional athletes. Conceivably, one would hold in awe a patient who achieved a perfect score on a highly competitive professional school entrance examination and gained acceptance into the country's top schools in her area of interest. As with any of the reactions that have been discussed, the problem is less with the occasional feelings of idealization that may arise within the consultant, and more with an inability to be aware of the feelings and forestall their disruption of the therapy process.

## ETHNIC ISSUES

Related to, but not the same as, countertransference is the potential vulnerability of the sport psychiatrist consultant to underestimate the role of the social construct of race in the life of his professional athlete of color. As previously stated, a substantial percentage of professional athletes are of African-American descent. It is vitally important that those treating the professional athlete of color have basic multicultural competency as well as comfort with and awareness of their personal feelings about race. In remarks made to the British Association of Pakistani Psychiatrists in Birmingham, the President of the Royal College of Psychiatrists underscored this point by cautioning that one of the greatest challenges facing the College is the possibility of institutional racism in "both the practice of psychiatry and the structures of our psychiatric profession … Young black males tell us that they are wary of psychiatric services that do not seem sympathetic to them; they feel, with some justification, that they are more likely to be perceived as 'dangerous' than their white counterparts. They are loath, therefore, to come forward early when treatment might be most effective and the consequences complete the vicious circle" [27]. In a reply to the president's remarks, a member of the college wrote, "No doubt some psychiatrists hold racist attitudes, as do many other people. However, the president's suggestion that psychiatrists in this country allow any racial views they may privately hold to influence their professional practice is unjustified and offensive" [27].

Though written about British psychiatry, the point is useful for discussion. We live in a system in the United States in which racial matters ignite passionate discussion. No one wants to be labeled racist, and no one wants to receive treatment that feels racist. Despite efforts to provide competent care that is bias-free, many athletes of color express concerns about experiences with health care providers that they fear are influenced by racial attitudes. The idea that one can hold racist views privately but not manifest them professionally is naïve [28].

Comas-Diaz and Jacobsen [29] note, "Psychotherapy with ethnoculturally different patients frequently provides opportunities for empathic and dynamic stumbling blocks in what might be termed ethnocultural disorientation." If color matters in society, then color matters to clinicians, and it can impact therapeutic interactions. Discussions with therapists treating professional athletes reveal that the therapist is clearly attentive to the athlete's dialect, dress, and customs. More often than not, these three variables are highly correlated with the athlete's color. There are stylistic differences between black and white athletes. Also, matters such as hobbies, child-rearing practices, values, and providing financial support to the family of origin are often based in ethnic and cultural value systems, and the consultant must work to determine the impact of intervention in such areas. For example, urging an athlete to deny the requests of his family for homes, cars, money, and other material goods may be perceived as both absurd and culturally unacceptable by some athletes. For a therapist from a different ethnic background than the athlete, the athlete's willingness to subsidize the family of origin may seem unwise. This is an obvious cultural gulf that can be quite damaging to the therapeutic alliance.

Comas-Diaz and Jacobsen [29] caution that the therapist of color need be aware of the vulnerability he faces for intra-ethnic countertransference. They note the tendency of therapists from ethnic minority groups to often employ activist and supportive therapy with ethnic minority patients. They urge therapists to consider whether the mode of treatment is selected because the clinical conditions call for such an intervention or because of the therapist's unconscious identification with their patients. They urge therapists of color to be particularly aware of their vulnerability to alignment with patients of color. Thoughts of them (persons outside of the therapeutic dyad), and us (the therapist and athlete-patient) may be a warning to the therapist of color that some countertransference processes are present and are potentially correlated with the therapist's unresolved issues with oppression, discrimination, and status.

## RESOLUTION

As intimidating as it is to think that each interaction with the athlete and sports organization is a land mine, the work is both exciting and rewarding if appropriate steps are taken. First, work with highly visible, famous persons is overstimulating. The societal system in which we operate values fame. We are psychologically influenced by the views of society. Our best practice is not to ignore our attitudes, but to acknowledge the feelings within ourselves and obtain supervision if our work is compromised by our feelings. Anderson and colleagues [10] urge the sport mental health professional to review his work with "a disinterested peer."

Although the consideration of reviewing work with someone is useful advice, the consultant has a duty to protect the athlete/patient and the sports organization to which he consults. It is preferable to buy supervision from someone with a clear understanding of the processes involved in working with famous persons, rather than working with a disinterested peer whose initial disinterest will likely be transformed to interest by the consultant's data. It may well be that the ideal supervisor for the consultant working with professional athletes is someone who has some expertise in psychodynamic work in systems or social cognitive theory. The supervisory process need not result in any type of quasi-analytic process for the sports psychiatrist, but it would be helpful to have supervision with someone who is able to sort through the complexities of multiple systems operating simultaneously. It is important to grapple with the reciprocal process between the therapist system and the sports system.

Second, it is also important that consultants working with athletes remain flexible. Although there is unmistakable value in the directive to adhere firmly to the established frame and boundaries set at the start of treatment, it may be that the consultant needs to make a home visit or see a player in a nontraditional setting. The boundaries that must be established may well be within the therapist himself if the sports system requires that the consultant assume multiple roles.

It is imperative that the consultant clearly understand the expectations the club has for services and fully accept that he can work within the sports system. Clarification of roles, fees, confidentiality rules, and other key administrative parameters will facilitate a smooth working relationship [7].

## SUMMARY

Sport psychiatrists face a number of systemic and intra-psychic issues when treating professional athletes. Although only a modicum of literature exists to aid sport psychiatrists, there are several steps they may take to become an integral part of an athletic organization and to be successful in the treatment of the athletes themselves. The ability to delineate their role within the sports club is crucial to mental health professionals' organizational success. Equally important, it is incumbent upon sport psychiatrists to recognize and transcend intra-psychic issues that occur between athlete and physician.

## References

[1] Bourgeois JA, Hilty DM, Klein SC, et al. Expansion of the consultation-liaison psychiatry paradigm at a university medical center. Integration of diversified clinical and funding models. Genl Hosp Psychiatry 2003;25(4):262–8.

[2] NCAA News online. November 8, 2004. Available at: http://www2.ncaa.org/media_and_events/association_news/ncaa_news_online/2004/11_08_04/front_page_news/4123n03.html. Accessed July 14, 2005.

[3] Macleod AD. Sport psychiatry. Aust N Z J Psychiatry 1998;32(6):860–6.

[4] Glick ID, Horsfall JL. Psychiatric conditions in sports; diagnosis, treatment and quality of life. Phys Sportsmed 2001;29(8):45–55.

[5] Begel D. An overview of sport psychiatry. Am J Psychiatry 1992;149:606–14.

[6] Tofler IR. Sport psychiatry. Child Adolesc Psychiatr Clin N Am 1998;7(4):697–935.

[7] Calhoun JW, Ogilvie BC, Hendrickson TP, et al. The psychiatric consultant in professional team sports. Child Adolesc Psychiatr Clin N Am 1998;7(4):791–801.

[8] Calhoun JW. Male developmental aspects of professional sports. Presented at the 44th annual meeting of the American Academy of Child and Adolescent Psychiatry Symposium on Developmental Issues in Childhood and Adolescent Sports. Toronto, Canada, October 14–19, 1997.

[9] Petrie TA, Diehl NS. Sport psychology in the profession of psychology. Prof Psychol Res Pr 1995;26(3):288–91.

[10] Andersen MB, Van Raalte JL, Brewer BW. Sport psychology service delivery: staying ethical while keeping loose. Prof Psychol Res Pr 2001;32(1):12–8.

[11] Miller TW, Kraus RF, Adams J, et al. Sports medicine in the new millennium. A vision for 2020. Sports Med 1999;29(3):145–9.

[12] Burton RW. Psychiatric consultation to athletic teams. In: Begel D, Burton RW, editors. Sport psychiatry theory and practice. New York: W.W. Norton & Company; 2000. p. 229–48.

[13] Hunt J, McCollom M. Using psychoanalytic approaches in organizational consulting. Consulting Psychology Journal 1994;46(2):1061–87.

[14] Kilburg RR. Integrating psychodynamic and systems theories in organization development practice. Consulting Psychology Journal: Practice and Research 1995;47(1):28–55.

[15] Matheny AC, Zimmerman TS. The application of family systems theory to organizational consultation: a content analysis. Am J Fam Ther 2001;29:421–33.

[16] Bandura A. A social cognitive theory of personality. In: Pervin L, John O, editors. Handbook of personality. 2nd edition. New York: Guilford Publications; 1999. p. 154–96.

[17] Fuqua DR, Kurpius DJ. Conceptual models in organizational consultation. J Couns Dev 1993;71:607–18.

[18] Langs R. The adaptational-interactional dimension of countertransference. Technique in transition. New York: Jason Aronson; 1978. p. 501–36.

[19] Binder JL, Strupp HH, Schacht TE. Countertransference in time-limited dynamic psychotherapy. Contemporary Psychoanalysis 1983;19(4):605–23.

[20] Eastwood J, Spielvogel A, Wile J. Countertransference risks when women treat women. Clin Soc Work J 1990;18(3):273–80.

[21] Art R, Herron WG. Psychoanalysis and the disenfranchised: countertransference issues. Psychoanal Psychol 2002;19(1):149–66.

[22] Moore RA. Some countertransference reactions in the treatment of alcoholism. Psychiatry Dig 1965;26(11):35–43.

[23] Harty MK. Countertransference patterns in the psychiatric treatment team. Bulletin of the Menninger Clinic 1979;43(2):105–22.

[24] Tyson RL. Countertransference evolution in theory and practice. J Am Psychoanal Assoc 1986;343(2):251–87.

[25] Avialable at http://sports.yahoo.com/nba/preview?gid=2004110316. Accessed July 14, 2005.

[26] Wahl CW, Schimel JL, Feiner AH. Psychoanalysis of the rich and famous. Journal of Contemporary Psychoanalysis 1974;10(1):71–84.

[27] Bronks IG, Shooter M. Institutional racism in British psychiatry? Reply to Ian Bronks' letter for the Bulletin. Psychiatry Bulletin 2003;27(4):155.

[28] Spurlock J, Norris DM. The impact of culture and race on the development of African Americans. In: American Psychiatric Press review of psychiatry. Washington (DC): American Psychiatric Press; 1991. p. 594–607.

[29] Comas-Diaz L, Jacobsen FM. Ethnocultural transference and countertransference in the therapeutic dyad. Am J Orthopsychiatry 1991;6(13):392–402.

Clin Sports Med 24 (2005) 943–958

# CLINICS IN SPORTS MEDICINE

ELSEVIER
SAUNDERS

## Professional and Collegiate Team Assistance Programs: Services and Utilization Patterns

David R. McDuff, MD*, Eric D. Morse, MD,
Robert K. White, MA

*Division of Alcohol and Drug Abuse, Department of Psychiatry, University of Maryland School of Medicine, 710 West Pratt Street, 3rd floor, Baltimore, MD 21201, USA*

Every federal agency and most large businesses have cost-free, work site-based programs to improve employee morale and productivity through leadership consultation, training, and worker personal problem interventions [1–4]. Some professional sports organizations and university athletic departments have followed industry's lead by hiring psychiatric consultants or sport psychologists, or by offering assistance services to players, team staff, and organizational leaders [5–9].

Major league baseball (MLB) requires each of its 30 teams to have an active employee assistance program (EAP). In an effort to standardize program staffing and services, MLB's medical advisor disseminated a set of practice guidelines in 2003 [10]. The National Football League (NFL) does not require individual team assistance programs, but rather facilitates the development of assistance services to players and families by developing health plan networks of qualified local participating providers. Recently, however, the NFL's Office of Player and Employee Development created an employee assistance staff position to encourage the creation of more typical cost-free assistance programs [11]. Some Division I university athletic departments, including those at Penn State, Ohio State, Purdue, and the University of Tennessee, offer combined sport psychology and counseling services to teams and individual student athletes and coaches [12]. These services are usually in addition to those offered at student health or campus counseling centers.

To address all important areas, assistance programs for sports teams should offer a broad set of services in some or all of the following areas: substance abuse prevention, stress recognition and control, tobacco cessation, mental illness management, injury rehabilitation, performance enhancement, and cultural awareness and support [13–25]. Common core functions are the same as for

* Corresponding author. *E-mail address:* dmcduff52@yahoo.com (D.R. McDuff).

0278-5919/05/$ – see front matter
doi:10.1016/j.csm.2005.02.001

industry EAPs, and include: (1) problem assessment; (2) short-term problem resolution; (3) referral and monitoring; (4) crisis intervention, including critical incident debriefing; (5) organization and supervisory consultation; (6) use promotion through outreach visits and educational seminars; and (7) program evaluation [1].

Team assistance programs (TAPs) are an effective way to address typically low annual behavioral health use rates for athletes and coaches [16,23,26]. A regular presence of assistance program staff at practice or before games dramatically increases annual use rates to 10% or higher. By working closely with the team's physicians, trainers, and strength and conditioning staff, TAPs generate new referrals and make follow-up visits or monitoring easier.

The University of Maryland School of Medicine's Department of Psychiatry has run comprehensive TAPs for two professional sports organizations since 1996. This same model was used to develop services at two University of Maryland, National Collegiate Athletic Association (NCAA) Division I athletic programs. This article describes the history, organizational structure, direct services, typical activities, referral sources, and use patterns over 9 years for the professional teams and 3 years for one of the university programs. Extremely high use rates of 15% to 30% annually by players and team staff were achieved through regular on-site visits by TAP staff throughout the year. Strong linkages with each team's medical staff by the group's four sport psychiatrists built trust and ensured a steady stream of referrals. By offering performance enhancement training, initial resistance to seeking assistance for problems is reduced.

## HISTORY AND PROGRAM DESIGN
### Professional Teams
In 1996, two professional sports organizations independently requested proposals for team assistance services that emphasized substance abuse prevention and early intervention for personal problems and workplace stress. One was relocating and wanted to replicate a very successful program that had high satisfaction and use rates. The other was looking to replace an ineffective program that operated exclusively by linking team members and other staff to off-site providers through telephone self-referral. Both teams eventually contracted for free, confidential services that covered all employees and family members. A general six-visit limit, including the initial intake evaluation, was established for both. Regular team assistance advisory program meetings involving the general managers, directors of player development, head trainers and team physicians, and our group's staff were held at least semiannually. At these meetings, policies were approved and trends in use were reviewed.

To ensure that the services would be actively used, both teams contracted for comprehensive services and aggressive outreach approaches. In the first year and thereafter, the assistance program staff had a strong presence at preseason training. As the playing season began, staff members made once- or twice-weekly visits to the training facilities for practice or to the stadiums before games. At each visit, staff members would interact with key members of the coaching and medical staffs to provide consultation and solicit referrals. Group talks on various performance-related topics, such as life balance, stress control, supplement use, substance abuse, mental skills, relationships, and anger management, were given. Players and staff would often self-refer after one of these talks.

While at the training facility or the stadium of a team, most of the assistance program staff time was spent in the training room or conditioning areas. Many informal contacts were made with players and other team staff members who were receiving treatments for injuries or working on strength and fitness. Managers and coaches were approached casually in their offices or on the field as they prepared for practice or games. Assistance team staff also traveled periodically with the team for out-of-town games. This allowed for extensive interaction with players and team staff while traveling or at the team hotel. Front office staff members were also seen informally during team drop-in visits, or more formally during or after supervisory training or open seminars. An office for evaluation and intervention was made available near the training areas and locker room. This on-site approach worked much better than trying to get players and team staff to go off-site to private offices.

While at practices or before games, assistance staff had extensive interactions with the team's primary care physician, orthopedist, chiropractor, dentist, nutritionist, and strength staff. Because on-site TAP visits usually lasted 3 to 5 hours and occurred more than 20 times in a year, there was ample time to develop great trust by discussing topics and players of mutual concern.

## University Athletics

In 2002, a Division I university athletic department in Maryland established a TAP. A campus primary-care sports medicine physician, who also serves as the head team physician for one of the professional teams, facilitated its development using the professional TAPs as a model. The TAP coordinator (a sports psychiatrist) assembled an interprofessional staff of on-campus resources, including a sport psychologist, an eating disorder counselor, and a substance abuse counselor at the Counseling Center; a career counselor the Career Counseling Center; a former eating disorder nurse at the Women's Center; a nutrition and health promotion counselor at the Health Education Office; and a domestic violence counselor in the Abused Person Program. The director of the athletic department's academic support program was recruited to join the TAP, in the event a student athlete needed assistance with a learning disorder or attention deficit disorder. The idea that the athletic department would have a point person based in the training room to coordinate care was particularly appealing. Before the TAP's development, the Director of Sports Medicine had been frustrated with low Counseling Center show and retention rates, and with restrictions on feedback.

Once the members of the TAP were recruited, a brochure was designed and presented to sports medicine physicians and trainers. It was posted in the training room for student athletes to see. The TAP was presented annually to all coaches at a monthly compliance meeting. At the beginning of the 2002–2003 season, a letter attached to a screening questionnaire introduced the TAP to each student athlete. The TAP sport psychiatrist also met each incoming freshman and transfer student athlete while giving lectures in a required health and human behaviors course. Referrals were possible to any TAP staff member.

## STAFFING AND SERVICES

### Professional Teams

The authors' group uses an interprofessional, culturally diverse team of mental health and substance abuse experts. The team consists of three psychiatrists, one psychologist, three clinical social workers, and one certified chemical dependency counselor. Each team member is assigned responsibility for a specific service area or outreach to one of the eight teams. Six specific service areas were developed after the first few years: (1) substance abuse prevention, (2) tobacco cessation, (3) stress control for individuals and families, (4) cultural support, (5) psychiatric treatment, and (6) performance enhancement.

Substance abuse prevention is the most active service area, because most of these referrals come from league or team urine testing. In addition to the common drugs of abuse (marijuana, stimulants, opioids, cocaine, ecstasy, and phencyclidine [PCP]) testing is also done for supplements, adulterants, anabolic steroids, and alcohol. Every positive test is medically reviewed for justified use, and an intake is scheduled for confirmed positive tests. Referrals also come from alcohol or drug-related behavioral problems such as partner violence or arrests [9–11,17,19,20]. Most cases are for substance misuse or abuse rather than dependence.

Because 30% to 40% of athletes and coaches on these teams use spit-tobacco products (primarily moist snuff), tobacco cessation became an important focus. The most successful approach for case identification thus far results from linkages with the team dentist at the time of the preseason physical examination [18]. At that time, a dental assistant asks current users to fill out a form that asks about the pattern of tobacco use and indicators of nicotine dependency. If the dentist identifies an oral lesion or an "at-risk" user, then a referral is made for those wanting information or intervention.

Stress control services focus primarily on relationships, parenting, financial and legal problems, traumatic events, and grief [13–16]. These services extend to immediate family members and even to extended family members in distant cities, especially if a team member is worried and distracted. Marital or relationship strain, with or without partner violence, is common. Staff provides couples counseling and support following relationship strain, aggression, or breakups. Because many players and team staff have infants or school-aged children, parenting issues such as discipline or learning often surface. Spouses travel or move frequently, and are often alone in distant cities without adequate support networks. Losses of family members or close friends are more difficult, because of geographic separations and a strong shared sense of family that teammates and coaches develop.

Cultural support services developed because of the high percentage of foreign-born players in baseball. Today 30% or more of players on most teams are Latinos. Communication, acculturation, and complex family problems are addressed. Our group has a Dominican-born psychiatrist who translates all presentations and documents into Spanish. He travels frequently to the developmental leagues in the Caribbean to meet younger players, so that he can interact with them over several seasons in order to facilitate assimilation and acculturation.

Mood, anxiety, sleep, impulse control, and attention deficit disorders are the most common problems in this population [23]. Psychiatric evaluation and treatment is provided on-site at the training facility. Careful attention is paid to the use of alcohol, stimulants, and steroids, because these are common inducers or exacerbators of insomnia, nervousness, inattention, and irritability [21,22]. Psychotropic medications are chosen carefully, and the dosages are adjusted slowly in order to avoid negative effects on temperature regulation, sweating, level of alertness, or fine motor coordination [27]. Stimulants for attention deficit disorder must be prescribed with caution, and only after a rigorous diagnostic evaluation, so as to avoid their misuse as performance-enhancing substances [21]. Because of the concern about medication side effects, nonmedication approaches such as time management, positive sleep hygiene, relaxation training, meditation, massage, and biofeedback are often used first.

Many professional athletes are reluctant to discuss personal problems, even if on-site assistance is readily available. They will, however, readily engage in discussions of strategies to improve performance in practice and games. After several years of offering more typical problem-based assistance, the authors' group added mental toughness training services [12]. One of the assistance team's psychiatrists, along with clinical social workers who had strong backgrounds in stress medicine and clinical hypnosis, sought additional training in sports psychology. They began to offer biofeedback-assisted skills training for relaxation, concentration, attentional shifting, visualization, intensity regulation, goal setting, positive self-talk, and precompetitive routine development [28]. Although initial meetings start with a mental skills focus, discussions commonly drift to lifestyle and stress barriers to peak performance.

## University Athletics

The staff consists of a sport psychiatrist and psychologist; a nutritionist; substance abuse, career, and domestic violence counselors; and an eating disorder specialist. The TAP sport psychiatrist is available on-site in the training room for an afternoon each week. He sees student athletes for performance enhancement, stress reactions, relationship difficulties, substance use prevention, mental health concerns, sleep and attention problems, and partner violence. Other TAP staff members focus on substance abuse prevention, nutrition, disordered eating, women's issues, and team motivation and mental skills training.

Student athletes, trainers, sports medicine physicians, the chiropractor, coaches, and academic support staff have access to the sport psychiatrist's schedule. Records are kept in separate folders locked in the director's office. Athletes understand that access to these is limited to the TAP and sports medicine staffs. TAP notes are written with as much discretion as possible. The trainers write prescribed medications and dosages in the general medical record. Only one athlete refused treatment because of this arrangement, and she was given a referral to a preferred provider in her insurance network.

Appointments are scheduled on Wednesday afternoons in 1-hour sessions for intakes and half-hour sessions for follow-ups. The schedule is usually full. No-shows are limited by training staff reminder calls on Wednesday mornings. Some urgent problems are dealt with over the phone. The sport psychiatrist works with teams on performance enhancement, mental skills, positive self and team talk, and communication skills or conflict resolution between teammates and coaches in early morning, evening, or weekend times.

As with the professional athletes, many student athletes are reluctant to seek treatment unless initially asking for performance enhancement. The one notable exception is the self-referrals that come in after the "disordered eating" lecture given in health education class by the sport psychiatrist each semester. Athletes usually walk in the following week with a chief complaint of "I think I have an eating disorder."

Sessions with the sport psychiatrist involve the use of one or more of the following therapeutic techniques: performance enhancement training; diagnostic screening; motivational interviewing; cognitive behavioral therapy; talk therapy; work on stress and time management, including proper sleep hygiene; substance use prevention; and careful, conservative medication management. All those requesting treatment are seen.

## PROGRAM USE
### Professional Teams

The overall annual use rates for both organizations are impressive, averaging nearly 20% for baseball and 15% for football. The use rate is computed by adding the number of different employees or family members seen in a year and dividing by the total number of employee family units in the organization. The authors' group averaged 7.2 visits per intake in football, and 2.7 visits for each individual seen in baseball. The maturity and long-term nature of the NFL substance abuse program and a greater numbers of complicated family cases among football team staff explains this difference. All four major target groups (players, team staff, front office, and family members) were solidly represented in most years.

Players represent the largest percentage of those seen, averaging just more than 70% for baseball and 50% for football; however, they make up 50% and 43% of the total number of employees, respectively. This active use is not surprising, because the most attention was given to player services. The percentages of team staff of the total of those seen were about equal for baseball and football (13% versus 14%), but more family members were seen in football than baseball (21% versus 7%). Supervisory referrals were more common in baseball than football (41% versus 24%). The greater urine drug testing frequency in minor league baseball as compared with football may explain this. Trainers and team physicians facilitated most of the self-referrals of players or team staff, whereas others resulted from team visits. Not surprisingly, substance abuse prevention was the most common primary problem, totaling about 30% of intakes for both sports.

In baseball, the player use rate rose steadily over the first 3 years from 10% to 21%, and has averaged nearly 40% over the last 6 years. Regular 4-day visits to spring training and regular clubhouse visits before games during the season have built trust and kept use rates high. The authors' group averages about 15 clubhouse visits per year for the major league team, and about 4 for each of the seven minor league teams. At many of the minor league visits, we give clubhouse talks on such topics of interest as alcohol or stimulants and athletic performance, stress control techniques, or mental skills for baseball. These talks are very popular, and usually generate many questions and new referrals (Table 1).

The overall and player baseball use rates for 1999 and 2003 stand out when compared with all other years. With overall rates of more than 30% and player rates of 58% and 45%, respectively, these 2 years merit further discussion. In 1999, with the support of a new general manager and the major league and AAA managers, we greatly expanded our performance enhancement and tobacco cessation services. This was also the first year for more comprehensive cultural

**Table 1**
TAP service volumes and utilization patterns for baseball: 1996–2004

| Baseball | 1996 | 1997 | 1998 | 1999 | 2000 | 2001 | 2002 | 2003 | 2004 |
|---|---|---|---|---|---|---|---|---|---|
| Intakes | 24 | 38 | 64 | 131 | 76 | 92 | 100 | 142 | 84 |
| Visits | 36 | 135 | 227 | 306 | 207 | 225 | 243 | 392 | 291 |
| Athlete utilization rate | 10% | 18% | 21% | 58% | 35% | 37% | 36% | 45% | 28% |
| Job Class | | | | | | | | | |
| Player | 18 | 33 | 39 | 107 | 65 | 69 | 66 | 95 | 51 |
| Team staff | 01 | 01 | 07 | 15 | 07 | 07 | 16 | 28 | 13 |
| Front office | 02 | 04 | 07 | 01 | 02 | 03 | 10 | 08 | 12 |
| Family | 03 | 00 | 11 | 08 | 02 | 08 | 06 | 06 | 08 |
| Other | — | — | — | — | — | 05 | 02 | 05 | — |
| Total intakes | 24 | 38 | 64 | 131 | 76 | 92 | 100 | 142 | 84 |
| Referral type | | | | | | | | | |
| Self | 11 | 18 | 49 | 66 | 43 | 42 | 74 | 82 | 57 |
| Supervisory | 13 | 20 | 15 | 65 | 33 | 50 | 26 | 60 | 27 |
| Primary problem | | | | | | | | | |
| Sub prevention | 12 | 9 | 7 | 26 | 35 | 30 | 23 | 38 | 32 |
| Relationships | 07 | 03 | 22 | 34 | 07 | 14 | 22 | 13 | 17 |
| Performance | 00 | 10 | 06 | 20 | 08 | 08 | 08 | 22 | 03 |
| Stress/psych | 03 | 01 | 09 | 27 | 07 | 08 | 16 | 28 | 20 |
| Career | 02 | 02 | 02 | 03 | 02 | 07 | 05 | 14 | 05 |
| Tobacco | — | — | 05 | 09 | 07 | 13 | 09 | 00 | 02 |
| Other | — | 02 | 01 | 01 | 06 | 12 | 17 | 04 | 05 |
| Cultural support | — | — | 02 | 11 | 04 | — | — | — | — |
| Grief | — | — | — | — | — | — | — | 23 | — |

support services. These expansions led to 30% more clubhouse visits. The increased availability allowed more players to easily access services for relationship concerns and their mood and anxiety disorders.

The high use rate for 2003 has tragedy as a partial explanation. In spring training, a major league team player died unexpectedly of ephedrine-related heat stroke after collapsing on the field the day before. In the days, weeks, and months that followed, many players and team staff sought assistance for grief and anxiety. More than 30 individuals received grief counseling or therapy for recurrent waves of emotion that surfaced each time the death received additional publicity. The assistance program arrived within 24 hours to assist the organization's response to the loss. Four team members stayed 5 days, and along with a baseball chaplain, helped organize several clubhouse meetings for the players and staff, and a memorial service. In addition, support services were provided to the player's and spouse's families. In addition to increased workload from the player's death, this was also the busiest year ever for substance abuse prevention. Stimulants and alcohol were seen more often than before as the organization adopted a more aggressive approach to urine drug testing, with teams being tested five rather than four times that season. Our staff members also wondered whether the stress of the loss resulted in heavier drinking.

In football, the player and family member use rates have fluctuated from year to year. In the first 5 years, substance abuse prevention intakes were more common for players, whereas in the past few years psychiatric disorder and performance enhancement visits have increased. The decline in substance abuse intakes follows a policy shift in football and other professional sports to sanction first before sending for counseling or rehabilitation. This is especially true when players test positive for performance enhancing substances such as anabolic steroids or stimulants. The reasons for increased psychiatric disorders in recent years are not entirely clear, except that we are seeing more cases of attention deficit disorder and depression. Many of these athletes were diagnosed in college, and some came to the team already on medications. Performance enhancement service use has also increased recently. This is because of an increased general interest in this service among younger players. Many more are being exposed to mental skills training in college, and are interested in continuing this work. In addition, we have placed a stronger emphasis on tracking the emotional and behavioral adjustment of injured players. During prolonged rehabilitation periods, some players are electing to work on mental skills improvement (Table 2).

Family member use rates have also varied significantly from year to year. Most of these cases involve spouses or adolescent and young adult children of team or front office staff. The head team physician or trainer refers them. The most common reasons for referral are mood, anxiety, somatization, or substance use disorders. Front office staff have also been regular users of the group's services over the years. One of the team physicians, who also serves as the primary care provider to these staff, makes most of the referrals. Tobacco cessation, family stress, and generalized anxiety are the most common problems.

**Table 2**
TAP service volumes and utilization patterns for football: 1997–2004

| Football | 1997 | 1998 | 1999 | 2000 | 2001 | 2002 | 2003 | 2004 |
|---|---|---|---|---|---|---|---|---|
| Intakes | 21 | 22 | 29 | 23 | 33 | 36 | 44 | 28 |
| Visits | 207 | 253 | 305 | 206 | 219 | 248 | 262 | 246 |
| Athlete utilization Rate | 13% | 9% | 18% | 16% | 25% | 14% | 28% | 20% |
| Job class | | | | | | | | |
|   Player | 11 | 08 | 15 | 11 | 21 | 12 | 24 | 17 |
|   Team staff | 02 | 06 | 04 | 03 | 03 | 06 | 06 | 05 |
|   Front office | 02 | 05 | 04 | 04 | 02 | 06 | 05 | 01 |
|   Family | 06 | 03 | 06 | 05 | 07 | 12 | 09 | 05 |
| Total intakes | 21 | 22 | 29 | 23 | 33 | 36 | 44 | 28 |
| Referral type | | | | | | | | |
|   Self | 08 | 11 | 21 | 17 | 22 | 28 | 37 | 25 |
|   Supervisory | 13 | 02 | 08 | 04 | 11 | 08 | 07 | 03 |
| Primary problem | | | | | | | | |
|   Sub prevention | 13 | 05 | 09 | 06 | 14 | 09 | 08 | 02 |
|   Relationships | 06 | 08 | 06 | 02 | 07 | 13 | 10 | 04 |
|   Performance | — | — | 02 | 04 | 03 | 01 | 13 | 10 |
|   Stress/psych | 02 | 09 | 10 | 09 | 06 | 09 | 11 | 09 |
|   Career | — | — | 01 | — | 02 | — | — | — |
|   Tobacco | — | — | — | 02 | — | 03 | 02 | 03 |
|   Other | — | — | 01 | — | 01 | 01 | — | — |
|   Cultural support | — | — | — | — | — | — | — | — |
|   Grief | — | — | — | — | — | — | — | — |

## University Athletics

Only individual sessions with the sport psychiatrist in the training room office are in the use data. Neither formal sessions with other TAP members nor informal advice by the sport psychiatrist are included. Unlike the professional TAPs, the university TAP is focused only on student athletes. Service data for 3 years are found in Table 3.

Most referrals were self-referrals, followed by referrals from trainers, team physicians, and coaches. Some athletes were seen repeatedly. In fact, 22 athletes initially seen in 2002–3 were seen again in 2003–4. A total of 69 different student athletes were seen over 3 years. Visits averaged five per intake, although some athletes were seen once or twice and others more frequently. No significant gender use rate differences were noted. Few athletes were seen in 2002 because

**Table 3**
University TAP service volumes and use rates: 2002–2004

| Year | Intakes | Visits | Total athletes | Use rate |
|---|---|---|---|---|
| 2002 (3 mos) | 6 | 10 | 354 | 1.7% |
| 2002–2003 | 43 | 224 | 328 | 13.1% |
| 2003–2004 | 47 | 201 | 322 | 14.6% |

the sport psychiatrist's time was used primarily for staff recruitment, presentations, and coaches' meetings.

Identifying a primary problem for individual athletes was not always possible. Therefore, if athletes had two or more significant problems, each was included in the common problem list in Box 1 below. Interestingly, two athletes had three problems together—"the overdoer triad," which includes an eating disorder, obsessive compulsive disorder, and exercise dependence [29].

## STRATEGIES

There are few published articles describing practical strategies to increase athletes' use of lifestyle management, stress control, mental health, or substance abuse prevention services [7–9,13,16,18,23]. Even fewer can be found for sports psychiatry/psychology and sports medicine linkage strategies, except in the area of injury rehabilitation [5,7,24,30–32]. This is despite the fact that some sports

---

**BOX 1: TOTAL PRESENTING PROBLEMS: 2002–2004***

Performance enhancement (23)

Stress reaction to injury/rehabilitation (9)

Depression (9)

Attention deficit disorder (8)

Substance use (7)

Eating disorders (7)

Post-concussive syndrome (4)

Obsessive compulsive disorders (4)

Stress reaction to break-ups (3)

Generalized anxiety (3)

Grief (3)

Domestic violence (3)

Exercise dependence (3)

Learning disorder (2)

Insomnia (2)

Panic disorder (2)

Bipolar disorder (2)

Anger management (2)

Dysthymia (1)

Social phobia (1)

Specific phobia (1)

* Some athletes had more than one presenting problem.

medicine staff are not comfortable with diagnosis and intervention in these areas [33]. Finally, the authors were only able to locate one published report of a sports-specific EAP, and this was in the horse racing industry, for jockeys and back stretch personnel [9].

Over the past 9 years the authors' group provided comprehensive behavioral health and performance enhancement services for two professional teams and more recently for two Division I athletic programs. These TAPs were modeled after typical, aggressive-outreach EAPs seen in industry [1,3,4]. We have been able to achieve high use rates and develop solid sports medicine linkages through a number of different strategies. We believe that the following ten strategies are essential for good outcomes.

## Provide Services On-Site

Regular attendance at off-season fitness sessions, preseason training camps, practices, and games allows for longitudinal interactions with players, coaches, and sports medicine personnel, and the development of trust. The training room is a good environment for brief interactions about lifestyle concerns and performance. More in-depth discussions often follow. Use flows from a physical presence and a "walking around" style of interacting. Collaborative relationships with sports medicine personnel are built from case reviews and discussions about substance prevention, sport psychiatric, and performance topics.

## Hire a Diverse Staff

The stigma associated with mental illness, substance abuse, or lack of mental toughness makes many athletes reluctant to seek assistance [23,26]. A staff that is diverse in gender, ethnicity, professional discipline, and competencies allows for team members and staff to have a choice. The experience of the authors' group has been that it is hard to predict which athlete will be attracted to which provider, because these decisions are often made on the basis of appearance, culture, or perceived competency. We try several times each year, but especially during preseason, to expose players and coaches to our entire staff. After every such meeting each staff member gets approached.

## Connect with Preseason Physicals and Injured Athletes

The preseason physical evaluation is a good time to ask about past or current concerns with sex, stress, anxiety, aggression, substances, tobacco, depression, or performance. A recent review by Joy et al [34] recommends that inquiries of this sort become standard practice. The authors have helped revise or construct screening questions in these areas for inclusion in preseason and postseason physicals. Supportive interactions with injured athletes are also important. Severe athletic injuries, especially those requiring surgery or prolonged rehabilitation, often produce emotional distress and lowered self-esteem [35,36]. Return-to-play and retirement decisions relating to injury, especially head injury, are now more clinically, socially, politically, and legally complicated [37–39]. Consequently, an expert panel of sports medicine physicians recently recommend that return-to-play processes be formalized, and that psychosocial issues be routinely addressed [37].

## Give Prevention Talks

Staff members from the authors' group regularly give brief 10 to 20-minute pre- and in-season talks to athletes and coaches. Tying the topic to athletic performance is critical to getting their attention and stimulating discussion. The most popular topics are supplements, alcohol, tobacco, stress, and mental skills training. Our group's sport psychiatrists stay current on athletic performance, and on psychoactive drugs and supplements such as amino acids, creatinine, prohormones, stimulants, and androgenic steroids [40–42]. Our staffers often collaborate with the team's sports nutritionist and strength and conditioning staff when preparing these talks. After every prevention talk, our group gets active discussion and requests for further assistance.

## Offer Tobacco Cessation Services

The adverse health effects, the inconvenience of using, and pressure from family, teammates, and the league cause athletes and coaches to be very interested in tobacco cessation. Our group's staff members routinely distribute quitting guides [43] or collaborate with the team dentist during preseason physicals to assess and intervene [18]. In addition, the team's primary care sports medicine physicians routinely ask about use, and support quitting by referring athletes to our program. Studies have shown that brief interventions can reduce spit-tobacco use in athletes [44]. Our experience has shown that athletes and coaches do better if they can find effective substitutes for their tobacco. These have included nicotine and non-nicotine gum, candy, herbal dips, aromatic hardwood branches, plastic cigar tips, and others. Continuous monitoring, encouragement, and craving coping strategies are needed to present slips or relapses.

## Offer Performance Enhancement Services

The authors' group has modeled these services after the approaches recommended by Dorfman and Kuehl in *The Mental Game of Baseball* [28]. Our staff members work collaboratively with the player and coach to identify major barriers to performance (ie, divided attention, negative self-talk, poor emotional control, pregame arousal, inability to let go of mistakes). We develop goal-oriented improvement plans and monitor progress over a season. We ask athletes to systemically record information about thoughts and emotions (positive and negative) during competition, using a mental training log as recommend by Porter [45]. We review these and our plan every three to five games, teaching relevant basic mental skills along the way. We often identify and resolve high-stress situations or other problems in the course of this work.

## Provide Critical-Incident Stress Management Services

Sports organizations occasionally experience traumatic events or unexpected tragic losses. Several recent ephedrine-related deaths in football and baseball are examples. Critical incidents such as these have the potential to disrupt individual or team functioning. Organizational leaders are expected to respond to such challenges by offering comprehensive support services for all employees. TAPs with critical incident stress management or traumatic grief expertise will likely be called on for planning and direct assistance during and after a critical incident [46,47]. The authors' group was involved in such a critical incident in 2002. The existence of a positive working relationship with the team's management, coaches, and players made the initial response more effective. Longitudinal follow-up of many individuals for a year was necessary. Key lessons learned were: (1) know the organization and its people; (2) get involved within 24 hours; (3) collaborate with a chaplain; (4) work in pairs and debrief regularly; (5) create a formal support plan with the general manager, manager, and team physician; (6) facilitate role definition, especially for a media spokesperson; (7) establish linkages with the league's medical advisors; and (8) give extra support to the medical and conditioning staff.

### Know Something About Fitness and Supplements

Over the last decade, supplement use by professional and collegiate athletes has increased dramatically [22,40,41]. Although it is true that most athletes are looking to gain a competitive advantage, they are still concerned about false claims, long-term side effects, and contamination. It is therefore possible to engage many in active discussions of these issues. Current factual information about policy and the risks and benefits is most helpful. Whether presented in preseason talks or in printed materials that are posted in the clubhouse or locker room, coaches and players are interested. Collaboration with the team physicians, trainers, strength staff, and nutritionists is necessary to ensure a consistent message. The more knowledge TAP staff have about exercise physiology, cardiovascular fitness, and speed, strength, and flexibility training, the more credibility they will have with supplements.

### Think About Sleep, Jet Lag, Chronic Fatigue, and Burnout

Professional and collegiate sports training and competition are now year-round ventures. The notion of an "off-season" is a thing of the past. It is therefore critical to monitor athletes for sleep and stress recovery. Military studies have demonstrated that approximately 6 hours of continuous sleep a night are needed for ongoing operational effectiveness. Long seasons can bring on chronic mental and physical fatigue and poor sleep, because of chronic injuries and performance pressure. Travel adds to the demands of competition, especially if it crosses two or more time zones or if circadian rhythms are disrupted [48,49]. In the last few years, our team's medical staff have received more requests for short-acting sleep medications. We have responded to this trend by conducting in-depth evaluations by TAP psychiatrists for repeat requestors. In these evaluations, we look for poor sleep hygiene, excessive stimulant or alcohol use, high stress levels, or sleep mood or anxiety disorders that might explain the insomnia.

## Reach Out to Family Members

Professional and collegiate athletes, team staff, and front office personnel work long hours and have frequent or prolonged family separations. Marital and relationship stability, parental support, and parenting may consequently suffer. The authors' group has found it useful to reach out to spouses, significant others, parents, and children. Many teams have organized gatherings of these groups. Formal presentations about TAP services or stress control topics often lead to new referrals. In addition, the authors' group actively involves key family members in new evaluations or ongoing assistance. For our professional teams, we have established national and international networks of certified assistance program providers who can respond quickly to crises by providing comprehensive evaluations and brief treatment.

## SUMMARY

TAPs that are on-site and link strongly with the medical staff can increase stress control and behavioral health services use. Although there are few sports EAP studies documenting a positive impact on performance, there are many in industry [1–3]. TAPs that offer free, comprehensive services to all team and front office staff members are most likely to have successful outcomes. Adding mental skills training to the service menu is attractive to players and coaches, and can be extended to the organization's executives and management staff. More descriptive papers of model programs and studies on TAP cost-effectiveness and performance outcomes are needed.

## References

[1] Employee Assistance Professionals Association. What's an EAP? Available at: www.eapassn.org/public/pages/index.cfm?pageid=507. Accessed March 6, 2005.

[2] Office of Personnel Management. Employee assistance program. Available at: www.opm.gov/ehs/eappage.asp. Accessed March 6, 2005.

[3] White RK, McDuff DR, Schwartz RP, et al. New developments in employee assistance programs. Psychiatr Serv 1996;47:387–91.

[4] Zarkin GA, Bray JW, Karuntzos GT, et al. The effect of an enhanced employee assistance program (EAP) intervention on EAP utilization. J Stud Alcohol 2001;62:351–8.

[5] Calhoun JW, Ogilvie BC, Hendrickson TP, et al. The psychiatric consultant in professional team sports. Child Adolesc Psychiatr Clin N Am 1998;7:791–802.

[6] Burton RW. Psychiatric consultation to athletic teams. In: Begel D, Burton RW, editors. Sport psychiatry: theory and practice. New York: W.W. Norton & Company; 2000. p. 229–48.

[7] Anderson MB, Brewer BW. Organizational and psychological consultation in collegiate sports medicine groups. J Am Coll Health 1995;44:63–9.

[8] Anderson MB, Van Raalte JL, Brewer BW. Sport psychology service delivery: staying ethical while keeping loose. Prof Psychol Res Pr 2001;32:12–8.

[9] Schefstad AJ, Tiegel SA, Jones AC. Treating a visible problem within a hidden population: a working sports EAP in the horse racing industry. Employee Assistance Quarterly 1999; 14:17–32.

[10] Major league baseball's minor league drug prevention and treatment programs and major league baseball's joint drug prevention and treatment program. Available at: www.mlb.com. Accessed April 1, 2005.

[11] National Football League. Office of the vice president of player and employee

development. Available at: www.nfl.com/player-development/story/6190917. Accessed March 5, 2005.

[12] Gentner NB, Fisher LA, Wrisberg CA. Athletes' and coaches perceptions of sport psychology services offered by graduate students at one NCAA Division I university. Psychol Rep 2004;94:213–6.

[13] Raglin JS. Psychological factors in sport performance: the mental health mode revisited. Sports Med 2001;31:875–90.

[14] Iso-Ahola SE. Intrapersonal and interpersonal factors in athletic performance. Scand J Med Sci Sports 1995;5:191–9.

[15] Baker J, Cote J, Hawes R. The relationship between coaching behaviors and sport anxiety in athletes. J Sci Med Sport 2000;3:110–9.

[16] Pinkerton RS, Hinz LD, Barrow JC. The college student athlete: psychological considerations and interventions. J Am Coll Health 1989;37:218–26.

[17] Miller TW, Adams JM, Kraus RF, et al. Gambling as an addictive disorder among athletes: clinical issue in sports medicine. Sports Med 2001;31:145–52.

[18] Walsh MM, Greene JC, Ellison JA, et al. A dental-based, athletic-trainer mediated spit tobacco cessation program for professional baseball players. J Calif Dent Assoc 1998;26:365–72.

[19] Miller BE, Miller MN, Verhegge R, et al. Alcohol misuse among college athletes: self-medication for psychiatric symptoms? J Drug Educ 2002;32:41–52.

[20] Greene GA, Uryasz FD, Petr TA, et al. NCAA study of substance use and abuse habits of college student athletes. Clin J Sport Med 2001;1:51–6.

[21] Hickey G, Fricker P. Attention deficit hyperactivity disorder, CNS stimulants and sport. Sports Med 1999;27:11–21.

[22] Pope HG, Katz DL. Psychiatric and medical effects of anabolic-androgenic steroid use. A controlled study of 160 athletes. Arch Gen Psychiatry 1994;51:375–82.

[23] Glick ID, Horsfall JL. Psychiatric considerations in sports: diagnosis, treatment and quality of life. Phys Sportsmed 2001,27(0).1 ?.

[24] Ahern DK, Lohr BA. Psychosocial factors in sports injury rehabilitation. Primary care of the injured athlete, part II. Clin Sports Med 1997;16:755–68.

[25] McAllister DR, Motamedi AR, Hame SL, et al. Quality of life assessment in elite athletes. Am J Sports Med 2001;29:806–10.

[26] Schwenk TL. The stigmatisation and denial of mental illness in athletes. Br J Sports Med 2000;34:4–5.

[27] Baum AL. Psychopharmacology for athletes. In: Begel D, Burton RW, editors. Sport psychiatry: theory & practice. New York: W.W. Norton & Company; 2000. p. 249–59.

[28] Dorfman HA, Kuehl K. The mental game of baseball. 2nd edition. South Bend (IN): Diamonds Communications, Inc.; 1995.

[29] Morse ED. Eating disorders in athletes. Presentation given at the International Society for Sport Psychiatry's scientific session at the American Psychiatric Association annual meeting. New York, New York, May 2, 2004.

[30] Brewer BW. Role of the sports psychologist in treating athletic injuries: a survey of sports medicine providers. Journal of Applied Sport Psychology 1991;3:183–90.

[31] Heil J. Sport psychology, the athlete at risk and the sports medicine team. In: Heil J, editor. Psychology of sport injury. Champaign (IL): Human Kinetics; 1993. p. 1–13.

[32] Larson GA. Psychological aspects of athletic injuries as perceived by athletic trainers. The Sport Psychologist 1996;10:37–47.

[33] Vaughan JL, King KA, Cottrell RR. Collegiate athletic trainers' confidence in helping female athletes with eating disorders. J Athl Train 2004;39(1):71–6.

[34] Joy EA, Paisley TS, Price R, et al. Optimizing the collegiate preparticipation physical evaluation. Clin J Sport Med 2004;14:183–7.

[35] Smith AM, Scott SG, Wiese DM. The psychological effects of sports injuries. Coping. Sports Med 1990;9:352–69.

[36] Johnson U. Coping strategies among long-term injured competitive athletes. A study of

81 men and women in team and individual sports. Scand J Med Sci Sports 1997;7: 367–72.

[37] McFarland EG. Return to play. Clin Sports Med 2004;23:xv–xxiii.

[38] Cantu RC. Recurrent athletic head injury: risks and when to retire. Clin Sports Med 2003;22:593–603.

[39] McCrea M, Guskiewicz KM, Marshall SW, et al. Acute effects and recovery time following concussion in collegiate football players. JAMA 2003;290:2556–63.

[40] Schwenk TL. Psychoactive drugs and athletic performance. Phys Sportsmed 1997;25:1–9.

[41] Consumer Reports. Health and fitness. Drugs and supplements. Dangerous supplements 5/04. Dangerous supplements: still at large. Available at: http://www.consumerreports. org. Accessed April 1, 2005.

[42] Jones AR, Pinchot JT. Stimulant use in sports. Am J Addict 1998;7:243–55.

[43] Severson HH. Enough snuff. 6th edition. Eugene (OR): Applied Behavior Science Press; 2001.

[44] Walsh MM, Hilton JF, Ellison JA, et al. Spit (smokeless) tobacco intervention of high school athletes results after 1 year. Addict Behav 2003;28:1095–113.

[45] Porter K. The mental athlete. Champaign (IL): Human Kinetics; 2004. p. 26–7.

[46] Ruzek J, Watson P. Early intervention to prevent PTSD and other trauma-related problems. PTSD Research Quarterly 2001;12:1–8.

[47] Shear K, Smith-Caroff K. Traumatic loss and the syndrome of complicated grief. PTSD Research Quarterly 2002;13:1–8.

[48] Manfredini R, Manfredini P, Fersini C, et al. Circadian rhythms, athletic performance, and jet lag. Br J Sports Med 1998;32:101–6.

[49] Waterhouse J, Edwards B, Nevill A, et al. Identifying some determinants of jet lag and its symptoms: a study of athletes and other travelers. Br J Sports Med 2002;36:54–60.

Clin Sports Med 24 (2005) 959–971

# CLINICS IN SPORTS MEDICINE

ELSEVIER
SAUNDERS

# The Sport Psychiatrist and Golf

Terrence P. Clark, MD[a], Ian R. Tofler, MB, BS[b],
Michael T. Lardon, MD[c],*

[a]Department of Psychiatry and Behavioral Sciences, James H. Quillen College of Medicine,
East Tennessee State University, 52 Dogwood Lane, Mountain Home, TN 37684, USA
[b]Charles R. Drew University of Medicine and Science/University of California, Los Angeles, 1731 East 120th Street,
Los Angeles, CA 90059, USA
[c]Department of Psychiatry, School of Medicine, University of California at San Diego, 3750 Convoy Street, #318,
San Diego, CA 92111, USA

G
olf is a mentally challenging game. The sport psychiatrist knowledge-able in the game of golf is well-positioned to consult to competitive golfers. Golf is the only sport in which practice and competition take place in different environments: the practice range and the golf course. Additionally, no other sport has world-class, top-30 players ranging in age from 19 (Sergio Garcia, 1999) to 50 (Jay Haas, 2005). This broad age range speaks to the fact that aging world-class golfers can compensate for physical deterioration with mental maturation. Most significant, however, and warranting the authors' discussion here, are issues of time management.

The sport of golf is uniquely challenging because its duration, interrupted pace of play, and excessive amount of idle time make the competitor vulnerable to external and internal distracters [1,2]. A golf round of 18 holes takes 4 to 5 hours to play, weather permitting. A golf swing lasts only about 3 seconds; thus the professional player swings the club for a total of about 3 1/2 minutes in an entire 4 1/2-hour round! The pre-shot routine takes about 30 seconds, resulting in the professional golfer having greater than 3 1/2 hours of idle time during the heat of competition. This excessive down time can lead to obsessive thinking and distraction, as well as amplification of pre-existing negative self-perceptions, performance anxiety, panic, and affective overarousal [1,2].

To perform well, competitive golfers must have a trustworthy pre-shot routine, as well as other strategies to deal with these inevitable distracting thoughts, emotions, and doubts. They also need a sound psychological and philosophical belief system contextualizing the meaning of winning and losing.

The ultimate reason many, but not all, people play games is to win. On the golfing circuit, a competitive golfer rarely wins most of his tournaments. Stuart Walker [3] contends that it is even more difficult to win if a player is investing

* Corresponding author. E-mail address: drlardonsoffice@cox.net (M.T. Lardon).

0278-5919/05/$ – see front matter
doi:10.1016/j.csm.2005.04.001

his sense of self-worth or ego in the outcome. He contends that playing a game for narcissistic or ego purposes is "playing a game within a game" [3]. A more mature competitive philosophy is to play to win, yet to at the same time to acknowledge that losing is a possibility. This competitor enjoys matching his expert skills against other highly skilled competitors, and can derive pleasure from the process of performing well, even without always winning.

Renowned golf teacher David Leadbetter [4] comments that golf is like "mental chess," and that the mental component is possibly the toughest part of playing golf. The mental chess of golf is the challenge of how well a player focuses on the shot at hand, rather than being taken off-task by thoughts, emotions, or poorly controlled physiological arousal.

The protracted pre-performance time can lead the athlete to experience potentially counterproductive cognition, such as overevaluating the importance or risks of the next shot [1,2]. This in turn may lead to self-doubt and fear of failure. At times of heightened pressure in competition, an athlete may experience difficulty ridding his mind of negative thoughts. These thoughts can lead to impaired performance, including the athlete doing exactly what he is trying to avoid [5,6]. Examples are a basketball player trying not to throw a second air ball from the free-throw line in basketball and doing just that, or a golfer trying not to hit a ball into a water hazard and then doing so. Wegner [5] theorized that such behavioral enactment represents an "ironic process." Alternatively, Beillock et al [7] demonstrated that trying not to imagine landing a ball short results in an increased incidence of hitting the ball long. Thus, ironic processes may not just result in enacting the unwanted action, but may lead to over-compensation. The sport psychiatrist can help the athlete interrupt ironic processes by first recognizing when they occur, and then developing strategies to lessen cognitive and emotional overload. Prompt and effective management allows the golfer to attend to the task of preparing to hit his next shot [5,6].

Confidence and trust are the cornerstones to succeeding in competitive golf [7]. The study of confidence is best described by Albert Bandura's work on self-efficacy [8]. Confidence is a state of mind marked by freedom from uncertainty coupled with a sense that a desired task will be accomplished. Confidence is based upon one's past experiences and performances. It is also dependent upon vicarious experience, good preparation, and established, solid routines. A competitor rediscovering confidence based on vicarious experience is exemplified by the experience of Rich Beem, who in 1995 had quit playing golf and took a job selling cell phones in Seattle. In 1996 Paul Stankowski, with whom Beem had competed in college, won the Bell South Classic. An inspired Beem felt that if Stankowski could succeed, he could certainly do it as well. Beem has since won three Professional Golfers' Association (PGA) Tour events, including the 2002 PGA Championship [9].

## THE PRE-PERFORMANCE ROUTINE

A consistent pre-performance or pre-shot routine is essential in sports activities that are self-paced, such as competitive golf, target shooting, or shooting free throws in basketball [1,2]. Such a routine can help the competitive golfer's resilience under pressure. He can invest his attention in a well-established pre-shot routine rather than allowing distractions such as thinking about the importance or prestige of a tournament. This permits the competitor to access a cognitive, emotional, and psycho-physiological state that optimizes his chances of hitting an excellent shot. Once confidently settled by his pre-shot routine, the elite golfer customarily imagines the shot, focuses his attention on a relevant external cue or thought, executes with a quiet mind, and then evaluates the quality of the execution [2]. This structured approach enables the performer to stay well-focused, or sometimes to approach or remain in a state of "flow" or "the zone."

Elite athletes, including golfers, often describe their best performance as being "in the zone" [10,11]. Flow [12] is a research-verified state that is closest to the phenomena of playing in the zone in sports or other activities [12]. Flow is a state experienced in a task-oriented activity. The individual may experience a sense of absorption, loss of self-consciousness, an almost dissociative detachment, power, pleasure, altered perception of time (usually slowing), and a sense of control and unity.

Researchers at the University of California, San Diego (UCSD) and Scripps Research Institute [13] hypothesized that the zone state may be a manifestation of an adaptive dissociation, and that similarities exist between the zone, hypnosis, and dissociation. They characterized the athletic zone as having four essential components: (1) enhanced attentional focus, (2) time slowing, (3) sense of detachment, and (4) super-normal performance. They define enhanced attentional focus as consisting of multiple cognitive components, including general alertness and the ability to sustain and select where attention is directed. They conceptualize dissociation as a mental separation of components of experience which would normally be processed together that is seen in trauma and in highly stressful situations, as well as in some psychiatric disorders. Hypnosis is defined as an enhancement of focal concentration with suspension of peripheral awareness. Its components include absorption, which is the tendency to become fully involved in a perceptual experience, and suggestibility, which allows heightened responsiveness to the environmental stimuli. The researchers noted that hypnosis has been used as a model for dissociative states. Neuroelectric measures, such as electroencephalography (EEG) and event-related potential (ERP) techniques, have been used to assess these phenomena, with findings that suggest that the same attentional mechanisms are affected by hypnosis and dissociation [14]. Given these relationships and the clinical observation that certain individuals may inherently be more susceptible to dissociative states, they hypothesized that the zone, in the context of athletic performance, could be measured by neuroelectric evaluation. The researchers [15,16] used clinical histories, neuropsychological assays, and neuroelectric measures on three groups of individuals. The experimental group was composed of highly accomplished athletes (among the best in the world in various sports). Two control groups were used; one was physically conditioned and one was not. Although early results suggested that the highly accomplished athletes may in fact have some neurophysiologic trait differences (decrease in delta brain wave activity), clear brain wave changes (increase in P300 amplitude and decrease in delta band) were seen in both this group and the physically conditioned control group in contrast to the unconditioned control group. Interestingly enough, amphetamines have been suggested to heighten hypnotic induction, and highly hypnotizable individuals have been shown to have higher cerebral spinal fluid levels of homovanellic acid (HVA), a dopamine metabolite [17,18]. UCSD researchers Lardon and Polich [15] raised the question of whether elevated levels of dopamine are implicated in the athletic zone phenomenon. They further suggested that because dopaminergic medicines are useful in treatment of attention deficit hyperactivity disorder, predominately inattentive type (ADHD-1), then the zone is possibly in some way the inverse of ADHD-1.

## BEYOND CHOKING—THREE DISTINCT FORMS OF PERFORMANCE FAILURE

"Choking" is a colloquial, pejorative term used to convey the phenomenon of acute performance failure under perceived stress; however, acute performance failure is not a homogenous phenomenon. In golf there appear to be at least three distinct, although sometimes overlapping, entities that produce acute performance failure. In an attempt to establish a consistent nomenclature the authors will name these three entities panicking, choking, and the "yips." All three of these phenomena are exacerbated by stress, but they differ in their characteristics. Neuroscience theories of memory and learning are helpful in understanding their etiologies. Explicit (declarative) memory governs the recollection of facts, events, and associations. In contrast, implicit memory deals with procedural memory that does not require conscious awareness; for example, one is able to recall how to ride a bicycle or play the piano after many years of not performing either function [18]. Explicit (declarative) memory appears to be centered in the part of the brain called the hippocampus. When an individual experiences severe stress, there is secretion of epinephrine and glucocorticoids. Severe stress responses can harm and, over time, produce atrophy of the hippocampus, preventing consolidation or retrieval of conscious explicit memory [19]. The individual often experiences this as the mind going blank, something psychologists call perceptual narrowing. The stress response, with concomitant impairment in explicit memory, may hinder one's ability to think clearly during intense competition, leaving the athlete to rely on instinct alone. In summary, when an athlete is exposed to excessive autonomic hyper arousal and panics he turns to his "instinct" and temporarily loses his ability to think critically.

An excellent example of this panic phenomenon in golf occurred in the 1999 British Open, when Jean Van de Velde had a three-shot lead going into the final hole. Those watching the event acknowledged that all Van de Velde needed to do on the dangerous 18th hole at Carnoustie was to hit three conservative iron shots, two-putt for bogey, and receive his first Claret Jug trophy as British Open Champion, with a shot to spare. Van de Velde made a critical strategic error, however; by relying on instinct, he chose his driver to tee off on the final hole. He compounded this poor decision with another unnecessarily aggressive play by taking a two iron, going for the green, and hitting into the water. His poor judgment continued when he took off his shoes and went into the water to hit his third shot. Finally, he regained his senses, took a penalty shot and made a great eight-foot putt to force a playoff, which he eventually lost. The famous image of Van de Velde going into the water to hit the ball haunts golf fans to this day. It would be reasonable to assume that his mind went blank, and that he relied on instinctive behaviors and lost his ability to think about what shots he needed to attain his goal. This type of performance failure the authors will call panicking, as in Malcolm Gladwell's original description [20]. In contrast, Ben Hogan had a two-shot lead playing the 72nd hole of the 1951 Masters. He hit a perfect drive and then strategically hit his next shot 30 yards short of the green, chipped to four feet short of the hole, and made the putt to secure victory. In fairness to Van de Velde, Hogan was able to think so clearly because he had the experience of twice before losing his chance at victory in the Masters by hitting the ball beyond the hole on this very same green, and three-putting on both occasions [21]!

In contrast, Gladwell [20] posits that choking is not about reversion to instinct but rather about the loss of instinct or the loss of previously mastered motor programs. Motor programs that are normally implicit (are not in conscious awareness) partially reside in the deep brain structures, the basal ganglia and the cerebellum. In conditions of severe stress when an individual chokes, the explicit memory system takes over. An individual who has had mastery of certain motor execution programs (such as a golf swing) starts to consciously think about his swing, thus resulting in loss of fluidity and kinesthetic touch. In a sense, the athlete becomes a beginner again, because he starts to rely on a learning system that is no longer implicit, subconscious and automatic. This is often termed "explicit monitoring" [22].

In their 1993 study of the electroencephalographic patterns of golfers before putting, Crews and Landers [23] found that the best putters had a distinctive bimodal brain-wave pattern in the seconds leading up to the putt. It was noted that the left side of the athletes' brains (which controls logical and analytical processing) was active. Then, just before the subject putted, the left side quieted and the more intuitive right side (which controls spatial orientation, timing, and balance) became more active. The study authors hypothesized that chokers exhibit a different pattern, in which their left brains never shut down. They then raised the question of whether or not this situation led to a possible obstruction preventing the "passing of the baton" to the right frontal-parietal brain hemispheres [23].

In another interesting study [22], Beilock and Carr at the Department of Psychology at Miami University in Oxford, Ohio hypothesized that limiting putting time would actually help execution by preventing skilled golfers from allocating too much attention to task control and guidance. In their experiment, they demonstrated that golfers were more accurate under speed instructions.

They reported that speed instruction aided the performance of several golfers by preventing over-thinking about execution. Their research has also shown that expert swing execution does not require constant monitoring, and that limiting the time experts have to over-think prevents interference with performance and execution of various shots. These two studies [22,23] support the notion that in choking, individuals lose their capacity to access implicit learned motor programs. Thus, they start to over-think and rely on explicit (conscious) learned models, resulting in acute performance failure.

An excellent example of this choking phenomenon was evident in the final round of the 1996 Masters, when Greg Norman had a six-shot lead against Nick Faldo. Norman, the number one golfer in the world at that time, poorly executed a number of shots, which was markedly uncharacteristic of him. He did not panic and make a variety of poor choices, as Jean Van de Velde did in our example. Rather, Norman was unable to properly execute shots that he had previously shown mastery of. In essence, Norman lost his instinct and "touch," and was probably thinking too much, resulting in acute performance failure.

A third type of acute performance failure is often known as the "yips." An example of the yips occurred on the final hole of the 1989 Masters, when Scott Hoch missed a simple 30-inch putt needed to win. Eyewitnesses were shocked wondering how he could yip a short putt that would have won the Masters. He had not three-putted for the entire tournament [24]! The phenomenon of the yips is often referred to as a focal dystonia [25–27]. Dystonia is characterized as a paroxysmal movement disorder in which an unwanted muscle contraction, or twitch, leads to an involuntary movement. In golf, it is seen most commonly in putting, but also is apparent in other shots. Symptoms of the yips, such as jerks during execution of shots, often result in miss-hits. This phenomenon has derailed the illustrious careers of Johnny Miller, Ian Baker-Finch, and Mark O'Meara, as well as being the bane of the average golfer.

The neurophysiology of focal dystonias has been best elucidated by Dr. Jonathan Mink [28]. He postulates that the basal ganglia (the area of the brain where implicit learning resides) is organized to facilitate voluntary movements and to inhibit competing movements that interfere with the desired movement. The idea is that in the basal ganglia there are various motor programs that operate on the subconscious level. When an athlete experiences the yips, or a focal dystonia, the pathways that govern the inhibition of competing motor programs break down. This results in the overriding of the original motor program. Therefore, instead of the individual making one smooth stroke engaging the appropriate motor program, the smooth stroke is interrupted with a twitch. Two motor programs are operating simultaneously, leading to miss-hit shots. The neuroanatomy of the basal ganglia and concomitant neurophysiology are currently of great research interest in the neuroscience community. It appears clear that stress causes release of the activating neurotransmitter glutamate, which in turn causes release of dopamine in basal ganglia pathways that may result in the disinhibition of competing motor programs. This is the reason why yips become more pronounced under stressful circumstances.

The renowned golf teacher, Hank Haney, has recently written a series of articles [29–31], starting in the August 2004 issue of Golf Digest, about overcoming the yips with both drivers and putters. Haney describes his own personal problems with the yips over his 20-year golf career, and relates how he has had success in helping Mark O'Meara regain his putting abilities and his elite golf ranking. Haney's premise is that stroke repetition is not effective. His intervention is to make a small change in the individual's grip, thus engaging a slightly varied stroke and subsequent new motor program. The idea is that by engaging a new motor program, one is able to avoid the phenomenon of a competing motor program overriding the stroke. This "new" practice has resulted in successfully resurrecting the career of Mark O'Meara and a variety of other elite players; however, longitudinal studies and long-term results are still needed to confirm the temporal efficacy of this intervention.

## TREATMENT OF PERFORMANCE FAILURE

Although a more comprehensive approach to treatment is beyond the scope of this article, it is important to initially recognize these different causes of acute performance failure so appropriate treatment can be chosen (Fig. 1). The panic phenomenon is best treated with relaxation techniques, breathing techniques, centering techniques, and by learning to use process cues. If panic attacks become recurrent and generalize outside of specific situations, psychopharmacotherapy with selective serotonin reuptake inhibitors (SSRIs), serotonin and norepinephrine reuptake inhibitor (SNRIs), and low-dose benzodiazepines may be useful. The choking phenomenon described is best addressed by using desensitization techniques coupled with attentional shift techniques, promoting instinctive execution of shots. The yips appears to be most effectively treated through making slight modifications in the golfer's swing or grip, thus engaging a

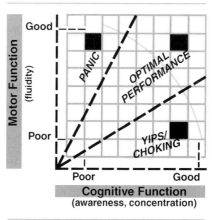

**Fig. 1.** Acute performance failure graph.

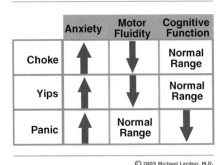

**Fig. 2.** Acute performance failure table.

different motor program that has not yet been overrun by the disinhibition of competing motor programs. In addition, there have been anecdotal reports of successful pharmacologic treatment of the yips with beta-blockers such as propranolol (Figs. 1,2) [25].

## THE ROLE OF THE SPORT PSYCHIATRIST IN GOLF

The role of the sport psychiatrist in golf, as in many other sports, is still being defined. The term "sport psychologist" has almost become a catchall that includes everything from motivational speakers to an athlete's personal guru to research scientists. To understand the role of the sports psychiatrist and other mental health professionals on the PGA Tour, it is helpful to think of a mental health continuum curve (Fig. 3).

Most sport psychologists on the PGA Tour are educators rather than clinically trained mental health professionals. They have certain technical skills or knowledge related to enhancing sports performance and they attempt to teach athletes these skills [32]. In academic and professional circles, the work of performance enhancement is often referred to as "applied sport psychology," and it is premised on the assumption that the athlete is mentally healthy, highly motivated, and

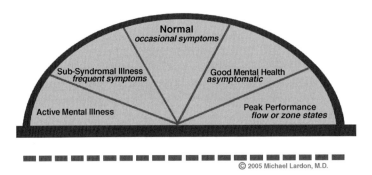

**Fig. 3.** Mental health well-being continuum.

possesses the mental and physical gifts required to compete at a high level. Applied sport psychology takes individuals who are in the normal range of the mental health performance continuum and tries to advance them into the peak performance realm (move them to the right hand side of the curve) (see Fig. 3). One challenge for applied sport psychologists lies in the assumption that all athletes are mentally healthy and fall into the so-called "normal" range of the mental health continuum. Indeed, depending on an athlete's genetics, biology, and current and past life stressors, any athlete can move along the mental health continuum at different times in his athletic career. It becomes critical for the applied sport psychologist to recognize when an individual is experiencing suboptimal mental health, such as all degrees of clinical depression, anxiety, and other psychiatric disorders. If such a mental health problem occurs, the applied sport psychologist must refer the athlete to the appropriate clinician for treatment, which requires rudimentary knowledge of psychopathology. If the problem is not adequately recognized, the athlete will not only continue to suffer a potentially life threatening condition unnecessarily, but is also impeded from deriving benefit from any kind of performance-enhancement techniques.

An example illustrating this dilemma is an elite golfer who developed panic attacks while playing. He subsequently sought the help of various sport psychologists who were unsuccessful in helping him find his optimal performance, essentially because they used sports enhancements techniques (ie, visualization, mental rehearsal, and relaxation), without recognizing the underlying psychopathology of a panic disorder.

He continued to compete, and the stress, in conjunction with a lack of understanding that he had developed a treatable medical/psychiatric illness, exacerbated his symptoms. He subsequently developed a phobic response to competing in front of crowds, despite having already won multiple times under similar circumstances. He continued his circuit of sport psychologists and motivational gurus for approximately 1 year before a renowned coach finally recognized that he was likely suffering from some form of psychiatric illness. By the time the sport psychiatrist was finally consulted, the individual had developed a full-blown panic disorder, with an entrenched agoraphobia circumscribed to competitive play. Through pharmacologic intervention and cognitive-behavioral education, the athlete's panic attacks have ameliorated. The current treatment has been focused on exposure therapy to address his phobic response; however, his confidence has been severely impaired. It is worth noting, that if the panic attacks had been recognized immediately and concurrently treated, this erosion of confidence could have been minimized or even prevented.

Psychiatrists may also have inherent clinical challenges treating the professional golfer. An excellent example of this challenge is exemplified by an elite female golfer who had been a multiple winner on the Ladies Professional Golf Association (LPGA) Tour and developed depressive symptomatology. She was sufficiently psychologically-minded to bypass her family physician and seek help from a local psychiatrist. Unfortunately, this local psychiatrist was not well versed in the athletic world and, in particular, golf. The psychiatrist placed the golfer on the mood stabilizer oxcarbazepine, in addition to trazodone for sleep and mood stabilization. She reported that her depression had lifted, but that she experienced morning grogginess and subtle balance and coordination problems. She felt this might be related to her psychotropic medications. Ironically, she did not seek alternatives because she trusted her psychiatrist. This example highlights the problems associated with a patient's positive transference toward her doctor, and the need for specialized psychopharmacologic expertise when treating the elite athlete.

In general, the authors recommend three pharmacologic principles. First, there are no superior medicines within comparable classes that specifically benefit the elite athlete. Fundamental and sound psychopharmacology is the rule. Athletes, like everyone, have individual and idiosyncratic biology and side-effect profiles, requiring customized tailoring of their medication regimens. Second, many athletes are very sensitive to medications, perhaps related to naïve receptor habituation, fitness, and dietary issues. They may show response or performance-related side effects at dosages that are normally considered homeopathic. During titration phases, and occasionally maintenance periods, one may require dosages smaller than the manufacture's smallest aliquots. Last, although it is critical to meticulously ask the athlete about any potential side effects, it is important to recognize that expectations often play a powerful role in determining outcome. The savvy physician will give and gather information about medication efficacy and side effects in a manner that is comprehensive, yet uses the language of the athlete and is not overly leading.

## CONCERN ABOUT CREDENTIALING AND LICENSING

On the PGA Tour there are no clear credentialing guidelines for sport psychologists. This allows individuals who have neither doctorate-level training nor credentialing from the Association for the Advancement of Applied Sport Psychology (AAASP) to practice as professional therapists or performance-enhancement consultants. In fact, in Golf Digest's ranking of 26 sport psychologists, which they call the Mental Guru Directory [33], only three are listed as clinical or counseling psychologists. Four individuals listed have no graduate training in psychology, and one individual is an endocrinologist. It was never mentioned that these individuals possessed different skill sets. It is this confusion that adds to the difficulty in helping golfers to consult with the appropriate expert. Fortunately, there are good examples being set. The renowned sport psychologist Robert Rotella, PhD [34], makes it clear that he does not help athletes who have underlying psychological conflicts, but rather circumscribes his treatments and teaching to the field of performance enhancement. Unfortunately, this is not always the case.

## CURRENT CHALLENGES TO A MULTIDISCIPLINARY APPROACH

The elite golfer often has a team of health professionals that consists of a personal trainer, physical therapist, sport psychologist, sport medicine physician, orthopedic surgeon, and family doctor. The majority of athletes who suffer from

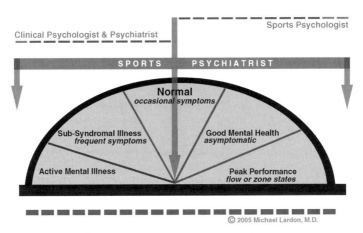

**Fig. 4.** Role of the sport psychiatrist.

psychiatric symptoms and require psychotropic medicine receive prescriptions from their family practice physicians, and this may be suboptimal due to their minimal psychiatric training. Occasionally, the health team oversteps its boundaries of clinical competence. A health care professional's unrecognized countertransference of wanting to appear more powerful, or conscious concerns of feeling threatened by losing control of the athlete's treatment, may prevent the athlete from receiving optimal mental health services. The psychiatrist, because of his medical training, can be the ideal candidate for functioning as a portal into mental health services. If the psychiatrist gains additional expertise in sport psychology, he will potentially be able to treat all mental health issues or make appropriate referrals (Fig. 4).

## THE FUTURE OF MENTAL HEALTH IN PROFESSIONAL GOLF

The AAASP is the largest applied sport, exercise, and health psychology organization in the world. This organization emphasizes appropriate clinical boundaries, confidentially, and the protection of athletes from exploitation. The group's ethical standards, which can be viewed on their Web site [35], state, "AAASP members trained in the sport sciences must be aware of their limitations in clinical and counseling psychology. Individuals from different training backgrounds must deliver services, teach, and conduct research only within the boundaries of their competence." The PGA Tour would benefit from adopting similar standards or requiring sport psychologists to be credentialed through organizations such as the AAASP. Likewise, psychiatry needs a fellowship in sport psychiatry that focuses on the art and science of psychopharmacology with elite athletes and the principles of applied sport psychology. Fellowship programs and credentialing organizations would provide the PGA Tour with the much needed resources to develop its own guidelines and regulations. Ultimately, the sport psychiatrist and psychologist, in addition to the professional golfer, will benefit.

## SUMMARY

The interrupted pace of golf provides a unique challenge for competitive golfer. Solid pre-performance routines provide excellent tools for managing common mental errors. Athletic zone states, which may be a subset of flow phenomena, may be understood by looking at models of dissociation and hypnosis. Acute performance failure occurs at even the highest levels of professional golf, and the authors posit three etiologies. Panicking is characterized by autonomic hyper-arousal, the player's mind going blank, and the player reverting to instinct. In contrast, in choking, an individual no longer relies on instinct but rather thinks consciously about what was previously a learned behavior (explicit monitoring), resulting in the loss of fluidity. And finally, the "yips" a more extreme form of choking, is characterized by the focal dystonia model. Sport psychologists and psychiatrists will benefit from staying informed about research in cognitive psychology, neuroscience, and applied sport psychology. The concept of a mental health continuum provides the sport psychiatrists and psychologist a guide to evaluate the golfer and refer to the appropriate expert. The authors contend to our sport medicine colleagues that professional golfers and athletes in general are well-served by consulting well-trained and experienced sport psychiatrists.

References

[1] Singer R. Pre-performance state, routines, and automaticity: what does it take to realize expertise in self-paced events. Journal of Sport and Exercise Psychology 2002;24:359–75.

[2] Singer R. Performance and human factors: considerations about cognition and attention for self-paced and externally paced events. Ergonomics 2000;43:1661–80.

[3] Walker S. Playing the racing game. In: Winning, the psychology of competition. New York, London: W.W. Norton & Company; 1980. p. 27–30.

[4] Leadbetter D. The mind game. In: 100% golf, unlocking your true potential. New York: Harper Collins Publishers Inc.; 2002. p. 173.

[5] Wegner D. Ironic processes of mental control. Psychol Rev 1994;101(1):34–52.

[6] Janelle C. Ironic mental processes in sport: implications for sport psychologists. The Sport Psychologist 1999;13:201–20.

[7] Beilock SL, Afremow JA, Rabe AL, et al. "Don't miss!" The debilitating effects of suppressive imagery on golf putting performance. Journal of Sport and Exercise Psychology 2001;23:200–21.

[8] Bandura A. Self-efficacy: the exercise of control. New York: W.H. Freeman; 1997.

[9] Netzer G. The way we live now. Encounter; what a year a win can make. New York Times Magazine. August 17, 2003. Section 6, p. 18.

[10] Diaz J. Finding the zone. Golf Digest 2004;55(7):134–45.

[11] Jackson S. Factors influencing the occurrence of flow states in elite athletes. Journal of Appled Sport Psychology 1995;7:138–66.

[12] Csikszentmiahalyi M. Flow, the psychology of optimal experience. New York: Harpers Collins Publishers Inc.; 1990. p. 43–70.

[13] Lardon M. Psychiatry grand rounds, University of California at San Diego, April 30, 2004.

[14] Spiegel D. Negative and positive visual hypnotic hallucinations: attending inside and out. Int J Clin Exp Hypn 2003;51(2):130–46.

[15] Lardon M, Polich J. EEG changes from long-term physical exercise. Biol Psychol 1996;44(1):19.

[16] Polich J, Lardon M. P300 and long-term physical exercise. Electroencephalogr Clin Neurophysiol 1997;103(4):493–8.

[17] Sjoberg BM. The effects of psychotomimetic drugs on primary suggestibility. Psychopharmacologia 1965;8:251–62.
[18] Spiegel D. Hypnotizability and CSF HVA levels among psychiatric patients. Biol Psychiatry 1992;31:95–8.
[19] Sapolsky R. Taming stress. Sci Am 2003;8:87–95.
[20] Gladwell M. The art of failure. The New Yorker 2000;21:84–92.
[21] Sampson C. Hogan. New York: Rutledge Hill, Bantam Doubleday; 1996. p. 151.
[22] Beilock SL, Carr TH. On the fragility of skilled performance: what governs choking under pressure? J Exp Psychol Gen 2001;130:701–25.
[23] Crews DJ, Landers D. Electroencephalographic measures of attentional patterns prior to the golf putt. Med Sci Sports Exerc 1993;25(1):116–26.
[24] Riley R, Hoch AS. In choke. Sports Illustrated 1989;70(25):62–5.
[25] Smith AM, Adler CH, Crews D, et al. The "yips" in golf: a continuum between a focal dystonia and choking. Sports Med 2003;33(1):13–31.
[26] Bawden M, Maynard I. Towards an understanding of the personal experience of the "yips" in cricketers. J Sports Sci 2001;19(12):937–53.
[27] Smith AM, Malo SA, Laskowski ER, et al. A multidisciplinary study of the "yips" phenomenon in golf: an exploratory analysis. Sports Med 2000;30(6):423–37.
[28] Mink JW. The basal ganglia and involuntary movements. Arch Neurol 2003;60:1365–8.
[29] Haney H, Rudy M. The secret issue: How I cure my driver yips. Golf Digest. August 2004. Available at: http://www.golfdigest.com/search/index.ssf?/instruction/gd200408 driveryips.html. Accessed March 25, 2005.
[30] Smith R, Rudy M. The chipping yips. Golf Digest. September 2004. Available at: http://www.golfdigest.com/search/index.ssf?/instruction/gd200409chippingyips.html. Accessed March 25, 2005.
[31] Haney H, Rudy M. How to beat the putting yips. Golf Digest. October 2004. Available at: http://www.golfdigest.com/search/index.ssf?/instruction/gd200410puttingyips.html. Accessed May 24, 2005.
[32] Nideffer R. The ethics and practice of applied sports psychology. Ann Arbor (MI): McNaughton Gunn; 1981. p. 11.
[33] Golf Digest. Mental guru directory, 2005. Available at: http://www.golfdigest.com/zone/. Accessed March 25, 2005.
[34] Rotella R. Golf is not a game of perfect. New York: Simon & Schuster Inc.; 1995. p. 19–29.
[35] Association for the Advancement of Applied Sport Psychology. Ethical code. Available at: www.aaasponline.org/governance/committees/ethics/standards.php. Accessed March 25, 2005.

Clin Sports Med 24 (2005) 973–977

# CLINICS IN SPORTS MEDICINE

# The Use of Relaxation, Hypnosis, and Imagery in Sport Psychiatry

Thomas S. Newmark, MD*, David F. Bogacki, PhD

*Division of Psychology, Cooper University Hospital, Robert Wood Johnson Medical School, 401 Haddon Avenue, 3 Cooper Plaza, Suite 307, Camden, NJ 08103, USA*

Hypnosis is a procedure during which a mental health professional suggests that a patient experiences changes in sensations, perceptions, thoughts, or behavior. Although there are many different induction techniques, most include suggestions for relaxation, or instructions to imagine or think about pleasant experiences or feelings of well-being [1]. The purpose of this article is to briefly describe the use of various methods of relaxation, hypnosis, and imagery techniques available to enhance athletic performance. Case studies are provided for illustration.

Various issues regarding all aspects of the clinical utility of hypnosis are beyond the scope of this article. The interested reader will find that the literature on hypnosis is replete with scientific debate about trance induction, depth of trance, hypnotic susceptibility, and the efficacy of hypnosis in various medical and research outcomes [2].

Athletes can use many characteristics of hypnotic trance to benefit their performance. The techniques described in this article facilitate learning new information that can be applied in competition, provide general relaxation to enhance performance, and assist in the rehabilitation of injury or pain.

The characteristics that these techniques have in common include relaxation, suggestibility, concentration, imaginative ability, reality testing, brain function, autonomic control, and placebo effect.

Hypnotic trance allows access to different functions of the brain. Two different aspects of brain function are of interest. First, hypnosis increases the opportunity to understand unconscious motivations of athletes. The unconscious motivations of the athlete are more accessible in a trance than in ordinary mental consciousness [3]. The writings of Freud and his collaborators suggest that gaining a greater understanding of the unconscious motivations of patients facilitates treatment goals. In this context, hypnosis is only part of an overall psychotherapy treatment plan.

Hypnosis also permits greater access to the functions associated with the right side of the brain. Gaining greater access to the functioning of the right

---

* Corresponding author. *E-mail address:* newmark-thomas@cooperhealth.edu (T.S. Newmark).

0278-5919/05/$ – see front matter
doi:10.1016/j.csm.2005.06.003

brain is useful in the mental training of athletes. The imaginative skill of the right brain can help make hypnotic imagery sessions more powerful and performance-enhancing.

It must be stressed that hypnosis is a tool with techniques. Hypnosis is not itself psychotherapy. Hypnosis has its limitations, and will not transform an average athlete into a superstar.

## HYPNOSIS AS A FORM OF RELAXATION

The most common function of hypnosis is the ability of a trance to facilitate relaxation. Feeling relaxed is the most frequently reported sensation after an athlete comes out of a trance. Using trance induction alone as a form of relaxation or using it as an adjunct to other performance-enhancing techniques is both recommended and widely practiced by sport psychiatrists and psychologists. Relaxation and stress reduction are keys to improved performance. For example, golf is a game in which calmness and concentration are vital.

Jacobson [4] recognized relaxation as teaching the body to recognize and eliminate any feeling of tension. His technique for achieving relaxation requires tensing and relaxing small muscle groups in a prescribed order. Most athletes can achieve relaxation after training a few muscle groups. When coaches who use this technique are appropriately trained in hypnotic and relaxation techniques, they will be better able to recognize the potential of relaxation techniques.

Suinn [5] has formalized Jacobson's relaxation procedure and called it visual motor behavior rehearsal (VMBR). After approximately four or five 20-minute practice sessions, an athlete can effectively use this technique. Suinn advises that athletes practice this technique daily for maximum effectiveness. Jacobson and Suinn designed techniques that focus on relaxing the body. In contrast, Benson [6] developed techniques that first focus on relaxing the mind, and then the body. After Benson's relaxation response (RR) is established, the right brain is more accessible to suggestions—as noted earlier, a characteristic of hypnosis. Suinn has noted that VMBR has improved the performance of skiers, golfers, and football players. Divers and gymnasts can employ this technique. It is a form of "mental rehearsal."

## IMAGERY TECHNIQUES TO ENHANCE PERFORMANCE

A substantial amount of research supports athletes' reliance on imagery. Imagery training has been used to increase time practicing, to set higher goals, and to increase adherence to training programs. Generally, research on imagery in sport performance enhancement has been positive.

The relaxed state facilitates most other uses of hypnosis, such as imagery, goal setting, pain alleviation, and controlling performance arousal and focus; however, athletes require a certain degree of alertness, and becoming too relaxed can be counter-therapeutic. Thus, an optimal level of readiness and relaxation is desirable.

Hanin [7] has termed this optimal state the zone of optimal functioning (ZOF). He conducted various research studies showing that many athletes find their optimal levels with low anxiety, others at moderate levels, and still others find a high level of anxiety as optimum [8]. These findings have significant implications for coaches who attempt to apply the highest possible level of arousal before competition. Athletes have described this state as being in a "zone." Basketball players can get into a zone, and their shooting is exceptional during this time.

Unestahl [9] has a different approach with his ideal performance state (IPS). In this technique, athletes are intensely focused on a limited number of task-relevant stimuli and dissociated from everything except these stimuli, almost like being in a tunnel. Perception in the IPS changes in several ways. The athlete experiences action as being slower and the stimuli imagined (golf cup, goal post) as being larger. Enjoyment is intense, pain is decreased, and action is experienced as effortless. Long-distance runners have described this state.

Imagery can be enhanced through the use of hypnotic trance. In a recent study [10] participants were asked to imagine a variety of situations: practicing a sport alone, practicing in front of others, watching a teammate make a mistake, and competing in an event. The participants imagined each situation in and out of a trance, and were asked to rate the vividness of the imagery on four dimensions. The results demonstrated that hypnosis enhanced the vividness of imagery.

## TECHNIQUES TO ENHANCE AUTONOMIC CONTROL

Another characteristic of the hypnotic trance is the ability to assist in the control of autonomic function, including blood pressure and blood flow. This control is important in recovery from injury, as well as in blocking the adverse reactions to anxiety. Athletes can be taught how to control autonomic functions through trance, and can apply the positive effects to enhance performance. Hypnotic techniques, biofeedback, and autogenic training may all be employed to facilitate the rehabilitation and healing process.

Recently the power of the individual for self-healing is becoming increasingly recognized. Much of contemporary psychosomatic medicine focuses on enlisting the aid of the patient in mobilizing the healing process, and hypnosis has a long history of energizing the healing forces within an individual. Hunter [11] emphasizes that the body and mind are in constant interaction.

Ievleva and Orlick [12] found that positive self-talk, goal-setting, and healing imagery enhance recovery from athletic injury. Hypnosis is valuable in mobilizing these curing forces within the athlete, and in uncovering psychological aspects in injuries that seem strictly physical.

## CLINICAL APPLICATIONS AND CASE STUDIES

To demonstrate the application of some of the techniques described above the following four cases are presented.

John was a 23-year-old man who was trying out for a professional football team. He was a wide receiver in college. He reported that during training camp he kept dropping passes that were thrown to him. He heard about hypnosis and wanted to see if it would help. Under hypnosis, he was provided with the image that he had stuck glue on the gloves that he was using. He visualized himself catching the pass with the help of the imaginary glue. The patient reported that this technique helped him overcome his acute slump and begin catching passes again.

Bob was a 15-year-old basketball player who sought hypnosis because of inaccurate shooting and ineffective defense. Under hypnosis, he was given the suggestion that whenever he shot the ball it would be a "76er ball," and would help his accuracy. He was also given the suggestion that whenever he looked at his wrist band his defense would become more active. A week later he reported that his shooting accuracy and defense had improved.

Jim was a 24-year-old amateur golfer who was having difficulty hitting the ball straight and putting. Under hypnosis, he was provided with visualization images that when he struck the golf ball, there was a magnetic force that directed the ball toward the hole. He visualized this imaginary magnetic force, resulting in improved performance.

Donald was a 17-year-old soccer player. He presented with problems controlling his anger during games; this led to him being ejected. Under hypnosis he was given the image that the soccer ball would become a "stay-in-the-game ball" and he would direct his anger toward the ball rather than other players. He stated that this helped him to control his outbursts.

In all of these cases, hypnosis was useful in overcoming an acute slump. The images, which were similar to visualization, were made more vivid by the forces that were suggested, and did help the athletes to overcome acute performance anxiety or slump. This technique seems to help in these particular situations. Hypnosis may help improve long-term performance, and it appears to be a useful tool in an acute slump situation. In each situation there were other issues involved, such as anxiety, depression, and family conflict, that were addressed in traditional therapy.

## SUMMARY

Hypnosis/VMBR can sharpen an athlete's focus and enhance performance or stop a slump. This mental rehearsal of success can give the athlete a mental edge in real competition.

References

[1] Begel D, Burton RW. Sport psychiatry: theory and practice. New York: W.W. Norton & Company; 2000.
[2] Kelly SF, Kelly RJ. Hypnosis—understanding how it can work for you. Toronto, ON: Addison Wesley Publishing Company, Inc; 1985.
[3] Liggett DR. Sport hypnosis. Champaign (IL): Human Kinetics; 2000.
[4] Jacobson E. You must relax. Chicago: University of Chicago Press, McGraw Hill; 1976.
[5] Suinn RM. Body thinking: psychology for Olympic champs. In: Suinn RM, editor. Psychology in sports: methods and applications. Minneapolis (MN): Burgess; 1976. p. 306–31.
[6] Benson H. The relaxation response. New York: Morrow; 1975.
[7] Hainin YL. Individual zones of optimal functioning (IZOF mode 1: an idiographic approach

to performance anxiety). In: Henschen KP, Strand WF, editors. Sport psychology: an analysis of athletic behavior. Longmeadow (MA): Movement Press; 1995. p. 103–18.

[8] Hainin YL. A study of anxiety in sports. In: Stravb WF, editor. Sport psychology: an analysis of athletic behavior. Ithaca (NY): Movement Press; 1980. p. 236–49.

[9] Unestahl LE. The ideal performance. In: Unestahl LE, editor. Sport psychology in theory and practice. Orebro (Sweden): Veje; 1986.

[10] Liggett DR. Enhancing imagery through hypnosis: a performance aid for athletes. Am J Clin Hypn 2000;43(2):14–28.

[11] Hunter M. Psych yourself in!: hypnosis and health. West Vancouver (Canada): Seawalk Press; 1987.

[12] Ievleva L, Orlick T. Mental links and enhanced healing: an explanatory study. The Sport Psychologist 1991;5(1):25–40.

Clin Sports Med 24 (2005) 979

# CLINICS IN SPORTS MEDICINE

ELSEVIER
SAUNDERS

## ERRATUM

# Erratum to "Thermophysiologic Aspects of the Three-Process-Model of Sleepiness Regulation" [Clin Sports Med 24 (2) (2005) 287–300]

Kurt Kräuchi*, Christian Cajochen, PhD, Anna Wirz-Justice, PhD

*Psychiatric University Clinic, Centre for Chronobiology, Wilhelm Klein Strasse 27, CH-4025 Basel, Switzerland*

In the April 2005 issue ("Sports Chronobiology"), in the article "Thermophysiologic Aspects of the Three-Process-Model of Sleepiness Regulation" by Kurt Kräuchi et al, Fig. 4 and Fig. 5 were cited incorrectly. The Fig. 4 data were originally from Kräuchi K, Cajochen C, Wirz-Justice A. Waking up properly: is there a role of thermoregulation in sleep inertia? J Sleep Res 2004:13:121–7; the Fig. 5 data were originally from Kräuchi K, Cajochen C, Wirz-Justice A. Melatonin and orthostasis: interaction of posture with subjective sleepiness, heart rate, and skin and core temperature. Sleep Res 1997;26:79.

DOI of original article title 10.1016/j.csm.2004.12.009.
* Corresponding author. *E-mail address:* kurt.kraeuchi@pukbasel.ch (K. Kräuchi).

0278-5919/05/$ – see front matter
doi:10.1016/j.csm.2005.07.001

Clin Sports Med 24 (2005) 981–997

# CLINICS IN SPORTS MEDICINE

## CUMULATIVE INDEX 2005

### A

Abdominal pain, 535

Abrasions, 582–583

Acclimatization, 696

Acetazolamide, in high altitude exposure, 427
  om high-altitude sickness, 714

Achievement by proxy, as distinct abuse,
  818–820
  as potential abuse, 818
  as risky sacrifice, 816–817
  objectification in, 817–818

Achievement by proxy distortion, 763–764,
  **805–828**
  and factitious disorder by proxy,
    814–815
  case vignette, and clinical strategies,
    823–825
  evolutionary historical perspective on,
    807–809
  families in, in stabilization/
    re-equilibration for, 806
  high potential for, 811–813
  mental health professional and, 822–823
  parental typologies in, 819, 820,
    821–822
  prior psychological and psychiatric
    research on, 809–810
  spectrum of, 820
  supportive behavior of, maintenance in
    families, 815–820
    normal range of, 815

Acne, 592

Acromioclavicular joint, arthrosis of, 191

Actigraphy, 452

Acute mountain sickness (AMS), 713, 714

Adolescents, and children, benefits and risks
  of sports participation for, 787–790
  children and, sleep and circadian
    rhythms in, **319–328**
  sporting participation for, 784

Aerobic capacity, menstrual cycle and, e61

Aerobic endurance, menstrual cycle and,
  e62–63

Age categories, in youth sports, e31

Aggression, and sport, **845–852**
  biological factors in, 846–847
  biopsychosocial model of, 846
  control of, 848
  learning to manage, 848–849
  meanings of, historically, 845
  observable, 845
  overly aggressive behavior and, 846
  psychological issues and, 847–849
  social issues and, 849–851

Air travel, and jet lag, implications for
  performance, **367–380**
  health consequences of, 372–373

Airway, upper, anatomy of, 330, 331

Alcohol abuse, and aggression, 847

Alcohol dependence, CAGE questionnaire
  in, 755
  diagnosis of, 755
    team physician in, 756
  effects of, 755

Alcohol use, motivation for, 886–887

Alcoholism, and substance abuse, 755–756
    among high school and college
      athletes, 755

Alertness-enhancing drugs, sports chronobiology and, 418–424

Allergic/anaphylactic conditions, exercise-
  associated, 513–517

Allergic contact dermatitis, 518–519

Allergic disorders, in athlete, **507–523**

Allergic rhinitis, 508–511
  allergens causing, 508–509
  allergy testing in, 511
  and athletic performance, e40–41
  in athletes, e39
  management of, e41–44, 509
  nasal obstruction in, 510
  pathophysiology and presentation of,
    e39–40

Allergy(ies), and Olympic athletes, e38–39
  diagnosis of, e37
  manifestations of, e37

*Note:* Page numbers of article titles are in **boldface** type.

pathophysiology of, e35–36
seasonal, medical treatment of, related to
    athletes, e42–43
    seasonal decrements in athletic
        performance and, **e35–50**
seasonal effects on athletes, e37
Allografts, osteochondral, in cartilage
    defects, 169
Amenorrhea, 623–626
Amphetamines, in attention deficit/
    hyperactivity disorder, 840–841
    use by athletes, 888–890
Anabolic steroids. See *Steroids*.
Analgesia, caffeine and, e8–9
Anaphylaxis, exercise-induced, 514–515
    food-dependent, 515–516
    treatment of, 516
    variant type, 516
Androstenedione, 726
Anemia, in athletes, 603, 604
Angioedema, 518
Ankle, and foot, osteoarthritis of, 65–66
    treatment of, 66
    degenerative joint disease of, 93
    replacement of, recovery following, 180
Anorexia, 753–754
    referral in, 754
    reverse. See *Muscle dysmorphia*.
Anorexia athletica, 753, 873
Anorexia nervosa, 753–754
Anterior cruciate ligament, effects on female
    of female hormones and, e66–68
    injury to, 40
    reconstruction of, in arthritic
        patient, 146
    tear of, osteoarthritis and, 192, 193
Antibiotics, 721–722
Antidepressants, in insomnia, 282
Antihistamines, in allergic rhinitis, 509
Anti-inflammatory drugs, nonsteroidal.
    See *NSAIDs*.
Anti-inflammatory sprays, in allergic
    rhinitis, 509
Anxiety, and "nerves", distinguishing
    between, 668
    definition of, 667
    normal, and anxiety disorder, differen-
        tiated, 748
    performance, 668
Anxiety disorder, in athlete, 748
Aortic stenosis, 469–470
Appendicitis, acute, 535

Applied sport psychology, 966–967
Applied systems theory, professional sports
    teams and, 932–933
Arachadonic acid, 74
Arachadonic acid derivatives, 74
Arrhythmogenic right ventricular dysplasia,
    472, 473
Arthritis, degenerative, of glenohumeral joint,
    dislocation of shoulder and, 47
    of distal radioulnar joint, 64–65
    of hip, arthroscopy in, 59–60
        early, osteotomy in, 59
    pisotriquetral, 65
    radiocarpal, after intraarticular distal
        radius fractures, 64
    reconstruction of anterior cruciate
        ligament in patient with, 146
Arthrography, CT, or MR imaging, of
    cartilage, 24–25
Arthropathy, of shoulder, incidence of, 47–49
Arthroplasty, abrasion, and microfracture, in
    knee, 144–145
Arthroscopic classifications, 133–135, 136
Arthroscopic lavage, debridement, in knee
    pain, 139, 140–141, 142–143
    in knee pain, 138–142
Arthroscopy, and high tibial osteotomy,
    146–147
    diagnostic, in knee pain, 135–138
    in osteoarthritis of knee, in athlete,
        **133–152**
        author's method of, 147–148
    of hip, in arthritis, 59–60
    of shoulder, rating of chondral damage
        for, 49
Arthrosis, surgical management of shoulder
    instability and, 50–51
Articular cartilage. See *Cartilage, articular*.
Artifacts, and inaccuracies in MR evaluation,
    23–24
Aspirin, in high-altitude headache, 713–714
Assistance programs, team, collegiate, design
    of, 945–946
        staffing and services of,
            947–948
        use of, 951–952
        critical-incident stress management
            sevices in, 954–955
        diverse staff for, 953
        family assistance in, 956
        fitness and supplement use
            information in, 955
        history and program design of,
            944–946

on-site services and, 953
preseason physicals and, 953–954
prevention talks in, 954
professional, approach for,
944–945
staffing and services of,
946–947
use of, 948–951
professional and collegiate, service
areas for, 943–944
services and utilization of,
**943–958**
strategies to increase use of,
952–956
sleep related problems and, 955
tobacco cessaion services and, 954
Asthma, chronic persistent, treatment for, 548
exercise-induced, diagnosis of, e46
pathogenesis and presentation
of, e45
seasonal considerations in, e45–46
in athletes, e45
management of, e46–e47
medications for use in, 722
prophylaxis of, e46
Atherosclerosis, 469
Athlete(s), alertness in, implications of caffeine
for, **e1–13**
child. See also *Child(ren)*.
and family, psychiatric interview
of, 797–801
elite, jet lag and, 371–372
family of, as influence on athlete's
life, 899
as source of support or pressure,
903–905
assessment of, 916–919
clinical assessment and treatment
of, 916
demands on, 899
developmental analysis of, 907–915
developmental events and,
902–903
developmental model for, 906–907
ethical issues in, 924–925
interactions of, 901–902
paradox of, 905–906
review of literature on, 901–906
treatment of, 919–924
challenge in, 923–924
education/prevention in,
921–922
imaging of cartilage of, **13–37**
obstructive sleep apnea in, 336–339
professional, and intra-psychic system,
933–934
and mental health professionals.
See *Mental health professionals,
and professional athletes*.

cognitive behavioral techniques
and, 934
countertransference issues and,
934–938
traveling, guidelines for adjustment
of, 367
Athletic participation, as therapy, 865–866
Athletic performance, implications of sleep
apnea for, **329–341**
of young people, sleep and circadian
rhythms and, **319–328**
seasonal decrements in, seasonal
allergies and, **e35–50**
seasonal variation in, e29–31
stimulants to enhance, 418–419
Atomoxetine, in attention deficit/hyperactivity
disorder, 837, 838, 839
Attention deficit disorder, stimulants for, 722
Attention-deficit/hyperactivity disorder, 670
Attention deficit/hyperactivity disorder,
758–759
and depressive disorders, 836
and psychiatric comorbidity, 835
and psychopharmacologic treatments,
**829–843**
and youth athlete, 833–836
case vignette of, 831–833
characteristics of, 830–831
"continuous chaos" sports for, 759
diagnosis of, 830
early symptoms of, 758–759
effects on performance, 829, 834
pharmacologic treatment of, 836–839
treatment of, 834
Autonomic control, techniques to
enhance, 975
Axis I psychopathology, suicide in athletes
and, 860
Axonal injury, diffuse, 645–646

**B**

Bacterial infections, 574–576
Balance error scoring system (BESS), 639
Basal forebrain arousal system, 212–213
Behavioral studies, of memory and sleep, 303
Behavioral treatment, in insomnia, 380
to increase alertness after air travel, 377
Beta-hydroxy beta-methylbutyrate (HMB),
729–730
Binge/purgers, 754
Bioregulatory factors, maturation of, 321
Bipolar disorder, 668–669
in athlete, 747–748

Bleeding, gastrointestinal. See *Gastrointestinal bleeding.*

Bleeding tendencies, 601

Blisters, 583–584

Body temperature, measuring of, 705

Bone, Wolfe's Law of, 181

Brace(s), and orthotic, in degenerative joint disease with angular deformity, **93–99**
  knee orthoses, mechanical, 97–98
  "unloader," 98
  varus unloader, 95–96

Brain plasticity, sleep-dependent, 311–315

Breathing techniques, for sleep promotion, 350

Bright light treatment, **381–412**
  administration of, 399–401
  adverse effects and reactions to, 401–404
  alerting and antidepressant effects of, 388–398
  and bipolar disorder, 400
  studies in athletes, 390–391
  to adjust body clock, 374, 375
  wavelength considerations and, 384–385

Bronchitis, acute, background of, 541–542
  clinical manifestations and diagnosis of, 542–543
  cough in, 542
  treatment of, 543–544

Bronchoconstriction, exercise-induced, and vocal cord dysfunction, compared, 550
  background of, 545
  clinical manifestations of, 545–546
  diagnosis of, 546–547
  isolated, 548–549
  nonpharmacologic management of, 547
  pharmacologic management of, 548
  plus chronic asthma, 548
  treatment of, 547

Bronchospasm, exercise-induced, e28

Brugada syndrome, 473–474

Bulimia, definition of, 754

Bulimia nervosa, 754–755

Burnout syndrome, 791

### C

Caffeine, 730–731
  action during exercise performance, e6–7
  administration of, following caffeine abstinence, e3
  adverse effects of, e3, e4
  and analgesia, e8–9
  and exercise performance, e6
  and performance effects during extreme conditions, e5–6
  as countermeasure to post-lunch dips in performance, e20–21
  as stimulant, 424
  cardiovascular effects of, e7
  cognitive effects of, e5
  consumption of, physiology of, e1–4
  dependence on, e3
  effects on measures of alertness, e4–5
  effects on plasma free fatty acids, e7–8
  implications for alertness in athletes, **e1–13**
  in common drinks and foods, e2
  psychologic effect of, e9
  respiratory effects of, e7
  to increase alertness after air travel, 376–377
  withdrawal, e3–e4

Calluses, 584–585

Cancers, skin, 593

Carbuncles, 576

Cardiac concussion, 475

Cardiac death, sudden, 467–475

Cardiology, sports, common issues in, **463–476**

Cardiomyopathy, hypertrophic, 464, 467–468

Cardiopulmonary resuscitation, in hypothermia, 709

Cardiovascular system, effects of caffeine on, e7
  health of, exercise and, e26–27
  obstructive sleep apnea and, 332
  sex steroid hormones and, e55–56

Career termination issues, 761–762

Cartilage, articular, and osteoarthritis, basic science of, **1–12**
  injury to, 42–43
    in repetitive training and competition, 163, 164
    irrigation, debridement, and abrasion chondroplasty in, 164–165
    surgical management of, 164
    treatment of, comparative studies of, 169–171
  of elbow, imaging of, 28, 29–30
  of hip, imaging of, 27, 28, 29
  of knee, imaging of, 26–27
  of shoulder, imaging of, 30, 32
  of wrist, imaging of, 30
  therapy for, postoperative considerations following, 32–35

tissue composition and load transmission in, 3–4
defects of, in athletes, surgical management of, **163–174**
marrow stimulation techniques (microfracture) in, 165–166, 170
hyaline, basic science of, functional structure of, 1–3
imaging of, radiographic considerations in, 14
techniques in development for, 25–26
MR imaging of, 14–23
imaging of, in athlete, **13–37**
osteoarthritis, structure and biochemical changes in, 4–7

Catastrophic injury, definition of, 644

Cellulitis, 574–576

Cerebral edema, high-altitude (HACE), 712, 713, 714

Cerebrovascular disease, eye in, 690

Child and youth sports, benefits of, 787–790
for twenty-first century, developmental overview of, **783–804**
importance of, 783
risks of, 789–790

Child(ren), and adolescents, benefits and risks of sports participation for, 787–790
sleep and circadian rhythms in, **319–328**
high-achieving, and adult caregivers, relationship between, developmental tasks of, 810–813
neuropsychological readiness for sports, 785
school-age, maturation of sleep-wake homeostasis in, 321–322

Chlorotrichosis, 589–590

Cholinergic urticaria, 513–514

Chondral injuries, in active patients, 164
rating of, for arthroscopy of shoulder, 49

Chondrocytes, autologous, implantation of, in cartilage defects, 167–168, 170

Chondroitin, 75, 76–77

Chondromalacia, in osteoarthritis, 5, 6

Chondroplasty, abrasion, in injured articular cartilage, 165
irrigation, and debridement, in injury of articular cartilage, 164–165

Chromium, 733

Chronobiology, sports, **413–454**

Circadian rhythm(s), 368, 369–370
functional neuroanatomy of, 219–221
in performance, 371
of core body temperature, 288–290
post-lunch dips in performance and, e17–19
sleep and, and psychomotor vigilance performance, **237–249**
in children and adolescents, **319–328**
terminology and definitions of, 219

Circadian timing system, maturation of, in school-age children, 322–324

Clonazwpam, 670

Coaches, aggression and, 850
as role models and active stress inducers, 793

Coagulation disorders, 600–602

Cocaine, medical sequelae of, 419

Cognitive behavioral techniques, and professional athletes, 934

Cognitive behavioral therapy, in eating disorders, 878
in insomnia, 280

Cognitive development, and effect on sporting performance, 785

Cognitive relaxation, for sleep promotion, 351

Cold injuries, 703–712
prevention of, 710–711

Collagenomas, 592–593

Commotio cordis, 475

Computed tomographic arthrography, or MR imaging, of cartilage, 24–25

Concussion, 672–673
clinical manifestations of, 640–641
definition of, 637
long-term sequelae of, 644
NATA graded symptoms checklist for, 639, 640
postinjury assessment for, 641–643
preinjury education and assessment in, 637–640
return to play and follow-up in, 643–644
Standardized Assessment of Concussion and, 638, 639

Conjunctivitis, allergic, 483–484, 511–512
bacterial, 483
considerations in athletes, 484
viral, 483

Consultation-liason service psychiatrist, 929

Consulting room atmosphere, "holding environment" in, 745

Contact dermatitis, 590–592

Continuous positive airway pressure, nasal, 555–556

Core body temperature, 287
and skin temperatures, sleepiness in relation to, 290–298
circadian rhythm of, 288–290

Corneal abrasion, 684–685

Corns, 584

Coronary artery(ies), abnormalities of, 468–469
anomalous, 468–469

Corticosteroids, in osteoarthritis, complications of, 86
contraindications to, 86
indications for, 84–85
mechanism of action of, 84
preparations of, 85–86
intranasal, in allergic rhinitis, 509–510

Countertransference, 764–765
issues of, and professional athletes, 934–938

Creatine, 728–729

**D**

Death, causes of, among young athletes, 464

"Decision-making skills," 757

Decongestants, and allergic rhinitis, e44

Degenerative joint disease, of midfoot or ankle, foot orthotics in, 94–97
with angular deformity, orthotic and brace use in, **93–99**

Dehydration, mild, 701

Dehydroepiandrosterone (DHEA), 726

Delayed sleep phase syndrome and, 443

Dementia pugistic, 760

Depression, and "feeling down", distinguishing characteristics of, 667
in athlete, 746–747
nonseasonal, 396
seasonal, light and, 391–396
secondary to overtraining, 761
symptoms of, 666

Dermatitis, allergic contact, 518–519

Dermatology, sports, training room management of, **565–598**

Dermatophytes, 565–572
play restrictions in, 580

Dermatoses, inflammatory, 590–593
mechanical and environmental, 582–593

Desentization therapy, in allergies, 520

Dexamethasone, om high-altitude sickness, 714

Dextroamphetamine, in attention deficit/hyperactivity disorder, 832, 837

Diabetes, eye pathologies in, 690–691

Diabetic retinopathy, 690

Diarrhea, 531–532
acute exercise-induced, 531

Diet, in osteoarthritic knee, 103

Doping concerns, management of allergic rhinitis and, e41–44

Doping issues, in future, 733–734

Dreams, related to sports medicine physician, 762–763

Drug abuse, diagnosis of, team physician in, 756

Drug testing, oral contraceptive pills and, e75–76

DSM-IV Axis I psychiatric disorders, 847

Dysmenorrhea, e70

Dyspepsia, 530–531

Dysphagia, 527–528

**E**

Eating disorders, 628–631, 753–755
American Psychiatric Association diagnostic criteria for, 629–630
in athletes, characteristic patterns of, 874–875
comorbid mental illnesses and, 879–880
diagnosis of, 873–875
etiology of, 875–877
managing the risks, **871–883**
organization response and, 880–881
prevalence of, 871–873
symptoms of, 875
treatment of, 877–879
suicide in athletes and, 861–862
surveys for identification of, 631–632

Ehrlichiosis, 496–497

Elbow, articular cartilage of, imaging of, 28, 29–30
osteoarthritis of, 61
symptoms of, 61
treatment of, 61–62
replacement of, constrained or linked hinged elbow arthroplasty in, 180

Electrophysiologic disorders, 471–475

Emotional distress, in termination of athletic career, 674–675

Energy expenditure, seasonal variation in, e26, e27

Energy metabolism, sex steroid hormones and, e58

Environmental exposures, effects on athletes, e37–38

Environmental illness, in athletes, **695–718**

Ephedrine, 731

Epididymitis/orchitis, 499–500

Epilepsy, seizures and. See *Seizures, and epilepsy.*

Erysipelas, 574–575

Erythema ab igne, 589

Erythropoiesis, iron-deficient, 607

Erythropoietin, 732

Esophageal dysphagia, 527–528

Estrogen, e55, e58, e71
    and brain, e59

Exercise(s), acute, influence on sleep, epidemiologic studies of, 356–358
    aerobic, in osteoarthritic knee, 103–128
    allergic/anaphylactic conditions associated with, 513–517
    and cardiovascular health, e26–27
    benefits of, 194
    chronic, influence on sleep, epidemiologic studies of, 358–359
    effects on hematologic parameters, 602–603
    effects on sleep, **355–365**
    for hip mobilization, in osteoarthritic knee, 105–106, 110
    immunologic responses to, 507–508
    influence on sleep, epidemiologic studies of, 356
    physiological responses to, e27–29
    range of motion, in osteoarthritic knee, 104–105, 106–107
    seasonal rhythms and, **e25–34**
    seizures and epilepsy and, 652–653
    strengthening, in osteoarthritic knee, 105–107, 108–111

Exercise performance, caffeine and, e6

Eye(s), conditions of, training room management of, **681–693**
    effects of bright light treatment on, 402–403
    evaluation of, equipment for, 681
        patient history in, 681–682
    in cerebrovascular disease, 690
    inflammatory conditions of, retinal detachments in, 687
    innervation of, 682–683
    migraine headache and, 688–690
    nerve injury to, clinical findings associated with, 683
    pathologies of, in diabetes, 690–691
    problems of, in Marfan's syndrome, 691
    special medical conditions of, 687–692

trauma to, 683–687
    physical examination in, 682–683

## F

Facial fracture, eye in, 684

Family, of athlete. See *Athlete(s), family of.*

Family systems model, **899–928**
    adapting to change in, 918
    interaction patterns in, 918–919
    levels of cohesion and, 917–918
    levels of stress and, 916–917

Fantasy league, involvement in, pathological gambling and, 758

Female athlete triad, **623–636**
    identification and clinical correlates of, 631–632
    sports disciplines at risk for, 628

Firearms, suicide in athletes and, 863

Flexion contractures, about knee, 103–104

Fluvoxamine, in depression, 761

Focal dystonia, and golf, 964

Folliculitis, 576

Food allergies, 519

Foot (Feet), and ankle, osteoarthritis of, 65–66
        treatment of, 66
    orthotics for, in midfoot or ankle degenerative joint disease, 61–67

Footballers, Australian, osteoarthritis of knee in, 191

Frostbite, 709–712
    clinical features of, 711
    treatment of, 711

Fungal infections, 565–574

Furuncles, 576

## G

Gambline, pathological, and fantasy league involvement, 758

Gastroenteritis, 488–493
    bacterial, 489–492
    protozoal, 492–493
    viral, 489

Gastroenterology, sports, training room management of, **525–540**

Gastroesophageal reflux disease, 528–530

Gastrointestinal bleeding, differential diagnosis of, 533–534
    in runners, 533
    management of, 534
    mechanisms of, 533–534

Gastrointestinal disorders, associated with travel, 535–536

Gastrointestinal illnesses, 525

Gastrointestinal pathogens, 490–491

Gastrointestinal tract, miscellaneous disorders of, 535–536
    physiologic adaptations to exercise, 526–527

Gene therapy, doping through, 734

Glenohumeral joint, degenerative arthritis of, dislocation of shoulder and, 47
    loose suture anchor within, after treatment of shoulder instability, 50, 51
    osteoarthritis of, after treatment of shoulder instability, 50

Glucosamine, 75–77

Golf, acute performance failure in, 962–965
        treatment of, 965–966
    "choking" in, 962–965
    confidence and trust and, 960
    ego and, 959–960
    focal dystonia and, 964
    mental health in, future of, 969
    multidisciplinary approach to health management in, 968–969
    over-thinking in, 963–964
    panic phenomenon in, 962–963
    pre-performance routine and, 960–962
    pre-performance time in, counterproductive cognition and, 960
    sport psychiatrist and, **959–971**
    unique characteristics of, 971
    "yips" in, 964–965

Gonadotropins, and melatonin, sleep and, 325–326

Green hair, 589–590

**H**

Hallux rigidus, 66–67
    diagnosis of, 67
    treatment of, 67

Headache(s), 653–657
    assessment in, 653–655
    high-altitude, 713
    migraine, 655–656
        eye and, 688–690
    post-traumatic, 656
    primary exertional, 656–657
    tension-type, 656
    treatment of, 657
    with vascular origin, 689

Heart, athlete's, 466

Heat cramps, 698

Heat edema, 698

Heat loss, 704–705

Heat-related illness, 695–703
    minor, 698

moderate, 698–699
    pathophysiology for, 699
    prevention of, 701–703
    return to play following, 700–701
    risk factors for, 696, 697
    severe, 699–700

Heat stress, recognizing and addressing of, 702

Heat syncope, 698

Heat tetany, 698

Heatstroke, exertional, 699
    treatment of, 699–700

Hematologic disorders, in athlete, **599–621**
    inherited, 599–600

Hematologic parameters, effects of exercise on, 602–603

Hematoma(s), epidural, 645
    subperichondrial, 587

Hemolysis, intravascular, 604, 606–607

Hemophilia, 602

Hemorrhage, 585–587
    subarachnoid, 645
    subdural, 645
    subungual, 585–586

Hepatitis B virus, 502

Hernia, 535

Herniations, 587–588

Herpes gladiatorum, 577–578

Herpes simplex, 577–578
    play restrictions in, 581

Hiatal hernia, 535

High altitude, sleep at, monitoring of, 427–428, 445–446

High-altitude cerebral edema (HACE), 712, 713, 714

High-altitude headache, 713

High-altitude illness, 712–716
    neurologic syndromes in, 713–714
    pulmonary syndromes in, 713–714
    risk factors for, 712
    treatment of, 713–714

High-altitude pulmonary edema (HAPE), 712, 713, 715–716

Hip(s), arthritis of, early, osteotomy in, 59
    arthroscopy of, in arthritis, 59–60
    articular cartilage of, imaging of, 27, 28, 29
    osteoarthritic, type of sport and, 190
    osteoarthritis of, etiology of, 57–58
        symptoms of, 58
        treatment of, 58–60

replacement of, metal-on-metal and
    ceramic-on-ceramic implants
    for, 179
        new plastics and ceramics for, 178
    total replacement of, sports participation
        following, 175, 176, 177, 178
HIV, 502
Hives, 512
"Holding environment", creation of, in
    consulting room, 745–746
Homeostatic and circadian influences, on
    performance, 238–241
Homosexuality, suicide in athletes and, 862–863
Human growth hormone (HGH), 726
Humeral head, lesion of, in tennis player, 193
Hyaluronic acid, clinical safety of, 88
    efficacy of, 88–89
    for viscosupplementation, 87–88
    properties of, 86–87
Hydration, appropriate, 701–702
    guidelines for, 702
Hypercoagulable states, 600–602
Hypertension, 466–467
Hyphema, 685–686
Hypnosis, 973–974
    as form of relaxation, 974
Hypnotic trance, 973, 975
Hypnotics, in insomnia, 280–281, 282
    to induce sleep, 375–376
Hypobaric hypoxia, 712
Hyponatremia, exertional, 701–702
Hypothalamic arousal systems, 211–212
Hypothalamic-pituitary-ovarian axis, 226
Hypothermia, 703–704
    immersion, treatment of, 708
    management of, 706–708
        general measures for, 708
    mild, treatment of, 708
    moderate, treatment of, 708–709
    physiologic response to, 705, 706
    rewarming in, 707–708
    severe, treatment of, 709
    severity of, determination of, 705, 706
    signs and symptoms of, 706
Hypoxia/hypercapnia, nocturnal,
    consequences of, 554


Imagery techniques, to enhance performance,
    974–975
Imaging, of hyaline cartilage, techniques in
    development for, 25–26

Immunizations, for athletes, 536
Immunologic responses to exercise, 507–508
Immunotherapy, in allergies, 520
Impetigo, 574
    play restrictions in, 581
Infectious diseases. See also specific types
    of infections.
    athletes and, 477–478
    seasonality of, e38, e39
    training room management of, **477–506**
Infectious mononucleosis, 484–486
    return-to-play following, 485–486
Injections, for osteoarthritis in joints, and
    sports activity, **83–91**
Injury(ies), in sports, and osteoarthritis, 72–74
        NSAIDs in treatment of,
        74–75
    psychological reaction to, 673–675
    suicide in athletes and, 855–857
Insomnia, and sleep disruption, **269–285**
    athletic performance and, 275–278
    consequences of, 274–278
    daytime functioning and, 274–275
    epidemiology of, 272
    management of, 279–282
    objective assessments of, 273–274
    primary, 270
    recognition and diagnosis of, 269–271
    secondary, 270–271
    severity of, 272
    subjective assessments of, 273
    transient or chronic, 271–272
International Society for Sport Psychiatry
    (ISSP), 669
Intra-psychic system, and professional
    athletes, 933–934
Inversion recovery imaging, 17
Iron, 733
Iron deficiency, and anemia, 604
    causes of, 609–611
    diagnosis and treatment of, 611–612
    in athletes, 608–609, 611
Irritable bowel syndrome, 532–533

J

Jet lag, and air travel, implications for
    performance, **367–380**
    avoidance of, interventions for,
        377–378, 437–439
    behavioral approach to, 373–374
    cause of, 368
    light as treatment for, 385–388
    management of, 448–450
    melatonin and, 441–442
    observations in elite athletes, 371–372

pharmacologic approach to, 374–377
room light and, 439–440
travel fatigue and, 368

"Jock itch," 568–570

"Jogger's nipples," 582

Joint(s), degenerative disease of, in midfoot or
    ankle, foot orthotics in, 94–97
        with angular deformity, orthotic
            and brace use in, **93–99**
    injury(ies) of, as risk factor for
        osteoarthritis, 188–189
        during sports, 189–190
    osteoarthritis in, injections for,
        and sports activity, **83–91**
    other than shoulder, osteoarthritis of,
        after sports injuries, **57–70**

Joint replacement, total, sports after, **175–186**
        based upon anatomic location
           of arthroplasty, 183
        based upon level of impact
           loading, 182

## K

Knee, abrasion arthroplasty and
    microfracture in, 144–145
    articular cartilage of, imaging of, 26–27
    degenerative joint disease and, 93
    flexion contractures about, 103–104
    normal alignment of, 154
    osteoarthritic, in obesity, in diet and
        exercise in management of,
        102–112
        sport-type and, 190
    osteoarthritis of, after sports injuries,
        **39–45**
        arthroscopically confirmed, radio-
           graphic diagnosis of, 137
        athlete with, use of arthroscopy in,
        **133–152**
            author's method of,
            147–148
        clinical approach in, 156–159
        history taking in, 155
        imaging studies in, 156
        in Australian footballers, 191
        pathophysiology of, 153–155
        physical examination in, 155–156
        rehabilitation in, **101–131**
        sites of, 97
        surgery in, clinical results of, 159
            complications of, 159–160
            for lateral opening
                osteotomy, 158–159
            for medial opening wedge
                tibial osteotomy,
                157, 158
            preoperative planning for,
                156–157

osteotomies around, for young athlete
    with osteoarthritis, **153–161**
replacement of, new developments
    in, 179
sports injuries of, osteoarthritis after,
    **39–45**
total replacement of, sports participation
    following, 175, 177
varus and valgus deformities about, 103

Knee orthoses (braces), mechanical, 97–98

## L

Lacerations, 582–583

Laser in-situ keratomileusis (LASIK), 692

Learning, motor, and overnight sleep,
    303–308
    perceptual, and overnight sleep,
        308–309
    skill, daytime naps and, 309–311

Learning disabilities, 762

Lice, 579

Ligament laxity, menstrual cycle, and injuries,
    e65–68

Light, administration of, 398–401
    as circadian phase shifting agent,
        382–383, 384
    as treatment for jet lag, 385–388
    as zeitgeber, 382
    bright. See *Bright light treatment.*
    in entrainment and phase shifting,
        382–388
    room, jet lag and, 441–442
    seasonal depression and, 391–396

Long QT syndrome, 473–474

Lyme disease, 494–495

## M

Magnetic resonance imaging, evaluation
    using, artifacts and inaccuracies in,
    23–24
    of hyaline cartilage, 14–25
    or CT arthrography, of cartilage, 24–25

Malassezia, 572–574

Malignancy, light at night and, 403

Marfan's syndrome, 470–471
    eye problems in, 691
    physical characteristics of, 465–466

Marrow stimulation technique (microfrac-
    ture), in cartilage defects, 165–166, 170

Mast cells and basophils, mediators of, e36

Medication(s), common, used by athletes,
    719–724
    for treatment of attention deficit/
        hyperactivity disorder, 836–839

over-the-counter, supplements and, 758
possibly interacting with exercise or
environment, 723–724
potentially causing photosensitivity
reaction, 724
use of, and supplement use, by athletes,
**719–738**

Melatonin, e25
and gonadotropins, sleep and, 325–326
jet lag and, 441–442
to induce sleep, 376, 377

Memory, categories of, 302–303
sleep and, behavioral studies of, 303
stages of, 303

Memory representations, overnight
reorganization of, 312–315

Meningitis, aseptic, 486–487
diagnosis of, 487–488
treatment of, 488

Meniscectomy, partial, in patients with
osteoarthritis, 145–1460

Meniscus, tears of, 42

Menstrual cycle, e53
and aerobic capacity, e61
and aerobic endurance, e62–63
and anaerobic capacity, e63–64
and sport performance, **e51–82**
in different sports, e64–65
methodological considerations
and, e53–55
and strength, e60–61
hormonal modification of, e70–71
injuries, and ligament laxity, e65–68
manipulation of, oral contraceptive pills
for, e73–75
therapeutic considerations and, e68–69

Menstrual rhythm, functional neuroanatomy
of, 225–226

Mental health professionals, achievement of
proxy distortion and, 823–825
and professional athletes, alignment and,
935–936
defensive normalization and, 938
disavowal and, 936
disdain and, 936–937
envy and, 937–938
ethnic issues and, 938–940
flexibility and, 940
idealization and, 938
identification issues for, 934–935
in psychiatric distress in sports, 675–676
in sports medicine, 930

Mental illness, stigma attached to, 931

Metabolic/endocrinologic system, obstructive
sleep apnea and, 332–333

Methylphenidate, in attention deficit/
hyperactivity disorder, 832, 837

Migraine headache, 655–656
eye and, 688–690

Miliaria rubra, 698

Mitral valve prolapse, 470

Mob behavior, 850, 851

Molluscum contagiosum, 577
play restrictions in, 581

Mononucleosis, 484–486
return-to-play following, 485–486

Mood disorders, sleep/wake considerations in,
424–425

Morningness/eveningness, and post-lunch dip
propensity, e19–20

Mosaicplasty, in cartilage defects, 168–169

Motility disorders, 531–533

Motor relaxation, for sleep promotion,
349–350

Multiple Sleep Latency Test, 252
details of, 252–253
maintenance of wakefulness test
and, 258
relating scores to real life, 254–255
reporting results of, 253–254

Muscle dysmorphia, 757–758

Myocardial bridge, 469

Myocardial disorders, 467–468

Myocarditis, 468
viral, 479

**N**

Nap(ping), daytime, skill learning and,
309–311
effects on performance, 241–242,
429–431
recommendations for, 377–378,
432–433

Nasal obstruction, allergy-associated, 510–511

Neoplasms, 592

Neurapraxia, cervical, 646–649

Neurocognitive deficits, obstructive sleep
apnea and, 333

Neurologic conditions, in sports, management
of, **637–662**

Neuropsychiatry, 759–760

Neuropsychological issues, psychiatric issues
and, in sports medicine, **663–679**
prevalence and incidence of,
665–666

Nonsteroidal anti-inflammatory drugs.
See *NSAIDs*.

NSAIDs, 720–721
and nutritional supplements, use of, in
athletes with osteoarthritis, **71–82**
behavioral aspects of use of, 78–79
development of, 74
efficacy of, in osteoarthritis, 74–75
side effects of, 77–78

Nutritional supplements, and NSAIDs, use of,
in athletes with osteoarthritis, **71–82**
behavioral aspects of use of, 79
in treatment of osteoarthritis, 75
side effects of, 78

**O**

Obsessive-compulsive disorder, and
superstitious rituals, differentiated, 753
example of, 752–753

Olympic athletes, allergies and, e38–39

Oral contraceptive pills, e71, 721
and drug testing, e75–76
and injuries, e68
and performance, e71–73
prescription of, for menstrual cycle
manipulation, e73–75

Orbit, fracture of, 683

Oropharyngeal dysphagia, 527

Orthotic(s), and brace, in degenerative joint
disease with angular deformity, **93–99**
foot, in midfoot or ankle degenerative
joint disease, 94–97

Osteoarthritis, and articular cartilage, basic
science of, **1–12**
athletes with, use of NSAIDs and
nutritional supplements in, **71–82**
chondromalacia in, 5, 6
effect of, on joint structures, 7
evaluating and monitoring of, 194
following instability of shoulder, **47–56**
impact of, 192–194
on sports careers, **187–198**
in joints, corticosteroids in,
complications of, 86
contraindications to, 86
indications for, 84–85
mechanism of action of, 84
preparations of, 85–86
injections for, and sports activity,
**83–91**
traditional nonoperative
treatments for, 83
viscosupplementation in, 86–87
viscosupplements in, 87–88
molecular etiopathology of, 7–9
nutritional supplements in treatment
of, 75

of ankle and foot, 65–66
treatment of, 66
of elbow, 61
symptoms of, 61
treatment of, 61–62
of glenohumeral joint, after treatment of
shoulder instability, 50
of great toe, 66–67
of hip. See *Hip(s), osteoarthritis of.*
of joints other than shoulder, after sports
injuries, **57–70**
of knee. See *Knee, osteoarthritis of.*
of shoulder. See *Shoulder, osteoarthritis of.*
of wrist, 62–63
pain control in, 102
partial mensicectomy in patients with,
145–146
patient education in, 102
radiographic evidence of, and symptoms
of, 192
rehabilitation in, goal of, 101
knee and, **101–131**
risk factors for, 188–190
soccer and, 191
sport type and, 190–192
sports injuries and, 72–74
NSAIDs in treatment of, 74–75
young athlete with, osteotomies around
knee for, **153–161**

Osteoarthritis cartilage, structure and
biochemical changes in, 4–7

Osteochondral allografts, in cartilage
defects, 169

Osteochondral autografts, in cartilage defects,
168–169, 170

Osteochondral injuries, in active patients, 164

Osteochondritis dissecans, 28, 29, 32–32, 33

Osteoporosis, 626–628

Osteotomy(ies), around knee, for young
athlete with osteoarthritis, **153–161**
high tibial, arthroscopy and, 146–147
in early arthritis of hip, 59
lateral opening, for osteoarthritis of
knee, 158–159
medial opening wedge tibial, for
osteoarthritis of knee, 157, 158

Otitis media/externa, 481–482

Overtraining, 672, 760–761, 791
depression secondary to, 761
physiological symptoms of, 760–761

**P**

Panic attack, anticipatory anxiety and, 749
management of, 749
symptoms of, 748–749

Panic disorder, in athlete, 748–750

Parasites, 579–581
    play restrictions in, 581

Parents, aggression and, 849–850
    as role models and active stress inducers, 792–793
    pressure on young athletes, 904

Performance, post-lunch dips in. See *Post-lunch dips in performance.*

Periosteal grafting, in cartilage defects, 166–167

Personality disorders, and aggression, 849

Pertussis, acute bronchitis and, 542–543

Pharyngitis, 480

Photosensitivity reaction, drugs potentially causing, 724

Physical activity. See *Exercise(s).*

Physical and psychological symptoms, adverse, interactional and systemic contribution to, 792–794

Pisotriquetral arthritis, 65

Pityrosporum, 572–574

Pityrosporum folliculitis, 573–574

Pneumonia, 543
    complicated, 544
    treatment of, 544–545

Pneumothorax, spontaneous, background of, 556
    clinical manifestations of, 556–557
    diagnosis of, 557
    treatment of, 557–558

Pollen counts, e36

Polysomnography, obstructive sleep apnea and, 334–335

Postconcussion syndrome, 759–760

Posterior cruciate ligament, tears of, 41–42

Post-lunch dips in performance, **e15–23**
    caffeine as countermeasure to, e20–21
    circadian rhythms and, e17–19
    field studies of, e17
    laboratory studies of, e17
    morningness/eveningness and, e19–20
    research directions in, e21

Post-traumatic stress disorder, 751–752
    characteristics of, 752
    diagnostic features of, 751–752
    example of, 751

Posture, inverted, for sleep promotion, 346–348

Pre-participation screening, 463–467
    history taking in, 464, 465
    physical examination in, 465–466

Pregnancy, sport performance and, e76

Premenstrual syndrome, e69–70

Preparticipation physical examination, atmosphere for, 745–746
    conditions revealed in, 746–762

Pressure to win, suicide in athletes and, 857–858

Professional sports teams, applied systems theory and, 932–933
    working with, ethnic issues and, 938–940
        resolution of, 940
        systemic issues and, **929–942**

Progesterone, e70, e71

Program coordinators, as important in child and youth sports, 794

Prohormones, 726

Prostatitis, 500–501

Protein, 727–728

Proteoglycan aggregate, 4

Proton density axial images, 16–17, 21

Pseudoanemia, dilutional, 604–606

Pseudoephedrine, as stimulant, 424

Psychiatric diagnosis, and referral, sports medicine physician and, 765
    and treatment, of athletes, **771–781**
        cases illustrating, 771, 774, 776, 777
        diagnostic issues in, 773–774
        goals of, 772
        inducing athletes to undergo treatment, 775–776
        methodology of, 772–773
        principles of, 771–778
        range of problems in, 774–775

Psychiatric illness, concept of immunity of athletes from, 853

Psychiatric interview fo child athlete and family, 797–801

Psychiatric issues, and neuropsychological issues, in sports medicine, **663–679**
    prevalence and incidence of, 665–666
    in training room, 666

Psychiatrist, sport. See *Sport psychiatrist.*

Psychodynamic psychotherapy, in eating disorders, 878

Psychomotor vigilance performance, measurement of, 239–240
    sleep, and circadian rhythms, **237–249**

Psychostimulants, in attention deficit/hyperactivity disorder, 837, 838

Psychotropic medication, 669

Pulmonary disorders in training room, **541–564**

Pulmonary edema, high-altitude (HAPE), 712, 713, 715–716

## R

Radiofrequency ablation/debridement, in cartilage defects, 166

Radioulnar joint, distal, arthritis of, 64–65

Radius, distal, intraarticular, fractures of, radiocarpal arthritis after, 64

Relaxation, hypnosis as form of, 974
    thermoregulatory after-effects of, sleep inertia and, 294–296

Respiratory system, effects of caffeine on, e7
    sex steroid hormones and, e56–57

Respiratory tract, upper, infections of, e28–29

Restless legs syndrome, exercise and, 359

Retina, injury to, 686–687

Retinopathy, diabetic, 690

Retirement, suicide in athletes and, 859–860

Rewarming, process of, 707–708

Rhinitis, allergic. See *Allergic rhinitis.*

Right ventricular outflow tract tachycardia, 474–475

Ringworm, 567–568, 569

Rocky Mountain spotted fever, diagnosis of, 496
    mortality rate in, 496
    risk factors for, 495

"Roid rage," 757

Rotator cuff, tears of, in throwing athletes, 191

Rugby, Australian, osteoarthritis of knee in, 191–192

Running, injuries related to, 190–191, 193

## S

Scabies, 579–580

Scaphoid, fractures of, nonunion advanced collapse of, 63–64

Scapholunate, advanced collapse of, 63

Seasonal rhythms, and exercise, **e25–34**
    functional neuroanatomy of, 226–228

Seizures, and epilepsy, 649–653
    assessment and management of, 650–652
    classification of, 649–650, 651
    exercise and, 652–653

Selective serotonin reuptake inhibitors, in eating disorders, 879

Sensory stimuli, withdrawal of, for sleep promotion, 350

Sex steroid hormones, biological effects of, e55–60
    cardiovascular system and, e55–56
    respiration and vantilation and, e56–57
    substrate metabolism and, e58–59
    thermoregulation and, e57–58

Sexual abuse, suicide in athletes and, 863–864

Sexually transmitted diseases, 501–502
    Centers for Disease Control (CDC) and, 501–502

Shoes, in osteoarthritic knee, 113

Shoulder, arthropathy of, incidence of, 47–49
    arthroscopy of, rating of chondral damage for, 49
    articular cartilage of, imaging of, 30, 32
    dislocation of, and degenerative arthritis of glenohumeral joint, 47
        osteoarthritis of shoulder and, 48, 49
    instability of, osteoarthritis following, **47–56**
        significance of osteoarthritis of shoulder after, 52
        surgery in, osteoarthritis of shoulder after, 51
        surgical treatment for, arthrosis and, 50–51
        treatment of, loose suture anchor within glenohumeral joint after, 50, 51
            osteoarthritis of gleno-humeral joint after, 50
        treatment of osteoarthritis of shoulder after, 52–54
    osteoarthritis of, after instability surgery, 51
        after shoulder instability, significance of, 52
        treatment of, 52–54
        and dislocation of shoulder, 48, 49
    replacement of, recent improvements in, 180

Sickle cell disease/trait, 599–600

Siesta naps, e15–16

Sinusitis, 480–481

Skin cancers, 593

Skin infections, 565–582
    play restrictions and regulations in, 580
    prevention of, 581–582

Skin temperatures, and core body temperature, sleepiness in relation to, 290–298

Skin warming/cooling, for sleep promotion, 348–349

Sleep, afternoon human propensity for, e15–16
  and circadian rhythms, in children and adolescents, **319–328**
  and melatonin and gonadotropins, 325–326
  and psychosocial factors, 320–321
  and wakefulness, functional neuroanatomy of, 205–210
  arousal from, consequences of, 554
  at high altitude, monitoring of, 427–428, 445–446
  chronotype for, 435–436
  circadian adversity and, 431, 442–443
  circadian markers for, 436–437
  circadian rhythms, and psychomotor vigilance performance, **237–249**
  conditions antagonizing, 346–350
  effects of exercise on, **355–365**
    antidepressant, 360
    anxiety reduction and, 359–360
    circadian phase-shifting, 361–362
    thermogenic, 360–361
  extra, study of, 263–264
  homeostatic adversity and, 428–431
  hormonal markers for, 437
  induction of, 431, 432–433, 446–447
  influence of, on thermoregulatory system, 293–294
  neural circuitry controlling, 344–345
  non-rapid eye movement, 206–208, 214, 345
  nonpharmacologic techniques for promoting, **343–365**
    at onset, 347
  overnight, motor learning and, 303–308
    perceptual learning and, 308–309
  physiologic foundation of, 344–345
  post-training, and brain activation, modification of, 311–312
  practice with, implications of sleep-dependent learning, **301–317**
  rapid eye movement, 206–207, 214–215
  refractory periods for, 434
  stages of, 206–208
    functional neuroanatomy of, 215–216
  too much, 266
Sleep apnea, background of, 552–555
  diagnosis of, 555
  exercise and, 359
  implications for sports performance, **329–341**
  obstructive, diagnosis of, 333–335
    health consequences of, 332
    in athletes, 336–339
    polysomnography and, 334–335
    prevalence and risk factors for, 330
    treatment of, 335–336

  pathophysiology of, 330–332
  symptoms of, 330
  treatment of, 555–556
Sleep debt, 258–261
  breakthrough experiment on, 259–260
  individual homeostatic sleep requirement and, 260–261
  or excess wakefulness, 261–262
  recovery from, 262
Sleep-dependent brain plasticity, 311–315
Sleep-disordered breathing, 553
Sleep disruption, insomnia and, **269–285**
Sleep extension, **251–268**
  and potential for enhanced athletic performance, 265–266
  study of, 262–263
Sleep gates, 433, 434
Sleep homeostat, 237
Sleep hygiene, in insomnia, 279
Sleep inertia, 242, 429
  avoidance of, 432–433, 447–448
  thermoregulatory after-effects of relaxation and, 294–296
Sleep loss, chronic partial, 256–258
  vulnerability to, individual differences in, 245–247
Sleep-promoting regions, 213–216
Sleep restriction, chronic, effects of, 242–245
Sleep tendency, daytime physiologic, relation to amount of sleep at night, 255–256
  quantifying of, 252–258
Sleep-wake cycle, 216–219
Sleep-wake homeostasis, and circadian timing system, 324–325
  maturation of, in school children, 321–322
Sleep-wake rhythm, and other biological rhythms, functional neuroanatomy of, **205–235**
Sleepiness, and alertness measurement, sports chronobiology and, 416–418
  and distal vasodilation, putative mechanisms involved in, 296–298
  circadian and homeostatic aspects of, 291–293
  definition of, 287
  in relation to core body temperature and skin temperatures, 290–298
  lying down-induced, related to relaxation-induced effects, 296
Sleepiness regulation, three-process-model of, thermophysiologic aspects of, **287–300**
Soccer, osteoarthritis and, 191

Social anxiety disorder, 750–751
  history taking in, 750
  injury revealing, 750
  symptoms of, 751

Sodium bicarbonate, 731

Special Olympics, 788

Spit tobacco, adverse health effects of, 891
  use by athletes, 890

Sport psychiatrist, and golf, **959–971**
  role of, 966–968, 969
  credentialing and licensing of, 968
  performance enhancement and, 966–967
  psychopharmacologic expertise and, 968

Sport psychiatry, relaxation, hypnosis, and
  imagery in, **973–977**
  case studies of, 975–976

Sports, adverse psychophysiological and
  somatoform effects of, 790–792
  child and youth. See *Child and youth sports.*
  in United States, social-historical
    perspective on, 794–795
  racial and gender report card and,
    794–795
  social roles of, 794

Sports careers, impact of osteoarthritis on,
  **187–198**

Sports chronobiology, **413–454**
  alertness-enhancing drugs and, 418–424
  consultation in, goals of, 415–416
  sleepiness and alertness measurement
    and, 416–418
  web-based resouces for information
    on, 451

Sports injuries, osteoarthritis of joints other
  than shoulder after, **57–70**

Sports medicine, mental health professionals
  in, 930

Sports medicine physician, psychiatrically
  aware, interviewing principles for,
  **745–769**

Sports parents interview, 763–764

Sports participation, benefits and risks for
  child and adolescent, 787–790
  effects on self-concept, 790
  moral developmental readiness for,
    786–787
  neuropsychological readiness for,
    785–787
  normal developmental readiness and,
    784–787
  physical and physiological readiness for,
    784–785
  social readiness for, 786

Sports performance, and alertness,
  homeostatic and circadian impairments
  in, 426

Sports psychiatry, and sports medicine
  specialists, interface between, 795–801

Sports teams, professional. See *Professional
  sports teams.*

Steroids, 725–726
  abuse of, 756–757
    as unrecognized problem, 757
    by athletes, 756–757
    emotions associated with, 756–757
    personality changes associated
      with, 756
    suicide and, 860–861
  and aggression, 847
  as addictive, 757
  reluctance of athletes to give up, 757
  use by athletes, 891–893

Stimulants, dependence on, treatment of,
  419–421, 422
    warning signs of, 421
  for attention deficit disorder, 722
  to enhance performance, 418–419
  use by athletes, 888–890
  use in sports, history of, 839–841

"Stinger," 646–649

Stress, athletes and, 664
  in young athlete, manifestations off, 791
  levels of, in athletic family, 916–917

Stressors, psychosocial, suicide in athletes
  and, 857

Striae, 588

Substance abuse, 670–672
  alcoholism and, 755–756
    among high school and college
      athletes, 755
  suicide in athletes and, 858–859

Substance use, in athletics, discussion of,
  893–895
    reasons for use, 885, 886
    sports psychiatry perspective on,
      **885–897**

Suicide, family history of, suicide in athletes
  and, 861
  in athletes, **853–869**
    cultural attitudes and, 863
    discussion of, 864–865
    etiology of, 855–864
    prevention of, 866–867
    studies of, 854
      results of, 854–855
  light treatment and, 403–404

Sunburn, 698

Supplements, over-the-counter medications and, 758
    use of, and medications use, in athletes, **719–738**
    used by athletes, 724–733
        detection of, 734
Suprachiasmatic nucleus, 221
    and peripheral oscillators, interaction between, 224–225
    at molecular level, 223–224
    efferent pathways, 222–223
    main afferent projections in, 221–222
Suture anchor, loose, within glenohumeral joint, after treatment of shoulder instability, 50, 51
Sweating, and exercise, e28

**T**

Talon noir, 586
Tennis player, lesion of humeral head in, 193
Tension-type headache, 657
Tetrahydrogestrinone, 734
Thalamocortical activating system, 210–212
Thalassemia, 600
Thermal injury, 589
Thermoregulation, 695–696, 704
    sex steroid hormones and, e57–58
Thermoregulatory system, influence of sleep on, 293–294
Thinking, self-evaluative, 785–786
Thinking process, versus outcome thinking, 786
Third-party payment, sports medicine physician and, 765
Thrombosis, effort, 612–614
Throwing athletes, rotator cuff tears in, 191
Tick-borne diseases, 493–497
    prevention of, 497
Tinea capitis, 566–567
Tinea corporis, 567–568, 569
Tinea cruris, 568–570
Tinea pedis, 570–571, 572
Tinea unguium, 571–572
Tinea versicolor, 572–573
Toe, great, osteoarthritis of, 66–67
Transference, and athlete's attitude toward doctor, 764
Travel, gastrointestinal disorders associated with, 535–536
Travel fatigue, and jet lag, 368
Turf burn, 583

**U**

Upper airway resistance syndrome, 329
Upper respiratory infections, diagnosis and treatment of, 478–479
    etiology of, 478
    participation guidelines in, 479–480
Urinary tract infections, 498–499
Urticaria, 512
    cholinergic, 513–514

**V**

Valproic acid, 669
Valvular diseases, 469–471
Ventricular tachycardia, 472–475
Verbal abuse, 850
Verruca vulgaris, 578–579
Verrucae, play restrictions in, 581
Violent behavior, 846
Viral infections, 577
Viscosupplementation, in osteoarthritis of joints, 86–87
Viscosupplements, in osteoarthritis of joints, 87–88
Vision correction surgery, 691–692
Visual motor behavior rehearsal, 974
Vitamins, 732–733
Vocal cord dysfunction, and exercise-induced bronchoconstriction, compared, 550
    background of, 549–550
    clinical manifestations of, 551
    diagnosis of, 551–552
    treatment of, 552
Von Willebrand's disease, 601

**W**

Wake maintenance zones, 431, 433, 435
Wakefulness, excess, sleep debt of, 261–262
Wakefulness/arousal promoting regions, 208–210
Warts, common, 578–579
Weight-lifter's hands, 584
Wolfe's Law of bone, 181
Wolff-Parkinson-White syndrome, 471
Wrist, articular cartilage of, imaging of, 30
    osteoarthritis of, 62–63

**Z**

Zero sleep debt study, 264–265

United States Postal Service
# Statement of Ownership, Management, and Circulation

| 1. Publication Title | 2. Publication Number | 3. Filing Date |
|---|---|---|
| Clinics in Sports Medicine | 0 2 7 8 - 5 9 1 9 | 9/15/05 |

| 4. Issue Frequency | 5. Number of Issues Published Annually | 6. Annual Subscription rice |
|---|---|---|
| Jan, Apr, Jul, Oct | 4 | $180.00 |

7. Complete Mailing Address of Known Office of Publication (Not printer) (Street, city, county, state, and ZIP+4)

Elsevier, Inc.
6277 Sea Harbor Drive
Orlando, FL 32887-4800

Contact Person
Gwen C. Campbell

Telephone
215-239-3685

8. Complete Mailing Address of Headquarters or General Business Office of Publisher (Not printer)

Elsevier, Inc., 360 Park Avenue South, New York, NY 10010-1710

9. Full Names and Complete Mailing Addresses of Publisher, Editor, and Managing Editor (Do not leave blank)

Publisher (Name and complete mailing address)

Tim Griswold, Elsevier, Inc., 1600 John F. Kennedy Blvd., Suite 1800, Philadelphia, PA 19103-2899

Editor (Name and complete mailing address)

Debora Dellapena, Elsevier, Inc., 1600 John F. Kennedy Blvd., Suite 1800, Philadelphia, PA 19103-2899

Managing Editor (Name and complete mailing address)

Heather Cullen, Elsevier, Inc., 1600 John F. Kennedy Blvd., Suite 1800, Philadelphia, PA 19103-2899

10. Owner (Do not leave blank. If the publication is owned by a corporation, give the name and address of the corporation immediately followed by the names and addresses of all stockholders owning or holding 1 percent or more of the total amount of stock. If not owned by a corporation, give the names and addresses of the individual owners. If owned by a partnership or other unincorporated firm, give its name and address as well as those of each individual owner. If the publication is published by a nonprofit organization, give its name and address.)

| Full Name | Complete Mailing Address |
|---|---|
| Wholly owned subsidiary of | 4520 East-West Highway |
| Reed/Elsevier, US holdings | Bethesda, MD 20814 |

11. Known Bondholders, Mortgagees, and Other Security Holders Owning or Holding 1 Percent or More of Total Amount of Bonds, Mortgages, or Other Securities. If none, check box ▸ ☐ None

| Full Name | Complete Mailing Address |
|---|---|
| N/A | |

12. Tax Status (For completion by nonprofit organizations authorized to mail at nonprofit rates) (Check one)
The purpose, function, and nonprofit status of this organization and the exempt status for federal income tax purposes:
☐ Has Not Changed During Preceding 12 Months
☐ Has Changed During Preceding 12 Months (Publisher must submit explanation of change with this statement)

(See Instructions on Reverse)

PS Form 3526, October 1999

| 13. Publication Title | 14. Issue Date for Circulation Data Below |
|---|---|
| Clinics in Sports Medicine | July 2005 |

| 15. | Extent and Nature of Circulation | Average No. Copies Each Issue During Preceding 12 Months | No. Copies of Single Issue Published Nearest to Filing Date |
|---|---|---|---|
| a. | Total Number of Copies (Net press run) | 2575 | 2500 |
| b. Paid and/or Requested Circulation | (1) Paid Requested Outside-County Mail Subscriptions Stated on Form 3541. (Include advertiser's proof and exchange copies) | 1561 | 1529 |
| | (2) Paid In-County Subscriptions Stated on Form 3541 (Include advertiser's proof and exchange copies) | | |
| | (3) Sales Through Dealers and Carriers, Street Vendors, Counter Sales, and Other Non-USPS Paid Distribution | 276 | 298 |
| | (4) Other Classes Mailed Through the USPS | | |
| c. | Total Paid or Requested Circulation [Sum of 15b. (1), (2), (3), and (4)] ▸ | 1837 | 1827 |
| d. Free Distribution by Mail (Samples, complimentary, and other free) | (1) Outside-County as Stated on Form 3541 | 92 | 96 |
| | (2) In-County as Stated on Form 3541 | | |
| | (3) Other Classes Mailed Through the USPS | | |
| e. | Free Distribution Outside the Mail (Carriers or other means) | | |
| f. | Total Free Distribution (Sum of 15d. and 15e.) ▸ | 92 | 96 |
| g. | Total Distribution (Sum of 15c. and 15f.) ▸ | 1929 | 1923 |
| h. | Copies not Distributed | 646 | 577 |
| i. | Total (Sum of 15g. and h.) ▸ | 2575 | 2500 |
| j. | Percent Paid and/or Requested Circulation (15c. divided by 15g. times 100) | 95% | 95% |

16. Publication of Statement of Ownership
☐ Publication required. Will be printed in the October 2005 issue of this publication. ☐ Publication not required

17. Signature and Title of Editor, Publisher, Business Manager, or Owner

*[signature]* Janet Zimmerman

Janet Zimmerman – Manager of Subscription Services

Date 9/15/05

I certify that all information furnished on this form is true and complete. I understand that anyone who furnishes false or misleading information on this form or who omits material or information requested on the form may be subject to criminal sanctions (including fines and imprisonment) and/or civil sanctions (including civil penalties).

## Instructions to Publishers

1. Complete and file one copy of this form with your postmaster annually on or before October 1. Keep a copy of the completed form for your records.
2. In cases where the stockholder or security holder is a trustee, include in items 10 and 11 the name of the person or corporation for whom the trustee is acting. Also include the names and addresses of individuals who are stockholders who own or hold 1 percent or more of the total amount of bonds, mortgages, or other securities of the publishing corporation. In item 11, if none, check the box. Use blank sheets if more space is required.
3. Be sure to furnish all circulation information called for in item 15. Free circulation must be shown in items 15d, e, and f.
4. Item 15h., Copies not Distributed, must include (1) newsstand copies originally stated on Form 3541, and returned to the publisher, (2) estimated returns from news agents, and (3), copies for office use, leftovers, spoiled, and all other copies not distributed.
5. If the publication had Periodicals authorization as a general or requester publication, this Statement of Ownership, Management, and Circulation must be published; it must be printed in any issue in October or, if the publication is not published during October, the first issue printed after October.
6. In item 16, indicate the date of the issue in which this Statement of Ownership will be published.
7. Item 17 must be signed.

*Failure to file or publish a statement of ownership may lead to suspension of Periodicals authorization.*

PS Form 3526, October 1999 (Reverse)

# *Changing Your Address?*

Make sure your subscription changes too! When you notify us of your new address, you can help make our job easier by including an exact copy of your Clinics label number with your old address (see illustration below.) This number identifies you to our computer system and will speed the processing of your address change. Please be sure this label number accompanies your old address and your corrected address—you can send an old Clinics label with your number on it or just copy it exactly and send it to the address listed below.

We appreciate your help in our attempt to give you continuous coverage. Thank you.

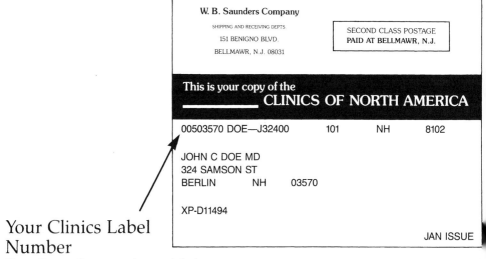

W. B. Saunders Company

SHIPPING AND RECEIVING DEPTS.
151 BENIGNO BLVD.
BELLMAWR, N.J. 08031

SECOND CLASS POSTAGE
PAID AT BELLMAWR, N.J.

**This is your copy of the**
**‗‗‗‗‗‗‗ CLINICS OF NORTH AMERICA**

00503570 DOE—J32400          101          NH          8102

JOHN C DOE MD
324 SAMSON ST
BERLIN          NH          03570

XP-D11494

JAN ISSUE

## Your Clinics Label Number
Copy it exactly or send your label
along with your address to:
**W.B. Saunders Company, Customer Service**
Orlando, FL 32887-4800
Call Toll Free 1-800-654-2452

Please allow four to six weeks for delivery of new subscriptions and for processing address changes.